ACOUSTIC TUMORS

Diagnosis

ing malady began nine months ago, with dizziness and a sense of rotation, and ringing noises with pulsation in the left ear. He soon noticed a difficulty in climbing stairs and that he "could not walk straight." This was followed by a marked unsteadiness of gait, ascribed to weakness of the left leg. Soon the left arm and hand became involved. Some suboccipital headaches; never severe: subsiding under iodides. Periods of diplopia, and for past month rapid failure of vision, with complete blindness five days before admission.

Treatment before admission.—A prolonged course of iodides. On *February 10* a trephine opening over left cerebellar hemisphere without incision of the dura; no relief. On *March 7* another opening over right cerebellar hemisphere with dura unopened. On *March 17* an osteoplastic flap over right cerebellar region with puncture and withdrawal of fluid: dura intact. On same day a small subtemporal decompression with incision of dura: wound not completely healed.

Positive neurological findings.—(A) *General pressure*. Optic atrophy with blindness secondary to choked disc. Protrusion of recent small subtemporal decompression. No present headaches or vomiting. No x-ray studies.

Deep reflexes exaggerated with possible increase in left over right: superficial plantar normal.

(B) *Localizing*. (1) *Cerebellar*. Nystagmus, coarser excursions to left. Conjugate movements to either side poorly sustained. A coarse ataxia of entire left side of astonishing degree. Gait and station impossible to test.

(2) *Extracerebellar. Cerebral nerves*. Vth—Hypaesthesia over entire left trigeminal field: areflexa cornealis. Jaw deflects to the left. VIth—Negative: history of diplopia. VIIth—Weakness of expressional movements on left: imperfect winking reflex. Taste not tested.

VIIIth—Complete left deafness. No x-ray; no caloric tests.

IXth, Xth, XIth,—Considerable dysarthria. XIIth—Tongue protrudes to left (probably from trigeminal motor palsy and deflection of jaw).

Clinical diagnosis.—Tumor of left lateral recess.

April 3, 1906. Operation.—Through a "cross-bow" incision giving a bilateral exposure with chief removal of bone on the left, the angle was well exposed. The growth, together with the cerebellar hemisphere, which had been covered by a protecting pledget of cotton, were both retracted to the right side so that the lesion, which at first was completely overlooked, was not seen until the search, which had been carried nearly to the auditory meatus, was about to be abandoned. A nodular, encapsulated, movable growth was finally disclosed. In the attempt to enucleate it intact, it was broken in two and possibly only about its lower half was removed. The upper fragment was left in place.

Post-operative notes.—The patient made a good surgical recovery despite a temporary increase in his dysarthria with some difficulty in swallowing. There was otherwise no change in the local neurological findings. The wound healed *per primam*. He was discharged *April 26, 1906*.

Pathologic note.—Sections of the tissue show for the most part a fibrous basis with some tendency in places to palisade and whorl formation. There are large areas of sparse round cells in a reticular meshwork. Many of these cells are large with abundant protoplasm containing a large nucleus, and they suggest ganglion cells.

Subsequent notes.—The patient was lost track of until the appearance of a paper by Dr. Julius Grinker in 1910, in which his case was reported. His death occurred suddenly while conversing over the telephone on *Dec. 2, 1909*, three years and eight months after the operation. "He had a peculiar seizure, in which he fell backward, striking the ground with his head and becoming unconscious." Coma supervened and he died two hours later.

Postmortem examination showed a recent hemorrhage filling the subarachnoid cyst around a large growth, obviously, from the photograph, an acoustic tumor. The growth was reported to be a "glioma."

Comment.—This is one of the few cases in which there was a definite history of local injury. In this respect the acoustic tumors differ from many other forms of intracranial tumor, particularly the endotheliomata, in which trauma so frequently figures as an apparent predisposing cause. The significance of the initial auditory disturbances was not appreciated when this patient was seen, and it is not improbable that they were of long standing and accompanied by vertiginous attacks. These matters were not thoroughly inquired into, and the fact of his unilateral deafness was only casually mentioned among the notes of the physical examination.

With our present experience it is quite possible that a total enucleation of this favorable tumor might have been accomplished.

Thus it can be seen that Cushing's first two cases were one fatality and one survival. The operative mortality rate in acoustic tumors reported by leading European surgeons of the time ran from 70 to 90%. Why, with this shocking mortality, were not all further attempts at acoustic tumor surgery abandoned? Why not let the patient live the remaining months or years before inevitable, sudden respiratory failure and death? Why perform a surgery with 80% chance that the patient would not live more than a few days?

Insight into the answers to these questions is given by Cushing in his discussion of his third acoustic tumor, operated in September, 1906. The patient was a 42-year-old woman with a 4-year history of deafness and a 3-year history of severe cerebellar ataxia, which made her bedridden. She had severe occipital headaches with marked suboccipital pain and tenderness. The patient had been given antiluetic treatment. Two years before surgery she had developed beginning loss of vision and blind spells. A year before surgery she had become completely blind and had lost most of her hearing, apparently due to pressure on the eighth nerve opposite the site of the lesion. A bilateral suboccipital craniotomy was done with intracapsular removal of a large portion of her tumor. She made a good postoperative recovery with marked lessening of headache and even some improvement in vision. The ataxia subsided, enabling her to walk about without assistance. Three years later she developed difficulty swallowing and died suddenly, apparently from respiratory failure.

Cushing commented, "In view of the advanced symptoms the results in this case were as good as might be expected—with three and a half years of fairly comfortable life. Had the operation been carried out a year before, when the diagnosis was first made, or even a few months earlier, so that the unfortunate woman might have enjoyed life with vision, the results would have been still more gratifying."

From this description we can conclude that acoustic tumor patients in the early 1900s were not properly diagnosed until they were extremely far advanced. Their suffering was intense, including headache, blindness, vomiting, dizziness, and ataxia. Only very few of these patients found their way to a medical center where a diagnosis of posterior fossa lesion could be established. The popular diagnosis at the time for any illness that the doctor could not explain was syphilis, since the Wasserman test had not yet been developed. In most instances patients were kept comfortable until their death by the use of opiates (e.g., laudanum), which were readily available over the counter. The first drug laws regulating narcotics did not come into being in the United States until 1914. These medications must have further depressed the respiratory function, mercifully hastening death due to pneumonia or respiratory failure.

Unless this bleak picture of the acoustic tumor patient is kept in mind, the brilliant contributions of Cushing and others cannot be adequately appreciated. Cushing's surgical approach at this time was purely palliative. He attempted to decrease the elevated intracranial pressure by decompression of the suboccipital area by partial removal of the tumor.

Eleven years after he had treated Case No. 3, he stated in his monograph,

> It has taken many years and much insistance to make the profession appreciate that a choked disc is a mechanical process due to tension which can be surgically relieved even though a localizing diagnosis cannot be made. It will doubtless take many years more to make them feel that it is somewhat disgraceful under these circumstances to permit a patient to become blind or even to allow the process to advance to such a stage that vision becomes impaired.

Thus, even in his early years Cushing was thinking about better diagnosis and increasing the awareness of doctors of acoustic tumors so that these patients could be referred for surgical relief at a much earlier stage. In addition, he and surgeons all over the world were thinking of better surgical techniques to lower the mortality of patients who presented for treatment. More on the diagnostic aspects later. Now let us examine the surgical ideas of the day.

In the early 1900s the radical mastoid operation had been perfected. A number of surgeons confined their activities to aural surgery. They also were involved with management of the draining of abscesses that had spread to the middle or posterior cranial fossa from the mastoid, and with management of lateral and sigmoid sinus thrombosis. It was only natural that neurologists enlisted the aid of these surgeons in surgical treatment of patients diagnosed with a posterior fossa tumor. The earliest attempts at tumor removal had been made through the Krause approach, which was a unilateral suboccipital approach, but it produced high mortality (5). In 1904 Panse reasoned that a more direct approach would be through the temporal bone (6). This operation was termed a translabyrinthine operation. Apparently it was a radical mastoidectomy with removal of all of the labyrinth, the cochlea, and the facial nerve. Apparently only a few of these procedures were performed, with high mortality due to hemorrhage from the venous sinuses surrounding the temporal bone or to the cerebrospinal leak through the mastoid cavity. This leak was extremely difficult to control with the iodoform gauze packing used at that time. In 1911 Quix of Utrecht excised a small tumor. The patient, who died 6 months later, was found to have only a partial removal of the tumor (7). However, as late as 1915, Zange and Schmiegelow had performed more operations with the translabyrinthine approach and were recommending its use (8, 9).

Later, the translabyrinthine approach was combined with the suboccipital approach and, in a few cases, the sigmoid sinus was also ligated. In 1913 Marx was able to find a record of only five combined translabyrinthine suboccipital approaches. One of the main causes of death of these patients was meningitis from the cerebrospinal fluid fistula through the radical mastoid cavity (10). The few patients who survived had partial removals, with little relief of increased intracranial pressure symptoms due to lack of decompression of the posterior fossa. These patients had facial paralysis that did not result from the partial suboccipital removal.

Cushing, in his description of the various procedures used at the time, prophetically states:

> It is, however, within the realm of possibility that in the case of a very early and minute tumor largely limited to the internal canal the translabyrinthine operation may in time become the operation of choice, but this will necessitate far more precocious and more exact diagnosis than we as yet are capable of.

Over the years, then, Cushing developed and standardized his bilateral suboccipital exposure combined with partial removal of the acoustic tumor. Cushing summarizes the advantage of the operation as he perfected it:

> From the outset this operation has seemed to possess certain advantages which are lacking in those heretofore described. Briefly, they lie in the wide bilateral exposure of the posterior surface of the cerebellum, and this, combined with the early evacuation of the cerebrospinal fluid, serves to promptly relieve the intracranial tension which in turn permits of sufficient dislocation of the hemispheres to expose the recess without jeopardizing the medullary centers or traumatizing the adjacent cerebellar lobe. Moreover, carefully planned haemostasis not only makes it possible to carry the procedure through in one session, but justified an exact reapproximation of the divided tissues in layers without drainage, thereby greatly lessening the risk of postoperative complications as well as giving the patient a sound and presentable neck. The large cranial opening, furthermore, serves as an effective palliative measure not only against the possible early edema but as a future decompression in view of almost inevitable continuance of the growth.
>
> Some of the imperfections of the operation, as it has been outlined, lie in its magnitude, the expenditure of time,—for one could hardly undertake two such procedures in a day,—and the fact that a partial intracapsular enucleation is advocated at the present time rather than an attempted complete extirpation. These, however, are drawbacks which must necessarily characterize all operations for tumors in this difficult region if they are undertaken with due precautions and respect for life.

Most attempts at total enucleation of the tumor at this time were done by inserting a finger through the suboccipital area and attempting to pull the tumor out piecemeal or totally. Bleeding from branches off the basilar artery was often profuse, leading to immediate fatality. If the patient did survive, he had a facial paralysis and involvement of the ninth, tenth, eleventh, and twelfth cranial nerves. Cushing therefore early abandoned attempts at total removal. He simply scooped out the center of the tumor with a curette and then placed Zinkers solution in the interior of the tumor to stop bleeding.

In 1911 Cushing developed silver clips. These obviously were a major advance in the control of intracranial bleeding (11). However, what was done in the first 17 years of the twentieth century to achieve better diagnosis of these tumors? A review of the case histories and findings of thirty verified and three unverified acoustic tumors in Cushing's book reveals that these patients presented at the Hopkins and Harvard clinics in the last stages of development of their brain tumor. Most patients had dysarthria; many had mental dullness that comes with elevated intracranial pressure. Soon after being seen, these patients became comatose. Most patients were so ataxic that they were bedridden, able to stand only with assistance. They had severe headaches, suboccipital discomfort, and impaired vision. Several were totally blind from elevated intracranial pressure. Cushing also mentions cerebellar crises that were "paroxysm of a most extreme and agonizing type, with retraction of the neck and back, respiratory difficulties, and altered pulse, a sense of impending death and often with loss of consciousness."

One can imagine Cushing at the bedside of these horribly ill patients. He must have been tempted to take a brief history from a relative about the duration of the headache and ataxia, to examine the optic fundi (the ophthalmoscope had been made portable and electric by Dennett in the early 1900s), and then to proceed with a general neurologic examination to determine the "localizing signs," which were recorded as cerebellar and extracerebellar. These measures obviously would have been enough to place the lesion in the posterior fossa and probably to determine the side of the lesion. However, he criticizes himself for his poor evaluation of Case 1, where, under clinical diagnosis, he simply states, "cerebellar tumor, presumable site not noted."

In reading Cushing's case histories, we see more and more careful documentation of the development of the patient's symptoms and more increasingly detailed neurologic evaluation. As new clinical tests became available, they were carefully evaluated and applied. Hearing tests were more than just a whisper in each ear; the tuning fork test and the Galton whistle test were used. The problems of masking in unilateral hearing losses obviously were appreciated and were discussed in his book:

> In reviewing the records it has been of interest to find that the first observer in going over the cerebral nerves has sometimes been confused regarding the question of deafness, and in a number of patients it was thought that bone conduction was present and, in some instances, air conduction also, when both were subsequently disproved. The absence of the latter, indeed, has only been absolutely certified in some patients by the complete deafness to external sounds which ensues when the unaffected ear is being irrigated in the course of the caloric tests. As Grey points out, the perception of after tones and the transmission of tones of the fork in the opposite ear somewhat interfere with the Rinne test and not infrequently, even with acoustic tumors of large size, the tones perceived by the unaffected ear are referred by the patient in part to the diseased side.

From 1906 to 1913 Barany published many articles on caloric testing (12–16). His work won him the Nobel prize in 1914. Cushing describes the first use of caloric tests in his Case 8, of September, 1910. The differentiation between labyrinthine unsteadiness and cerebellar ataxia was an important topic in neurologic circles of the day, and was fully discussed by Wilson and Pike in 1915 (17,18). X-ray had been discovered by Roentgen in 1895. Its first successful use in disclosing an intracranial tumor was in 1897, when Oppenheim detected the absence of the landmarks of the sella turcica and correctly diagnosed a tumor of the pituitary body. It was not until 1912, however, that Henschen reasoned from his study of autopsy cases of acoustic tumors that dilated porus acusticus should be visible by x-ray (19). Schuller, in a book on x-ray findings in patients with intracranial tumors, emphasized widening of the sinusoidal grooves and dilation of the siploetic vessels. The book described a lateral projection of the temporal bones called the Schuller position. This position was used to attempt to visualize the dilated porus acusticus. However, confusion often resulted because of superimposition of the external auditory canal and the internal auditory canal. Nevertheless, in 1913, in Case 12 of his monograph, Cushing mentions that x-rays of the porus acusticus are not conclusive. It was to be many years before x-ray techniques would be perfected to be of real value.

Over a period of 15 years, Cushing questioned not only his patients but also, I am sure, their relatives. He carefully recorded all of the myriads of details obtained—some relevant, some irrelevant. He did this not only for acoustic tumors but for all tumors he found in his large clinical practice. Gradually the chronology of symptoms of acoustic tumor began to form in Cushing's mind. His methods and conclusions were clinical research at its finest. At the end of his chapter on symptomatology, in his monograph titled "Afterword," he discusses his conclusions in brilliant simplicity:

> From the above group analyses of the individual symptoms, as well as from the story connected with the case histories, it can be gathered that the symptomatic progress of the average acoustic tumor occurs more or less in the following stages: First, the auditory and labyrinthine manifestations; second, the occipitofrontal pains with suboccipital discomforts; third, the incoordination and instability of cerebellar origin; fourth, the evidences of involvement of adjacent cerebral nerves; fifth, the indications of increase in intracranial tension with a choked disc and its consequences; sixth, dysarthria, dysphagia, and finally cerebellar crises and respiratory difficulties.

In several other places of the monograph Cushing emphasizes that unilateral hearing loss is the first symptom of an acoustic tumor, and that it is a symptom about which the patient must be carefully questioned:

> The chronology of symptoms in the foregoing series of cases makes it clear that the clinical diagnosis of an acoustic tumor can be made with reasonable assurance only when auditory manifestations definitely precede the evidences of involvement of other structures in the cerebellopontine angle.
>
> It would appear that patients rarely call attention to the premonitory auditory symptoms, which are either forgotten or are not associated with

> the subsequent and more incapacitating phenomena, and it is equally certain that the sequence is apt to be slighted by the questioner. On the other hand, a progressive unilateral loss of hearing, if unattended by tinnitus, may not be observed by the patient, and it is interesting to note how often, when it is observed, attention is called to the fact by disability in use of the telephone (cf. Cases XX, XXIV, XXV, and XXVIII).

Today, some 60 years later, it is unfortunate that we still see patients who have noted a difficulty in one ear while using the telephone, and who at that point are not carefully evaluated for an acoustic tumor.

Thus, Cushing made great contributions to early diagnosis of acoustic tumors. It was not until publication of his book in 1917 that his better diagnosis was appreciated by others in the medical profession. Cushing did not have the advantage that the next generation of surgeons was to have: referral at a less advanced stage in the development of the acoustic tumor. Therefore, during these years his attempts to lower the morbidity and mortality of this condition concentrated on improved surgical technique. His summary of the analysis of mortality with these cases is a masterpiece:

> (1) *The operative mortality*. This in the case of cerebellopontile-angle tumors, the majority of them as we have seen being acoustic tumors, has been variously estimated—though always high. This is so both for the cases assembled from miscellaneous reports in the literature as well as from the reports from individual clinics.
>
> Henschen in 1910 collected 43 cases with partial tumor removal of which only 8 lived for any length of time. Leischner's statistics gathered in 1911, including 10 cases from Eiselberg's clinic, gave a mortality of 70 percent. According to Fumarola, Krause had only 4 recoveries in a series of 30 angle tumors (86.6 percent mortality) and Eiselberg in 1912, 4 recoveries in 12 cases (66.6 percent mortality). Tooth's statistics of the operations with removal, complete or partial, of extracerebellar tumors during the years 1902 to 1912 at the National Hospital gave 24 cases with 17 deaths attributed to the operation (70.8 percent), whereas 11 out of 12 cases succumbed after a mere suboccipital decompression for tumor (91.6 percent). In the 70 cases of which Henschen found record between 1910 and 1915 there was a 68.7 percent mortality.
>
> Shocking as these figures are and desperate as the condition must be which justifies operation attended with such high risks, it must be acknowledged that they represent the experience of surgeons who at the time of their report had had but few cases, and whose later records would have been far better. After the first operation the surgical mortality in the writer's series of acoustic tumors was 100 percent. After the first 10 cases it was lowered to 40 percent, after 15 cases it had dropped to 33.3 percent, after 20 cases to 30 percent, after 25 cases to 24 percent, and after 30 cases to 20 percent; and it must continue to fall until it drops to 10 or 5 percent or better, even though the total figures must carry the burden of early inexperience.

In his preface Cushing summarizes the great difference between his era and the first era of acoustic tumor history, the nineteenth century, which was dominated by the principle of clinical observation and autopsy findings outlined by John Hunter. The second era, or, as I like to call it, the Cushing era, saw a transition to the ability to study surgical pathology rather than autopsy pathology.

> Whereas formerly occasional examples of the various types of tumor might have been made the subject of study, the opportunity of investigating the lesion except at autopsy was rarely given and then only as a terminal condition after the clinical picture had become more or less confused. Today the opportunity is given of verifying the lesion in an increasing number of cases at a much more early stage than has heretofore been possible, and the operating room has largely supplanted the postmortem laboratory as the source of material for study. This is merely a repetition of the story concerning lesions in many other parts of the body.

The most important legacy of the Cushing era was the elucidation of the chronology of development of symptoms of acoustic tumor patients. The speciality of neurosurgery was firmly established during this time, and the concepts and techniques of intracranial surgery were vastly improved. Great teachers of neurosurgery all over the world were now indoctrinating the next generation of surgeons. They were able to spend their entire careers in the field of neurosurgery, starting at the level of expertise where their teachers left off.

The next era of the acoustic tumor was to last from the beginning of World War I until after the end of World War II, when microsurgical techniques were introduced. During this time there were no dominating Cushings. Instead, many individuals contributed to the step-by-step progress in diagnosis and surgery that steadily improved the outlook of patients with acoustic tumors.

REFERENCES

1. Cushing, H. 1917. Tumors of the Nervus Acusticus and the Syndrome of Cerebellopontile Angle. W. B. Saunders Co., Philadelphia.
2. Henneberg and Koch. 1902. Über "centrale" Neurofibromatose und die Geschwülste des Kleinhirnbrückenwinkels (Acusticusneurome). Arch. F. Psychiat. xxxvi:251–304.
3. Virchow, R. 1858. Das wahre Neurom. Arch. f. Path. Anat. xiii:256–265.
4. Verocay, J. 1910. Zur Kenntnis der "Neurofibrome." Beitr. Pathol. Anat. Allg. Pathol. xlviii:1–68.
5. Krause, F. 1903. Zur Freilegung der hinteren Felsenbeinfläche und des Kleinhirns. Beitr. Klin. Chir. xxxvii:728–764.
6. Panse, R. 1904. Ein Gliom des Akustikus. Arch. Ohrenh. lxi:251–255.

7. Quix, F. 1915. Ein Fall von operierter Acusticus-Geschwulst mit Darstellung mikrophotographischer Lichtbilder und Besprechung der Operationstechnik. Monatsschr. Ohrenh. xlix:717–718.
8. Zange, J. 1915. Translabyrinthäre Operationen von Acusticus- und Kleinhirnbrückenwinkeltumoren. Berl. Klin. Wochenschr. lii:1334.
9. Schmiegelow, E. 1915. Beitrag zur translabyrinthären Entfernung der Akustikustumoren. Z. Ohrenh. lxxiii:1–21.
10. Marx, H. 1913. Zur Chirurgie der Kleinhirnbrückenwinkeltumoren. Mitt. a. d. Grenzgeb. d. Med. u. Chir. xxvi:117–134.
11. Cushing, H. 1911. The control of bleeding in operations for brain tumors, with the description of silver "clips" for the occlusion of vessels inaccessible to the ligature. Ann. Surg. liv:1–19.
12. Barany, R. 1906. Untersuchungen über den vom Vestibularapparat des Ohres reflektörisch ausgeosten rhythmischen Nystagmus und seine Begleiterscheinungen. Montsschr. Ohrenh. xl:193–297.
13. Barany, R. 1908. Operationsmethode zur Entfernung von Akustikustumoren. Z. Ohrenh. lv:414–415.
14. Barany, R. 1910. Die nervösen Störungen des Cochlear- und Vestibularapparates. Cf. v. Lewandowski: Handbuch der Neurologie, i:919–958, Berlin.
15. Barany, R. 1910. Spezielle Pathologie der Erkrankungen des Cochlear- und Vestibular- apparates. Ibid., iii:811–873, Berlin.
16. Barany, R. 1913. Die Ausführung der vestibularen Kleinhirnprüfung. Trans. Int. Cong. Med. (Lond.) Sec. XI:53–54.
17. Wilson, J., and Pike, F. 1915. Vertigo. JAMA lxiv:561–564.
18. Wilson, J., and Pike, F. 1915. The differential diagnosis of lesions of the labyrinth and of the cerebellum. JAMA lxv:2156–2161.
19. Henschen, F. 1912. Die Akustikustumoren, eine neue Gruppe radiographisch darstellbarer Hirntumoren. Fortschr. a. d. Geb. d. Röntgenstrahlen xviii:207–216.

ADDITIONAL REFERENCES

Toynbee, J. 1853. Neuroma of the auditory nerve. Trans. Pathol. Soc. (Lond.) vi:259–260.

Panse, R. 1904. Ein Gliom des Akustikus. Arch. Ohrenh. lxi:251–255.

Alexander, G. 1907. Zur Kenntnis der Akustikustumoren. Ztschr. Klin. Med. lxii:447–456.

Henschen, F. 1910. Über Geschwülste der hinteren Schädelgrube, insbesondere des Kleinhirnbrückenwinkels. Jena.

Wolff, H. 1912. Akustikustumor. Ein Beitrag zur Entstehung der Kleinhirn brückenwinkeltumoren. Beitr. z. Anat. Physiol. Path. u. Therap. d. Ohres v:464–466.

Henschen, F. 1915. Zur Histologie und Pathogenese der Kleinhirnbrückenwinkeltumoren. Arch. Psychiat. lvi:21–22.

Grey, E. 1915. Studies on the localization of cerebellar tumours. I. Posterior new growths without nystagmus. JAMA lxv:1341–1345.

Grey, E. 1915. Studies on the localization of cerebellar tumours. II. Staggering gait, limb ataxia, the Romberg test and adiodokokinesia. J. Nerv. Ment. Dis. xlii:670–679.

Grey, E. 1916. Studies on the localization of cerebellar tumours. III. The position of the head and suboccipital discomforts. Ann. Surg. lxiii:129–139.

Grey, E. 1916. Studies on the localization of cerebellar tumours. IV. The pointing reaction and the caloric test. AM. J. Med. Sci. cli:693–704.

Grey, E. 1916. Studies on the localization of cerebellar tumours. V. The cranial nerves. Bull. Johns Hopkins Hosp. xxvii:251–262.

Acoustic Tumors
Volume I, *Diagnosis*
Edited by W. F. House and C. M. Luetje

Chapter 3

A History of Acoustic Tumor Surgery 1917–1961, The Dandy Era

William F. House, M.D.*

Clinical Professor of Otorhinolaryngology, University of Southern California School of Medicine, Los Angeles; Research Director, Ear Research Institute, and President, Otologic Medical Group, Inc., Los Angeles

---

By the beginning of World War I all of the important elements in the management of acoustic tumors had come into being. Cushing had brilliantly elucidated the progression of symptoms of these lesions from the earliest unilateral hearing loss to death some years later caused by respiratory failure due to elevated intracranial pressure. Systematic neurologic examinations and the hearing and vestibular tests of the day were applied to these patients. X-ray of the temporal bone was beginning to be used.

On the surgical side, anesthesia had steadily improved since its discovery 75 years previously. The antiseptic principles of Lister, which made brain surgery possible, were being gradually replaced by the concepts of aseptic surgery. Decompression of increased intracranial pressure, introduced by Cottrell, was fairly well understood (1). The methods of handling of brain tissues and control of hemorrhage by the use of Horsley's bone wax and Cushing's clips were now widespread knowledge. Most importantly, neurosurgery had now become a specialty, so that diagnosis was linked to surgery and surgery to diagnosis, each putting pressure on the other for constant improvement.

This era of the acoustic tumor saga was to last 40 years, until the introduction of microsurgery techniques. It was to see the shift away

* Mailing address: 256 South Lake Street, Los Angeles, California 90057

from mere alleviation of symptoms and prolongation of life to an attempt in almost all cases to cure the acoustic tumor.

The next dominant figure to emerge on the pages of this history is Walter Dandy. He was a student of Cushing, and, after Cushing left for Harvard, he remained at Johns Hopkins Hospital. If Dandy's writings are any indication, he was brilliant, innovative, and very opinionated. Probably one of the greatest neurosurgical technicians of all time, he was able to accomplish surgical results far beyond those of his contemporaries. He lacked the painstaking clinical observation of Cushing, but he made up for this in brilliant surgical observation and innovation.

For reasons now somewhat obscured by time, these two men came into conflict, failing to recognize the great synergism of their contributions. Because of Cushing's careful documentation and widespread publication of the symptoms of acoustic tumor, these lesions were being universally recognized at a much earlier stage in their development. Recognition and proper diagnosis of acoustic tumors—in some cases before any evidence of increased intracranial pressure had occurred—made it necessary to modify the entire thinking regarding the surgical approach to this lesion.

Dandy's first great contribution was in 1918, when he introduced cerebral pneumography (2), which, of course, was of great importance in the localization and preoperative assessment of all intracranial masses.

By 1925 most acoustic tumors were diagnosed when their symptoms were unilateral progressive hearing loss, fifth nerve numbness, and elevated intracranial pressure. They were, however, rarely in the extremes of Cushing's cases. Obviously, an operation designed to decompress the posterior fossa and partially remove the tumor in order to give a few years of more comfortable life was inappropriate for these cases. Dandy correctly recognized that, if surgery was to be undertaken at this stage in the development of the acoustic tumor, the object of the surgery must be to cure the patient of his tumor and not merely to palliate his symptoms.

In 1915, when Dandy saw his first two cases, he apparently tried surgical decompression, which consisted of bilateral cerebellar exposure and opening of the posterior fossa dura (3). Both patients died within 12 hours. Both patients had elevated intracranial pressure but were conscious and in good physical condition at the time of the operation. He reasoned that the problem was the shift of both cerebellar hemispheres and the brainstem away from the tumor and, in addition, the pressure downward on the tentorium by the elevated intracranial pressure due to hydrocephalus. He recognized the block of the aqueduct of Sylvius but did not indicate whether he used a ventricular tap during this procedure. His article reveals him to be aware of this procedure:

> Krause (12, 1903) introduced a very useful procedure to reduce the excessive presssure which was nearly always present with cerebellopontile tumors. A trocar was passed through the tentorium into the lateral ventricle permitting the evacuation of its fluid. This procedure (ventricular puncture), in much more refined form, has come to be a most important item in all operations for tumors below the tentorium.

Cushing, in his 1917 monograph, also recommends this procedure in all of his surgical cases (4).

Dandy now goes on to state:

> In desperation, our next effort, total extirpation with the finger at one stage, then seemed the only alternative. It was, of course, merely a reversion to the well tried and fruitless method of Horsley, Krause, Eiselsberg and others. Nor was there reason to expect better results. After two initial successes, four deaths in succession showed the futility of further attempts.

Sudden traumatic removal of the tumor by this method resulted in what he calls an "excessive bleeding" controlled by packing with cotton and then attempting to find the bleeders to clip. He also placed small bits of muscle over the bleeders, as had been recommended many years previously by Horsley.

He next tried Cushing's intracapsular enucleation on three cases, resulting in one recovery and two later fatalities from meningitis, one on the fourth postoperative day and one of the forty-sixth day.

> Despite enthusiastic hopes (for intracapsular enucleation as introduced by Cushing), however, our first experiences with intracapsular enucleation were unfortunate in being less satisfactory than had been anticipated. Following an uneventful and quick recovery from the effects of the operation, the first patient 7 days later became listless and drowsy; vomiting, dysphagia and dysarthria appeared; and during the succeeding 3 days all symptoms became progressively worse and finally alarming. The late appearance of these symptoms seemed to exclude the postoperative complications which might have been expected, hemorrhage or infection, and suggested that in some way the reaction about the stump of tumor which remained was responsible for the condition. The wound was reopened and the shell of the tumor extirpated with the index finger. There was surprisingly little hemorrhage, which was readily controlled. The patient's condition then steadily improved. Diminished drowsiness was at once apparent, the vomiting at once ceased, and 5 days later she was able to swallow. From the result of this case it seemed logical to infer that if the shell of the tumor could in some way be removed at the first operation, this stormy and dangerous course following subtotal removal might be avoided.

Apparently, two more cases were then done in two stages, the second stage being the finger enucleation. This was followed by combining intracapsular enucleation with a finger enucleation of the partially removed tumor at one stage. Dandy now recognized that the finger enucleation was far too unreliable and often traumatic. Therefore, he developed a very painstaking removal of the capsule following extensive enucleation of the interior of the tumor. He describes it this way:

> The contents of the tumor are then curetted with the brainstem and cerebellum always fully exposed. Continuing this method, the capsule gradually becomes thinner and when drawn forward permits inspection of the cleavage line between the brainstem and capsule of the tumor. When the poles of the tumor have invaded the middle cranial fossa and the spinal canal, removal of their interior allows them to be easily withdrawn into the posterior fossa; such polar extensions of the tumor are least adherent to the brainstem. Gradually in this way the entire capsule is separated from the brainstem. As the capsule is cautiously retracted, several small blood vessels crossing from the brainstem or cerebellum are brought into view and double 'clipped' and the vessel divided. Practically all bleeding can be forstalled in this way.
> Removal of the capsule of the tumor in this way is necessarily very tedious and time consuming. The method employed is but the application of the fundamental surgical teachings of my former chief, the late Professor Halsted. By this great master every operation, whether unusual or commonplace, was performed with the utmost care. All tissues were handled with the greatest gentleness, the field unstained with blood, and a step was never taken blindly. Always his work was painstaking, the field of operation immaculate, and hemorrhage minimal. Time of operation was always subordinate to accurate and thorough performance.

By 1925, 9 years after he had entered practice, Dandy had treated twenty-three acoustic tumors. He had been able surgically to cure five successive patients. This was a truly monumental achievement. Dandy's next contribution was to modify the surgical approach to a unilateral cerebellar approach by gaining exposure through an incision of the outer cap of the cerebellum. This approach became the standard method of removal of acoustic tumors until the advent of microsurgery in 1961; it is well illustrated in Dandy's 1940 article (4).

Dandy's techniques obviously were brilliant, in that they lowered operative mortality and at the same time affected a cure. However, they did result in total loss of facial nerve function in virtually every case. In years to come there were attempts, especially by Olivecrona, to save facial nerve function by using Dandy's techniques (5, 6).

Over the years, as diagnosis was made earlier, many more tumors were seen before an elevated intracranial pressure had occurred. It became universally recognized and accepted that, in operating smaller tumors, the operative mortality was much decreased. At first this was believed to be simply because these patients had less preoperative edema of the brain, since they did not have elevated intracranial pressure, and therefore postoperative brainstem infarction was greatly reduced. Dandy recommended clipping and cauterizing of the vessels surrounding the tumor (7). Apparently there was no appreciation of the end-artery status of the anterior-inferior cerebellar artery.

In 1949 Atkinson published a careful study documenting his discovery that occlusion of the anterior-inferior cerebellar artery is the principal cause of operative fatality in acoustic neuroma surgery (8). Previously, brainstem infarction and cerebellar edema seen at the autopsy of patients shortly after acoustic tumor surgery were believed to be due to excessive manipulation of these structures during the surgical procedure. The condition of brainstem infarction and cerebellar edema was called malacia pontis.

Atkinson reviews the postoperative course of six patients who died from one to several days after removal of acoustic neuromas. In each case, either a thrombosis or surgical division of the anterior-inferior cerebellar artery was found. In one of the cases, the tumor was small, its size approximating a pigeon's egg. The anterior-inferior cerebellar artery was torn as it went across the inferior surface of the tumor. Atkinson noted necrosis of the pons and cerebellar peduncles in the area of distribution of the anterior-inferior cerebellar artery in each of these cases. Atkinson's observations explained a major cause of operative mortality but they did not result in changes in surgical technique, since magnification was not being used and since once an artery—the anterior-inferior cerebellar or any other—was torn, it had to be controlled by clipping or cautery.

Until now we have been telling the story of the acoustic tumor from the perspective of the pioneers who were contributing to its management. Let us now diverge to a description of the treatment of a typical acoustic tumor diagnosed during the time from the end of World War II until the advent of the microsurgical treatment in 1961.

World War II had greatly stimulated an interest in neurosurgery, with a large number of well-trained young neurosurgeons entering practice between 1945 and 1950. Almost all hospitals had a staff neurosurgeon considered capable of management of all neurosurgical problems, including cerebellopontine angle tumors. These specialists, who might have seen only two or three acoustic tumors in their practice, usually proceeded with surgical management upon presentation of a case. Twenty years earlier, when there were few neurosurgical clinics, a surgeon saw more cases and thus became more skilled in the techniques that had been so beautifully standardized by Dandy. It became widely recognized that the average neurosurgeon treated brain tumors, especially acoustic neuromas, with a higher morbidity and mortality rate than did the neurosurgeon who had gained great experience in large teaching centers.

After World War II most acoustic tumors were diagnosed by otologists. The surgical treatment of otosclerosis so firmly established by Lempert in the late 1930s had spurred careful evaluation of patients with hearing loss. Vestibular studies were now being commonly used in the evaluation of patients with dizziness. X-ray of the petrous pyramids, pioneered by Hinchen and perfected by Towne and others in the 1920s, had now become a standard practice (9). Unilateral hearing loss combined with facial numbness now equaled the diagnosis of acoustic neuroma in the minds of all otolaryngologists. These patients were routinely referred for surgical evaluation. In a growing number of cases unilateral hearing losses were carefully evaluated by x-ray and vestibular studies, enabling the discovery of tumors whose symptoms were still confined to the eighth nerve. It was at this point that a great dilemma arose: Should the patient be operated immediately, trading his partial hearing loss for a total hearing loss and a facial paralysis, and face a significant fatality risk from the surgery, or should the patient be observed for a few more years, enjoying a normal life without facial paralysis, until he developed more symptoms due to a larger tumor? At the later time of surgery, the patient not only would suffer postoperative facial paralysis, he would also run a much higher risk of operative mortality and morbidity due to the larger size of the tumor. In many cases the patient was observed for a few years until he had marked fifth nerve paresthesia and, usually, early papilledema. In 1950, watchful expectation was championed by Pennybacker and Cairnes; immediate surgery was championed by Dandy (10).

If all surgeons could have duplicated the 2.4% mortality that Dandy encountered in a particularly good run of 41 cases, then the early surgery demanded by otologists and neurosurgeons would have been justified. However, Dandy's lifetime mortality was 22.1% (11). Mortality figures for acoustic tumors for most surgeons at this time varied quite widely, seemingly in relation to the experience of the surgeon. When the results of a number of surgeons who were not doing a significant volume of tumors were compiled, the mortality figures were higher, as pointed out by Bloch and Nathanson in the Mount Sinai Hospital series (12). Their series of 64 cases had an overall mortality of 31%. Figures presented by the California tumor registry about this time were discouraging. They showed that from 1942 to 1962 various neurosurgeons in reporting hospitals operated on 85 cases. Thirty-one patients died within 1 month of surgery, representing a mortality of 36.5%. Another six cases died within 1 year, representing a 1-year mortality of 43.5%.

Pool, an experienced neurosurgeon, reported an operative mortality of 12.5% for 72 cases operated between 1950 and 1965 (13). Olivecrona, who reported a total of 415 acoustic neuromas operated between 1931 and 1960, was obviously the world's most experienced operator at that time. His overall mortality was 19.2% (6). Olivecrona conclusively pointed out (6) that his mortality was almost five times as high in large tumors as it was in the group he considered to be small tumors, or as he describes them, "hazel nut size." The difference was 4.5% mortality in the small tumors and 22.5% mortality in the large tumors.

The mortality, however, was not the only thing to be considered: in many cases a complete disabling due to severe ataxia and sometimes contralateral paresis made the patient incapable of caring for himself. This disabling occurred in 18% of survivors in a recent study compiled of 125 cases from the Ricks Hospital in Copenhagen (14).

Thus, in 1960, 60 years after the beginning of active interest in the diagnosis and surgery of acoustic tumors, it was clear that definitive diagnosis was far more advanced than definitive surgical treatment. The challenge was obvious. New surgical methods would have to be found that would allow us to take advantage of the low surgical mortality of operating on small tumors and at the same time to preserve facial nerve function. This challenge was met in the next era of the history of the acoustic tumor, through the applications of microsurgical techniques.

REFERENCES

1. Cottrell, B. 1899. Remarks on surgical aspects of a case of cerebellopontine tumor. Trans. Med. Chir. Soc. (Edinb.) xviii:215.
2. Dandy, W. E. 1918. Ventriculography following the injection of air into the cerebral ventricles. Ann. Surg. 68:5.
3. Dandy, W. E. 1925. An operation for the total removal of cerebellopontine angle (acoustic) tumors. Surg. Gynecol. Obstet. XLI:129–148 (Aug.).
4. Cushing, H. 1963. Tumors of the Nervus Acusticus and the Syndrome of Cerebellopontine Angle. Hafner Publishing Co., New York.
5. Dandy, W. E. 1969. The brain. In: Lewis' Practice of Surgery, p. 527. Harper and Row, New York.
6. Olivecrona, H. 1967. Acoustic tumors. J. Neurosurg. 26:6–13.
7. Olivecrona, H. 1967. The removal of acoustic neurinomas. J. Neurosurg. 26:100–103.

8. Atkinson, W. J. 1949. Anterior-inferior cerebellar artery. J. Neurol. Neurosurg. Psychiat. 12:137–151 (May).
9. Towne, E. D. 1926. Erosion of the petrous bone by acoustic nerve tumor. Arch. Otolaryngol. 4:515–519.
10. Pennybacker, J. B., and Cairnes, H. 1950. Results in 130 cases of acoustic neurinoma. J. Neurol. Neurosurg. Psychiat. 13:272–277 (No. 4).
11. Revilla, A. 1948. Neuromas of the cerebello-pontine recess: Clinical study of 160 cases including operative mortality and end results. Bull. Johns Hopkins Hosp. 83:47.
12. Bloch, J. M., and Nathanson, M. 1963. Results in acoustic neuroma surgery. J. Mt. Sinai Hosp. (New York) 30:217–227.
13. Pool, J. L. 1966. Sub-occipital surgery for acoustic neuromas: Advantages and disadvantages. J. Neurosurg. 24:483–492.
14. Thomsen, J. 1976. Sub-occipital removal of acoustic neuromas: Results of 125 operations. Acta Otolaryngol. 81:406–414.

Acoustic Tumors
Volume I, *Diagnosis*
Edited by W. F. House and C. M. Luetje

Chapter 4

A History of Acoustic Tumor Surgery 1961–Present

Michael E. Glasscock, III, M.D., F.A.C.S.*
Clinical Associate Professor of Surgery (Otology and Neurotology), Vanderbilt University School of Medicine, Nashville, Tennessee

Ronald L. Steenerson, M.D.†
Otologic Fellow, The Otology Group, P.C., Nashville, Tennessee (during the academic year 1976)

In the preceding chapters of this book, William F. House provides the reader with a fascinating account of the early history of acoustic tumor diagnosis and surgery. This chapter continues the account, encompassing the time from 1960 to the present.

The three giants in the field of acoustic tumor surgery in this century have been Harvey Cushing, Walter Dandy, and William House, the last being the leading authority on acoustic tumor surgery today. House's personal series is the largest ever accumulated; he has firmly established his place in medical history.

When a person has attained world-wide fame, his success is often seen as an overnight phenomenon resulting from an abundance of luck. In truth, most success stories are founded in hard work and years of preparation and sacrifice. Many times the individual has had to stand alone—to accept criticism, jealousy, and often open hostility.

New ideas in medicine have traditionally met great resistance. For William House, the early years were not easy ones. This modern era of

* Mailing address: 1811 State Street, Nashville, Tennessee 37203
† Mailing address: 2205 19th Street, Bakersfield, California 93301

acoustic tumor surgery began in 1956, when Dr. House made the diagnosis of a tumor in a young Los Angeles fireman. The man had very few symptoms—mostly unilateral hearing loss and tinnitus. He was referred to a local neurosurgeon for definitive treatment. At that time neurosurgeons did not operate upon cerebellopontine angle tumors unless they were producing symptoms of cranial nerve deficit (other than eighth), ataxia, or papilledema. The reason for this was the high morbidity and mortality rates associated with posterior fossa surgery as it was performed in the 1950s. Most surgeons would wait until the tumors were large and life-threatening before attempting to remove them. The young fireman was observed for 1 year following his diagnosis. At that time he developed fifth nerve findings, headaches, and papilledema. Surgery was performed by means of the suboccipital route without the benefit of microsurgical technique. The patient died on the third postoperative day.

During the next year Dr. House diagnosed two additional tumors. These patients survived their surgery, but both were left with major neurological deficits.

Simultaneously, Dr. House was in the process of developing the middle fossa approach to the contents of the internal auditory canal (1). He had used this procedure to section the vestibular nerve and to decompress the facial nerve. It occurred to Dr. House that he might be able to approach an acoustic tumor through the middle fossa and identify the facial nerve in the internal auditory canal. His plan was to trace the nerve into the posterior fossa and then remove the remainder of the tumor from the suboccipital route.

With these thoughts in mind, Dr. House contacted Dr. John B. Doyle, a Los Angeles neurosurgeon, and formed a surgical team. They aimed at developing a new technique for the removal of acoustic tumors that would lower morbidity and mortality.

The classic middle fossa approach as employed by neurosurgeons had always been performed with the surgeon in a seated position. Therefore, Doyle and House made some modifications to the Zeiss operating microscope and asked Mr. Jack Urban of the Urban Engineering Company to design a chair that the surgeon could use to rest his arms upon while operating. The first microsurgical removal of an acoustic tumor was performed on February 15, 1961. As a matter of fact, this was the first use of microsurgical technique in neurosurgery. A partial removal of the tumor was accomplished, and the patient later died in 1967 after two subsequent suboccipital procedures (2).

The initial eight cases in Dr. House's series were performed through the middle fossa between the dates of February, 1961, and May, 1962 (3).

At that time House and Doyle were removing a large part of the labyrinth to expose the posterior fossa. The main reason for choosing the middle fossa route was to be able to identify the facial nerve in the lateral extent of the internal auditory canal where there were boney landmarks.

It soon became apparent that the procedure was unsatisfactory, because very few of the tumors could be totally removed. It occurred to Dr. House that a direct approach through the mastoid and labyrinth might be a better choice, particularly since he and Doyle were already destroying the labyrinth.

Panse (4) had approached the cerebellopontine angle through the mastoid in the early 1900s, but without the aid of microsurgical technique or adequate instrumentation. In his procedure a radical mastoidectomy was performed and the facial nerve removed. There was, as one would expect, a great deal of difficulty with postoperative cerebrospinal fluid leak. Having become interested in the possibility of this approach, Dr. House performed a series of cadaver dissections in order to work out a method of exposing the internal auditory canal and cerebellopontine angle through the labyrinth. With the aid of magnification, the dental drill, and irrigation/suction, he was able to do so with preservation of the posterior canal wall, tympanic membrane, and facial nerve.

With the development of the translabyrinthine approach, a difference of opinion ensued between the two surgeons. This philosophical separation of ideas was the beginning of a long and continuing controversy concerning the best method of dealing with cerebellopontine angle lesions. The first translabyrinthine procedure was performed by House alone without the assistance of Doyle. In fact, there was a heated argument concerning the case just prior to surgery. However, House and Doyle continued to work together during this time period and did some cases as one-stage, some as two-stage, and a few from the suboccipital route using the microscope.

Obviously at this point there was some question whether the technique could be employed for the removal of larger tumors. In 1963, House and Doyle could no longer agree upon basic techniques. In July of that year Dr. William Hitselberger began to work with Dr. House, and they became a unique surgical team. After further cadaver dissections they began to employ the translabyrinthine procedure on a routine basis for tumors of all sizes. Dr. House's first 53 cases, most of which had been performed with Dr. Hitselberger, were reported in 1964 (3). Many of these cases were subtotal; as the surgeons gained experience, however, this percentage dropped (5).

Dr. Hitselberger worked diligently to learn temporal bone anatomy and surgical technique. He mastered the microscope and dental drill and became the first neurosurgeon to routinely perform mastoidectomy and labyrinthectomy surgery. His association with Dr. House and the translabyrinthine procedure, however, did not make him popular with his neurosurgical colleagues. During their pioneering years House and Hitselberger underwent close scrutiny by the Los Angeles neurosurgical community. At St. Vincent's Hospital, interdepartmental bickering and politics became a very real issue. At one point the administrator of the hospital had to lock Dr. House's charts in her personal office to keep them from hostile surgical committee members.

At national meetings translabyrinthine adversaries lambasted House and Hitselberger for their work. The neurosurgical community as a whole continued over the next few years to disagree vehemently with translabyrinthine surgery. Slowly, however, House and Hitselberger were able to win over a few neurosurgeons. One of these was a leading Los Angeles neurosurgeon, Dr. Henry Dodge. He reviewed their cases and helped them obtain credibility.

Other neurosurgeons across the country began to lessen the intensity of their attack but still continued to disapprove of transtemporal bone removal of acoustic tumors. In 1963, Dr. House offered a small, informal course on the diagnosis and surgical management of these lesions, and in 1965 he sponsored a large international symposium on acoustic tumor diagnosis and treatment.

Leading neurosurgeons, otologists, neurologists, and audiologists attended the 1965 meeting. For 5 days the subject was thoroughly covered by a wide range of disciplines. One of the most important aspects of that meeting was the overall summary of the advances that had been made in early diagnosis. The first monograph (3) had been published the preceding December, setting forth for the first time a logical, step-by-step method for early detection of acoustic tumors.

Cushing had been the first clinician (6) to recognize and to describe accurately the natural history of a cerebellopontine angle tumor. He noted that the most common initial symptoms were hearing loss and tinnitus. Lempert (7), who had popularized the use of the audiometer, was probably the father of modern otology due to his many innovative surgical techniques. House, with the advantage of sophisticated audiometric studies, pioneered the concept of a neuro-otologic evaluation for all patients presenting with unilateral tinnitus, unilateral hearing loss, or any form of spatial disorientation.

Many audiometric, vestibular, and x-ray procedures were in an explosive stage of development in the first half of the 1960s, spurred by the interest in early detection of acoustic tumors. Jerger (8) classified von Bekesy's work on adaptation of the acoustic nerve and established a practical method of reporting the results. The modified SISI (9) and the Tone Decay Test of Carhart (10) were also popularized during this period. More sophisticated vestibular studies were being advocated, and for the first time ENG was being discussed as a clinical method of investigation.

Of all the diagnostic studies available to the otologist, x-ray became the most valuable and accurate. Compere (11) advocated x-rays of the internal auditory canal performed with a special head unit that could be used in the physician's office. Dr. Robert Scanlan, a radiologist at St. Vincent's Hospital in Los Angeles, was responsible for the development of posterior fossa myelography as a means of detecting acoustic tumors. On a visit to the Mayo Clinic, he observed a posterior fossa study being performed and noticed that the internal auditory canal filled easily with iophendylate (Pantopaque). It occurred to Dr. Scanlan that it might be possible to outline a tumor at the internal auditory canal by this method (12). Upon returning to Los Angeles he discussed this possibility with Dr. House, and they began using the procedure on a routine basis. Later Dr. House was to combine this study with yet another new x-ray advancement, polytomography. Known as the polytome Pantopaque procedure (13), it involved a small amount (1 cc) of dye placed in the subarachnoid space and then maneuvered into the internal auditory canal without fluoroscopic guidance. The accuracy of the polytomograph made the diagnosis of small tumors extremely precise. Polytomography also had advantage of being performed as an outpatient procedure.

Two new diagnostic procedures have become popular within the past five years, and both are revolutionizing the diagnosis of acoustic tumors. One is brainstem evoked response audiometry (BERA) and the other is computerized axial tomography (CAT) (14).

The accuracy of BERA is astounding. Selters and Brackmann (15) have reported positive BERA in 39 out of 46 tumors, and recently John House (16) did the same with a larger series (143 out of 146). Other investigators (17) have had similar experiences. This topic is covered in greater detail in Chapter 10.

The CAT scanner has drastically changed neuroradiology. This procedure is basically non-invasive and is extremely accurate if the lesion is over 2 cm. It does have some limitations, however. First, if the individual is allergic to iodine, the study must be performed without enhancement. In most radiologists' experience, lesions in the cerebellopontine angle cannot be visualized, regardless of size, without the use of intravenous dye. Secondly, even with this adjunct, most tumors under 2 cm simply cannot be detected with this method. Therefore, the posterior fossa myelogram is still the procedure of choice in the diagnosis of small tumors. This situation may change in the future with more sophisticated scanners.

The historic international symposium in 1965 brought a new awareness of acoustic tumor diagnosis and surgical removal. Patients were no longer required to wait until their lesion was life-threatening before a surgical removal was attempted.

Neurosurgeons and otolaryngologists alike began to be more aware of early diagnosis, and the neurosurgical community across the country began to employ microsurgical technique in a wide variety of applications. Rand and Kurze (18) of Los Angeles advocated the use of the microscope for the suboccipital removal of acoustic tumors. Their technique required the removal of the posterior lip of the internal auditory canal with a dental drill. They became strong advocates of this procedure, and over the years the majority of neurosurgeons and a few otologists have adopted this method.

While the controversy continues, it is less heated and certainly no longer centers on House and Hitselberger. One reason for this is that these two surgeons have over the ensuing years trained many otologists who have gone out on their own to carry on the principles of transtemporal bone surgery (19–23). As these individuals have gained experience and reported their cases, it has become obvious that others could obtain similar results with the translabyrinthine approach. The number of translabyrinthine procedures currently performed must be well over 200–300 per year.

In the past 5 years there has been a great deal said about the advantages of the suboccipital route in the preservation of hearing. House, of course, was the first to routinely save the hearing by removing intracanalicular tumors from the internal auditory canal through the middle fossa. He was able to do this in five out of five attempts (24), but his success rate dropped to seven out of thirteen when he extended his indications to tumors outside the canal. Rand (25), Smith et al. (26), MacCarty (27), and Rhoton (28), have reported preservation of the cochlear nerve through the suboccipital route. Only Smith et al. have supplied the scientific community with adequate pre- and postoperative audiograms to back up their claims. Smith's results are impressive and he has backed down from some of his earlier statements concerning the best method of tumor removal. Glasscock and Hays (29) have now reported a series of tumor removals through the middle fossa with preservation of hearing. Certainly, in tumors under 2 cm it is possible to preserve the cochlear nerve; whether or not function is maintained depends upon preservation of the vascular supply to the cochlea.

As time goes on, it becomes more evident that there will continue to be two schools of thought about the best method for dealing with these lesions. There is no question that microsurgical technique has greatly improved the results one can expect from the classic suboccipital approach. With this technique, it is possible to preserve facial nerve function, and patients do not necessarily have ataxia postoperatively (depending upon the size of the tumor). There are many reasons why these authors personally prefer the translabyrinthine, middle fossa, and combined approaches, and all of these are documented (22,23,29). The fact remains that, if one takes an objective view and simply compares the results that have been reported in the literature, it is obvious that the transtemporal bone and combined procedures net the lowest morbidity and mortality rates. Unfortunately, at this time, 16 years after the pioneering work of William House, very few surgeons will report their results in a standardized method. Certainly neurosurgeons have been able to improve their statistics with microsurgical technique, but they continue in most instances to be extremely vague in their reports in the literature. Determining tumor size, for instance, continues to be a problem, since surgeons have a tendency to exaggerate the lesion they are dealing with. The CAT scanner may well dispense with this problem by providing an accurate assessment of the tumor dimensions prior to surgery.

If all surgeons dealing with these lesions would report all their results, including morbidity and mortality rates, we could obtain a better idea of what actual techniques are best for each size of tumor.

The translabyrinthine and combined approaches would seem, based upon the literature, to ensure the most favorable, functional results. The last 16 years have been exciting ones and have truly changed the course of acoustic tumor diagnosis and surgery. In the final analysis, William House and William Hitselberger are responsible for generating the interest that led to the field of microsurgical technique in neurosurgery.

William House's determination and perseverance against formidable opposition have finally brought him the recognition he deserves. Furthermore, his contributions have made us all better surgeons, so that we may better serve the needs of our patients with acoustic tumors and other cerebellopontine angle lesions. All of us, surgeons and patients alike, owe this man a great debt of gratitude. Thank you, Bill, from all of us!

REFERENCES

1. House, W. F. 1961. Surgical exposure of the internal auditory canal and its contents through the middle cranial fossa. Laryngoscope 71:1363–1385.
2. House, W. F. 1977. History of the development of the translabyrinthine approach. In: H. Silverstein and H. Norrell (eds.), Neurological Surgery of the Ear, pp. 235–238. Aesculapius Publishing Company, Birmingham, Alabama.
3. House, W. F. 1964. Report of cases; Monograph, transtemporal bone microsurgical removal of acoustic neuromas. Arch. Otolaryngol. 80:617–667.
4. Panse, R. 1904. Ein Gliom des Akusticus. Arch. Ohren. 61:251–255.
5. House, W. F. 1968. Partial tumor removal and recurrence in acoustic tumor surgery. In: W. F. House (ed.), Monograph II, Acoustic Neuroma. Arch. Otolaryngol. 88:86–106.
6. Cushing, H. 1963. Tumors of the Nervus Acusticus and the Syndrome of the Cerebellopontine Angle, ed. 2. Hafner Publishing Company, New York.
7. Lempert, J. 1963. Improvement of hearing in cases of otosclerosis: New one stage surgical technic. Arch. Otolaryngol. 67:233–258.
8. Jerger, J. F. 1960. Bekesy audiometry in analysis of audiometric disorders. J. Speech Hear. Res. 3:275–287.
9. Jerger, J., Shedd, J., and Harford, E. R. 1959. On the detection of extremely small changes in sound intensity. Arch. Otolaryngol. 69:200–211.
10. Carhart, R. 1957. Clinical determination of abnormal auditory adaptation. Arch. Otolaryngol. 65:32–39.
11. Compere, W. E. 1964. The radiographic examination of the petrous portion of the temporal bone. In: Book I of Radiographic Atlas of the Temporal Bone, First edition. American Academy of Ophthalmology and Otolaryngology, St. Paul, Minnesota.
12. Scanlan, R. L. 1964. Positive contrast medium (iophendylate) in diagnosis of acoustic neuroma. Arch. Otolaryngol. 80:698–706.
13. Glasscock, M. E., Overfield, R. E., and Miller, G. W. 1976. Polytomography in an otologic practice. South. Med. J. 69:1433.
14. Scott, W. R., Davis, K. R., Trevor, R. P., and Schneer, J. A. 1977. Computerized tomography of the cerebellopontine angle. In: H. Silverstein and H. Norrell (eds.), Neurological Surgery of the Ear, pp. 206–215. Aesculapius Publishing Company, Birmingham, Alabama.
15. Selters, W. A., and Brackmann, D. E. 1977. Acoustic tumor detection with electric response audiometry. Arch. Otolaryngol. 103:181–187.
16. House, J. W. 1977. Personal communication.
17. Clemis, J. 1977. Personal communication.
18. Rand, R. W., and Kurze, T. L. 1967. Micro-Neurosurgery in acoustic tumors (suboccipital transmeatal approach). Trans. Am. Acad. Ophthalmol. Otolaryngol. 71:682.
19. Maddox, H. E. 1969. Experiences in acoustic tumor surgery. Laryngoscope 79:652–670.

20. Clemis, J. D. 1971. Microsurgical treatment of acoustic neurinomas (results and complications). Laryngoscope 81:1191.
21. Montgomery, W. W. 1973. Surgery for acoustic neurinoma. Ann. Otol. Rhinol. Laryngol. 92:428–444.
22. Glasscock, M. E., and Hays, J. W. 1973. The translabyrinthine removal of acoustic and other cerebellopontine angle tumors. Ann. Otol. Rhinol. Laryngol. 82:415–427.
23. Glasscock, M. E., and Hays, J. W. 1977. Results and complications in the translabyrinthine removal of cerebellopontine angle tumors. In: H. Silverstein and H. Norrell (eds.), Neurological Surgery of the Ear. Aesculapius Publishing Company, Birmingham, Alabama.
24. House, W. F., Gardner, G., and Hughes, R. L. 1968. Middle cranial fossa approach to acoustic tumor surgery. In: W. F. House (ed.), Monograph II, Acoustic Neuroma. Arch. Otolaryngol. 88:83–93.
25. Rand, R. W. 1971. Suboccipital transmeatal microneurosurgical resection of acoustic tumors. Ann. Surg. 174:663.
26. Smith, M. F. W., Miller, R. N., and Cox, D. J. 1973. Suboccipital microsurgical removal of acoustic neurinomas of all sizes. Ann. Otol. Rhinol. Laryngol. 82:407.
27. MacCarty, C. S. 1975. Acoustic neuroma and the suboccipital approach (1967–1972). Mayo Clin. Proc. 50:15.
28. Rhoton, A. L. 1976. Microsurgical removal of acoustic neuromas. Surg. Neurol. 6:211.
29. Glasscock, M. E., Hays, J. W., Miller, G. W., Drake, F. D., and Kanok, M. M. 1978. Preservation of hearing in tumors of the internal auditory canal and cerebellopontine angle. Laryngoscope 88:43–55.

Acoustic Tumors
Volume I, *Diagnosis*
Edited by W. F. House and C. M. Luetje

Section II

PATHOLOGY

Chapter 5

Pathophysiology of Acoustic Tumors

Jose Bebin, M.D., Ph.D.*

Professor of Pathology (Neuropathology), University of Mississippi Medical Center, Jackson, Mississippi

---

The understanding of intracranial tumors arising from cranial nerves, such as those of the eighth nerve, includes the gross and microscopic appearance of the tumors, and the structural and functional changes, both focal and general, that these tumors produce in the nervous tissue, the vascular structures, and the meninges. Accordingly, the first part of this chapter briefly considers certain anatomical features of the eighth cranial nerve important to the understanding of neoplasms developing in that nerve.

* Mailing address: Department of Pathology, University of Mississippi Medical Center, Jackson, Mississippi 39216

DEVELOPMENT OF THE EIGHTH NERVE

The eighth nerve and its ganglia first become visible in the human embryo as a mass of epithelial cells, known as the acoustic-facial ganglion, which lies medial and ventral to the auditory vesicle. These cells subsequently migrate medially to lie between the auditory vesicle and the rhombencephalon. The facial portion is distinguishable early by its large and pale staining cells. The remainder of the triangular mass initially is undifferentiated but later divides into a dorsolateral vestibular ganglion and a dorsomedial cochlear ganglion. The cells of these ganglionic groups differentiate into two cell types: bipolar ganglion cells and the subcapsular satellites and Schwann cells of the sheaths of their fibers.

The vestibular ganglion cells send their processes to the auditory vesicle, followed shortly by the cochlear ganglion cells. From the other end of these bipolar ganglion cells, their processes extend into the rhombencephalon, forming the intracranial portion of the vestibular and cochlear divisions of the eighth nerve. The fibers of the vestibular nerve grow faster than those of the cochlear nerve. These fibers are accompanied by Schwann cells from the same source, but the axons outgrow them. Simultaneously, glial cells, astrocytes, and oligodendroglia from the brainstem migrate outward along the ingrowing axons, and these two types of covering cells meet at a variable distance from the brainstem. Because the vestibular fibers reach the brainstem earlier, the glial cells migrate further into the vestibular nerve. The junction or transition zone from neuroglia cells to Schwann cells is usually located more distally in this nerve production, which is, at this point, an excess accumulation of supporting cells and Schwann cells arranged irregularly between fibers and nerve cells.

ANATOMY OF THE EIGHTH NERVE

The eighth nerve, according to Henschen (1–3), is 17–19 mm long in men and 16–17 mm long in women. It extends from the cochlear and vestibular ganglia to the lateral recessus of the medulla. This nerve consists of two parts, preganglionic distal and postganglionic central portions. The latter is the larger and may be subdivided into a short intracanalicular portion lying within the internal auditory canal, a large free portion situated within the subarachnoid space (cisterna lateralis), and a short intramedullary portion terminating in the cochlear and vestibular nuclei.

The eighth nerve follows a medial and slightly downward course. There is usually a slight flexure at the point of entrance to the porus acusticus internus. On entering the brainstem, the nerve winds around the restiform body. The cochlear division passes over the restiform body, while the vestibular division passes medial and ventral to this structure.

The seventh and the eighth nerves are closely related during their course through the subarachnoid space and in the internal auditory meatus. The eighth nerve usually lies posterior and slightly caudal to the seventh nerve. From the cerebellar approach in posterior fossa craniotomy, the facial nerve may be hidden by the acoustic nerve. Although the facial nerve arises medial and slightly caudal to the roots of the eighth nerve, it becomes anterior to it and enters the internal auditory canal in a dorsal position. In addition to this crossing of the seventh and eighth nerves, there is also a crossing of fibers of the vestibular and cochlear divisions of the eighth nerve. This fiber crossing occurs in a spiral fashion. The cochlear fibers pass from behind, forward, and above the vestibular fibers. According to Skinner (4) the crossing is usually not apparent in sections of adult human nerves, but it is clearly shown in the embryo (Hiss, quoted by Skinner). As these nerves leave the brainstem, they lie closely applied to the cerebellum, in contact with the lateral recessus of the fourth ventricle and its fold of choroid plexus. The two portions of the eighth nerve, cochlear (auditory) and vestibular, may or may not be grossly identifiable since they frequently form a single nerve bundle. The facial nerve also consists of two roots, where it attaches itself to the lateral surface of the brainstem close to the caudal border of the pons. The motor root is larger and anterior to the mixed sensory and parasympathetic root (nervus intermedius), which is a rather small filament lying between the eighth and the seventh nerves. The nervus intermedius in some cases is attached to the eighth nerve.

The eighth and the seventh nerves pass laterally and slightly upward to enter the internal auditory meatus. As they cross the subarachnoid space, the facial nerve lies anterior to the eighth nerve with the nervus intermedius between the two.

The fundus of the meatus is divided into an upper and a lower portion by the transverse crest. In the upper portion is an anterior depression with an opening for the seventh nerve, and a posterior funnel-shaped depression that contains numerous openings for the branches of the superior vestibular nerve.

In the anterior lower portion, below the transverse crest, is a rounded depression, the cochlear area, with a series of small openings (tractus spiralis foraminosus) that transmit the bundles of the cochlear nerve directly to the cochlea. In the posterior portion of the same area, close to the transverse crest, lie the small openings for the inferior vestibular nerve fibers. These relationships are of great importance when considering the surgical removal of small intracanalicular tumors.

STRUCTURE OF THE EIGHTH NERVE

As originally noted by Henschen (1–3) and confirmed by Skinner (4), the eighth nerve, along with most of the other cranial nerves, may be divided histologically into a proximal and a distal part. The proximal part extends for an average distance of 8 mm in the seventh nerve and to 13 mm in the eighth nerve of men, 7 to 10 mm in women (2). This part contains, in addition to axons, neuroglia (astrocytes and oligodendroglia). The distal part has, on the contrary, the typical structure of a peripheral nerve: clearly discernible epineurium, perineurium, endoneurium, and Schwann cells enclosing the axons. It is this portion that is involved in neoplasms of the nerve.

Peripheral and central myelin sheaths are similar. Both consist of a spiral of plasma membrane derived from the myelin-forming cells—oligodendroglia in the central nervous system and Schwann cells in the peripheral nervous system. In the latter, the external surfaces of adjoining Schwann cells are separated from each other by the basal lamina that completely surrounds each Schwann cell and the collagen and reticulin fibers. In the central nervous system neither of the last two elements is present. At the junction between the distal and proximal portions of the nerve, the sheath of the axon changes so that on one side of the node the sheath is formed by the Schwann cell, and on the other side, by an oligodendroglia cell. The Schwann cells forming the peripheral internode abut onto a dome formed by the processes of astrocytes, the "fibrous cone" (Figures 1 and 2). As the axons enter the proximal portion of the nerve, they pass through this dome-shaped "fibrous cone." The basal lamina of the Schwann cells becomes confluent with the basal lamina that coats the astrocytic processes that form the dome (5). The epineurium becomes confluent with the dura matter as the nerve penetrates the meninges. Some think the perineurium continues with the pia-arachnoid, while others think that it disappears as the nerve roots in the subarachnoid space become covered by cells derived from the pia-arachnoid membrane.

ORIGIN OF ACOUSTIC TUMORS

The point of junction of the proximal glial and the distal Schwannic portions of the nerve usually lies near the porus acusticus internus, occa-

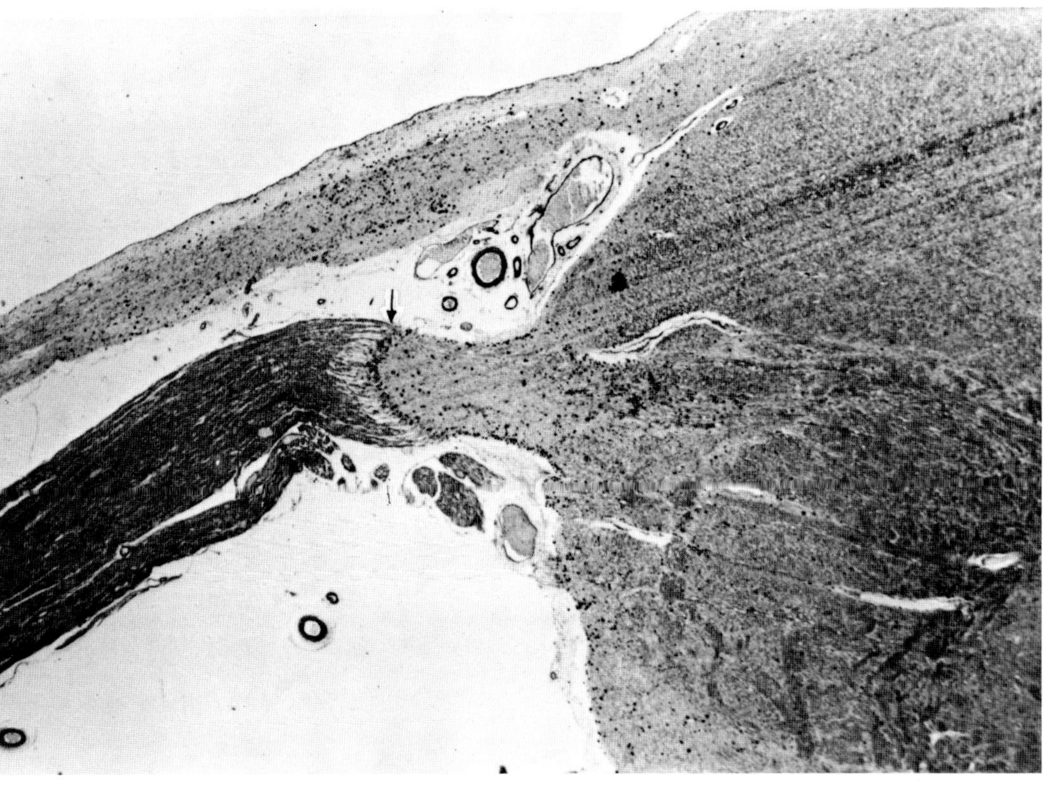

Figure 1. Structure of a cranial nerve (IX). The proximal glial portion meets the peripheral Schwannic portion at the "fibrous cone" (arrow) LFB-PAS. ×15

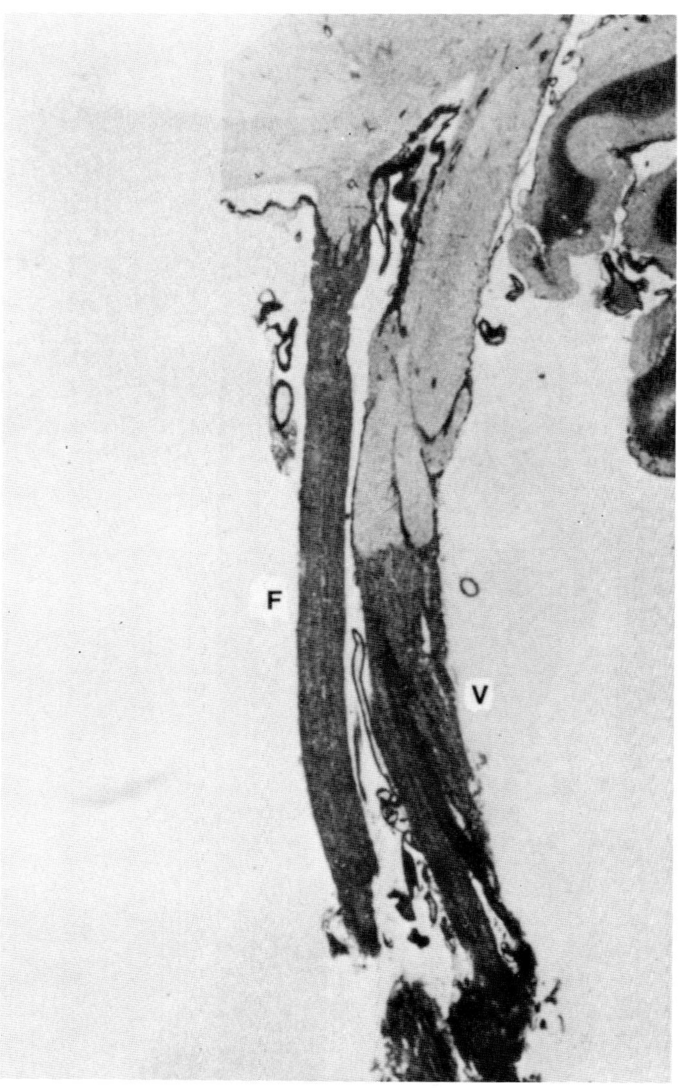

Figure 2. Section of the vestibular nerve (V) with the facial nerve (F) to left, showing the glial and Schwannic portions (2).

sionally more distal, close to the fundus, and, rarely, more proximal, outside of the temporal bone. This disposition may be slightly different on either side, and in the vestibular nerve it is more distal than in the cochlear nerve.

In the cochlear ganglion the subcapsular cells are regularly arranged and placed beneath the ganglion cells. In the vestibular ganglion there is a rich and excessive number of irregularly distributed cells resembling subcapsular cells and Schwann cells, which lie in a disorderly fashion between the ganglion cells. It is this apparent excess of Schwann cells in the vestibular ganglia and nerve that is thought to give rise to neoplasms (schwannomas) of this nerve.

It is not clear why the neoplasm should arise from the vestibular nerve, except that the vestibular nerve and ganglia tend to overproduce Schwann cells. In addition, the earliest tumors of this type found in the internal auditory canal take origin in the vestibular nerve (Henschen). Exceptions have been reported in the cochlear nerve (6–8). Several examples of small asymptomatic tumors found at autopsy have been published by De Moura et al. (9), who reported five asymptomatic acoustic tumors discovered among 140 processed temporal bones and referred to the another 31 tumors described previously in the literature. In a microscopic study of 250 temporal bones removed at autopsy, Hardy and Crowe (10) found six minute, asymptomatic schwannomas. Leonard and Talbbott (11) described four similar tumors found among 883 temporal bones in the Johns Hopkins Collection, and Schuknecht (12) found 3 small asymptomatic superior vestibular nerve schwannomas among 900 temporal bones collected at the Massachusetts Eye and Ear Infirmary. But it was Henschen (1) who first demonstrated their origin in the vestibular nerve. He studied four such cases in serial sections, among which was the case of a small intracanalicular tumor the size of a bean, which arose in the vestibular nerve. In the wax reconstruction of this tumor that he made (Figure 3), the facial nerve runs over the anterior surface of the tumor without being attached to it, and the well-preserved cochlear nerve appears as a thin broad band over the anterior lower aspect of the tumor. No significant changes were present in the spiral ganglion. The branches of the superior vestibular nerve were surrounded by the tumor-like cap and could not be separated from it, while the inferior branch of the vestibular nerve entered directly into the tumor mass. The vestibular ganglion was only partially involved by the neoplasm. As previously mentioned, in the vestibular nerve and ganglion, an excess of embryonic cells (precursors of Schwann cells and other cells) persists. It may well be that from this indifferent cellular material certain elements (Schwann cells) could give origin to the eighth nerve tumors (Henschen).

Pirsig et al. (13) found support for this hypothesis while examining 112 serially sectioned temporal bones of Wittmaak Collection in Hamburg. In 28 of these, the superior vestibular ganglion and nerve

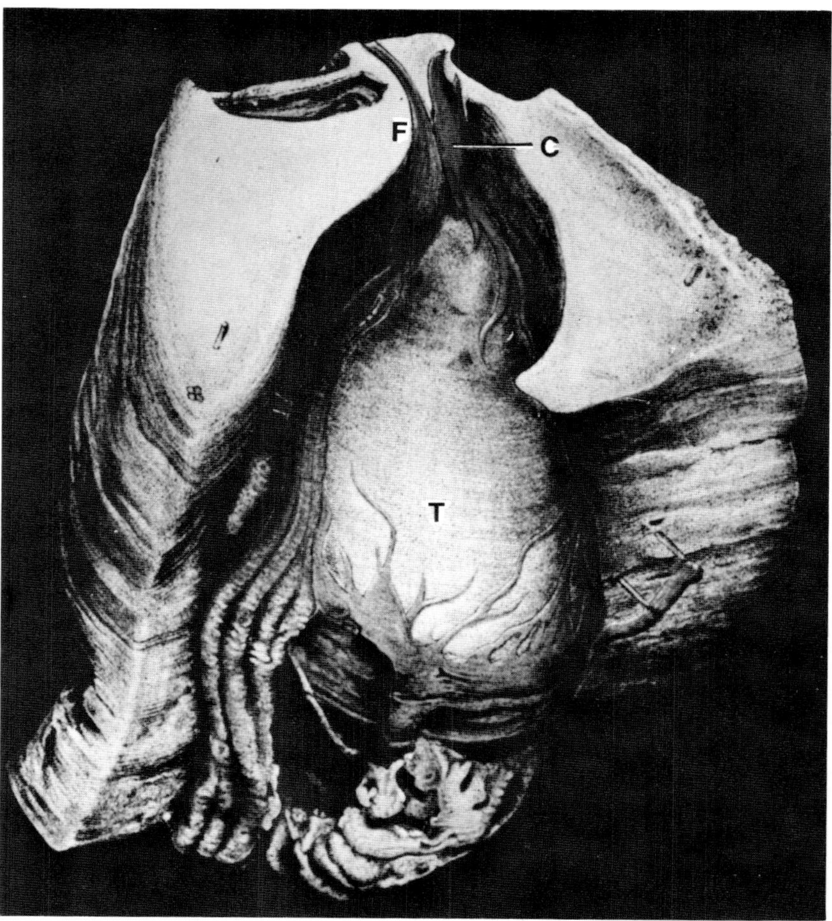

Figure 3. A: Henschen's wax reconstruction of a small acoustic tumor in the right internal auditory meatus. The tumor arose in the vestibular nerve. The facial (F) and the cochlear (C) are seen stretched at each side of the tumor.

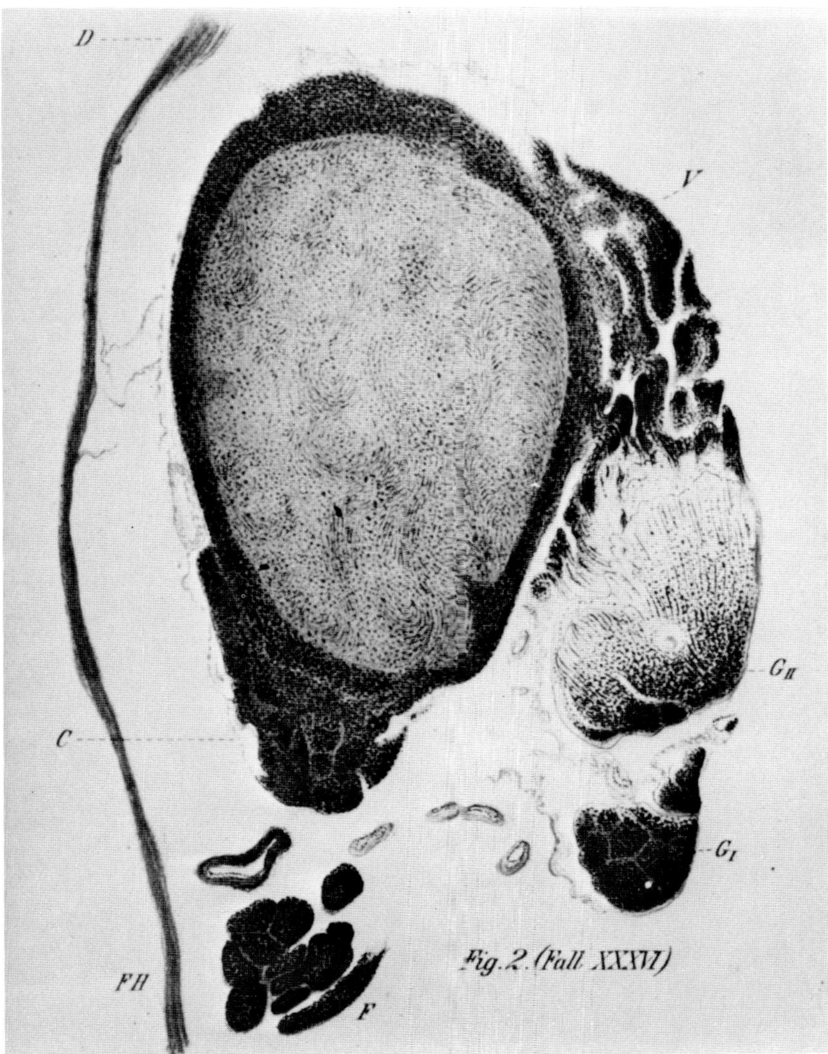

Figure 3B. Horizontal section of the tumor shown in 3A. The tumor arose in the inferior vestibular nerve (V); the facial (F) and the superior vestibular nerve (GI) are free of neoplasm (2).

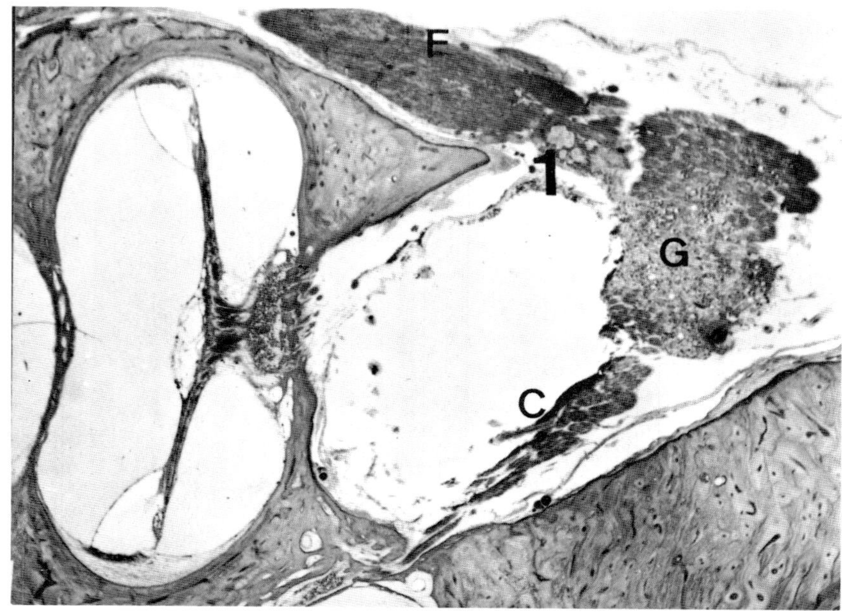

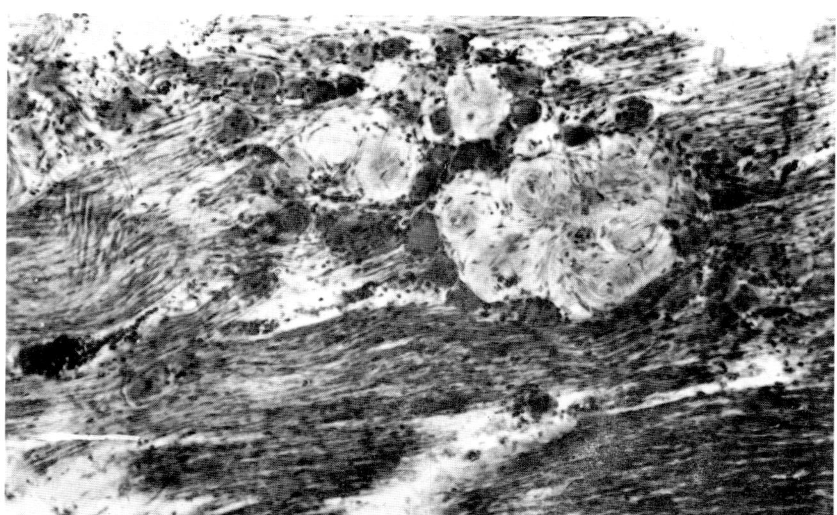

Figure 4. Top: Small cluster of ganglion cells and Schwann cells (1) near the left superior vestibular ganglion (G). Bottom: Higher magnification of area 1. (Courtesy of Prof. Pirsig.)

contain small nests of Schwann cells and "whorl-like formations" around eosinophilic bodies and ganglion cells, reminiscent of typical schwannomas. These structures were found only in the vestibular nerve and ganglion near the transverse crest, a common site of origin of vestibular schwannomas, and were considered to be the forerunners of vestibular schwannomas. The events that lead to production of neoplasm from this embryonic rest are not known (Figure 4).

The histogenesis of the nerve sheath tumors is dependent upon a proper concept of the histogenesis of the nerve sheath itself (14). Two schools compete for acceptance: the mesodermic theory, which considers that the acoustic nerve tumors are mesenchymal in origin and that they arise from endoneurial fibroblasts and should be called perineural fibroblastomas, and the neuroectodermic theory, which considers that these tumors are of Schwann cell origin and that they should be called schwannomas. Verocay (15), Masson (16), Stout (17), Rio-Hortega (18), and Russell and Rubinstein (19) support the neuroectodermic theory that these tumors are fundamentally composed of Schwann cells. Mallory (20), Penfield (21), and Tarlov (22) support the mesodermic theory. The application of in vitro tissue culture techniques to this problem by Murray and Stout (23) resulted in strong evidence in favor of the Schwann cell as the source of this neoplasm. However, recent application of the electron microscope to the study of this tumor has not clarified the problem of its origin. On the contrary, it has brought the controversy back to its beginning. Luse (24), Pineda (25), Poirier et al. (26), and Cravioto (27) favor the Schwann cell theory, whereas Raimondi and Beckman (28) maintain that the cell of origin is the fibroblast. We may conclude that most authors support the Schwann cell origin of tumors of the eighth nerve.

THE CEREBELLOPONTINE ANGLE (CPA)

Henneberg and Koch (29) introduced the term "cerebellopontine angle tumor." It refers only to an anatomical region, the site of the lesion; however, this term has been used for all tumors of this region and it has almost superseded the designation of acoustic tumor. The fact remains, as Cushing (30) so aptly stated, "By the time a tumor is present, the so-called angle has disappeared and its confines disordered beyond recognition."

The CPA may be considered a potential, rather than an actual, space. The pons and the medulla fit snugly into a gently sloping depression in the basilar portion of the occipital bone. When the flocculus of the cerebellum is prominent, it fits into a small depression in the posterior surface of the petrous pyramid caudal to the internal auditory meatus. The space between the brainstem, cerebellum, and the dura mater covering the petrous bone consists of a groove between the pons and the cerebellum, a groove between the medulla and the cerebellar tonsil, and an irregular cuboidal space between these two grooves. This space is bound medially by the inferior olive, rostrally by the caudal border of the pons, and caudally by the cerebellar tonsil. Its floor, in situ, is formed by the arachnoid crossed by the anterior inferior cerebellar artery (Figure 3) and other small arteries. Its roof is formed by the cerebellum and middle cerebellar peduncle. Its lateral wall is formed by the cerebellar tonsil and the flocculus, and it is crossed by the root fibers of the vagus and glossopharyngeal nerves (Figure 5). The arachnoidal floor is prolonged laterally into a cone that surrounds the roots of these nerves and then enters the internal auditory meatus. Thus, instead of being an angle, this irregular cisternal space resembles a tent, in which the seventh and eighth nerves provide a curving central support (Figure 6).

Loculated cerebrospinal fluid accounts for the superimposed "cyst" that often covers cerebellopontine angle tumors. Release and accumula-

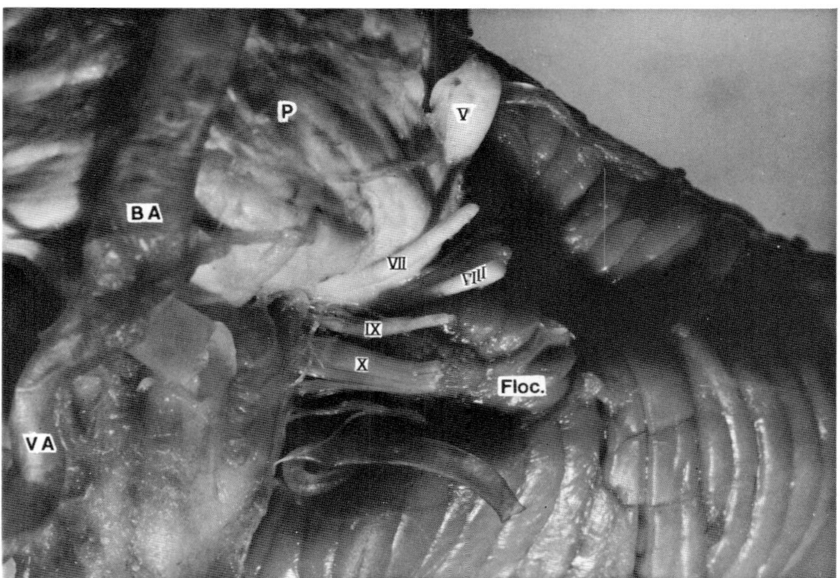

Figure 5. A view of the left cerebellopontine angle (CPA).

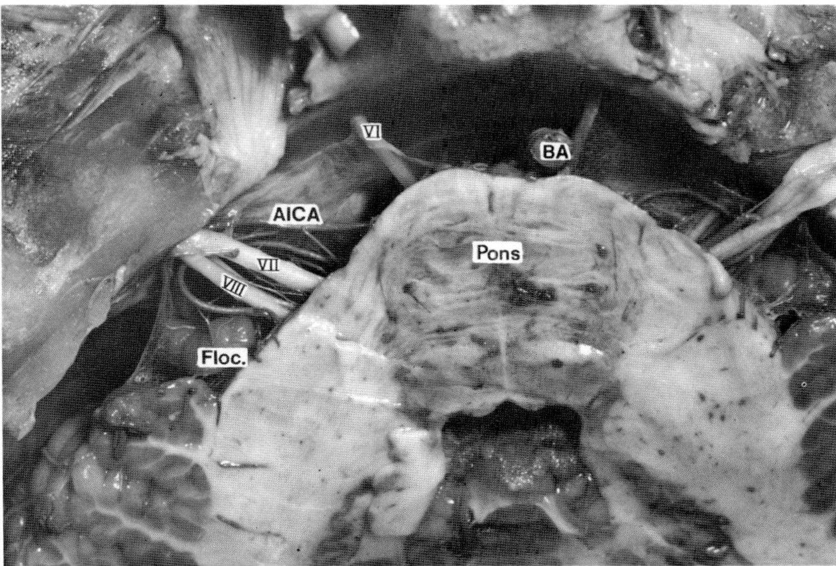

Figure 6. A view of the prepontine cisterns and the CPA after transection of the brainstem in situ. The neurovascular relations are clearly seen.

tion of fluid may cause fluctuation of symptoms in tumors occurring in this region.

TUMORS

Acoustic tumors vary greatly in size. Most, by the time they cause sufficient symptoms to oblige the patient to seek medical treatment, are rather large. Olivecrona (31) classified 415 cases operated in his clinic as follows: small size, no larger than a hazelnut (1.5 cm), usually situated at the porus acusticus internus; medium size, the size of a walnut (2.5 cm); and large tumors, the size of a ping-pong ball or larger (3.5 cm or more). He considered a tumor to be large when it extended from the tentorial incisura to the foramen magnum.

It is generally accepted that acoustic schwannomas are slow-growing neoplasms. The advanced age of 3 patients with small acoustic tumors, found in the study of temporal bones by Hardy and Crowe (10), seems to indicate that these tumors remain asymptomatic for a long time or may never reach a size sufficiently large to produce clinical symptoms. Olivecrona (32) observed that 50% of 83 patients remained asymptomatic after only a partial removal of the tumor. He concluded that the growth of these tumors is very slow or self-limited. Certain events within the tumor may alter this process; edema, cystic changes, or hemorrhages may lead to a rapid increase of volume and a corresponding increase of symptomatology.

Small tumors are usually 10–20 mm in size, spherical or fusiform, located in the internal auditory canal, and almost always in the vestibular nerve. Cases of this type were described by Toynbee (33), Panse (34), Henschen (2), and House and Hitselberger (35). Modern radiologic techniques have made possible the early detection of these tumors, with excision performed before they reach the posterior fossa. Panse (34) found at autopsy a small tumor of the eighth nerve in the internal auditory meatus that produced an enlargement of this opening. Henschen pointed out that this enlargement of the porus acusticus ought to be visible radiologically. Olivecrona found an enlarged internal auditory meatus in 80 to 90% of acoustic tumors. Fischgold et al. (36), in a radiologic study of 65 patients with acoustic tumors, found changes in the internal auditory meatus in 95%. In 75% of these, the changes observed were diagnostic of acoustic tumor.

Medium size and large tumors are encapsulated, frequently rounded or egg-shaped, with a smooth, somewhat nodular surface (Figures 7 and 8). Their size varies from 3 to 6 cm, and their color varies from grayish-pink to tan or yellow, depending on the vascularity of the tumor and the presence or absence of lipid degeneration within the tumor. Most of the acoustic tumors of this size consist of two portions: a stalk situated within the internal auditory meatus and a large extrapetrosal portion. Cruveilhier (37), in his admirable book *Anatomie Pathologique du Corps Humain*, illustrates the case of an acoustic tumor protruding from the porus acusticus internus and lodged in the CPA.

Tumors of this size without a stalk are rare. They arise from the intracranial (extrapetrosal) portion of the nerve. In rare instances the tumor is entirely intrapetrosal. The tumor fully occupying the internal auditory meatus enlarges and erodes its walls. When the tumor originates in the extrapetrosal portion of the nerve, the internal auditory meatus remains normal. Tumors in the earlier stages of their intracranial growth are confined to the space between the petrosal pyramid, the floor of the posterior fossa laterally, and the tentorium cerebelli above. Medially they tend to insinuate into the cerebellopontine angle, between the brainstem and the cerebellum. Tumors of this size are likely to produce the classical CPA syndrome.

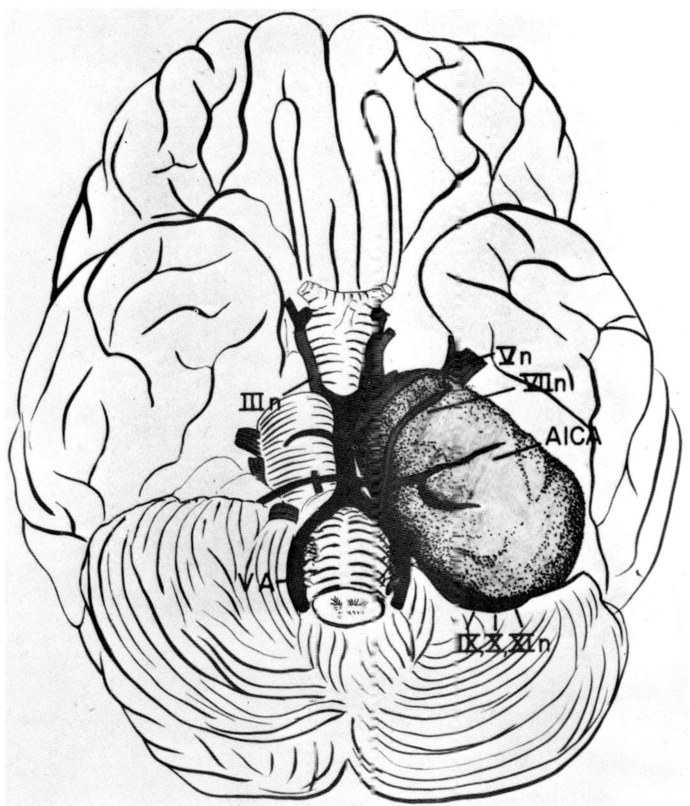

Figure 7. Basal view of the brain with an acoustic tumor in the left CPA. Note the stretching of the fifth, seventh, ninth, tenth, and eleventh nerves, the compression of the pons and cerebellar pressure cones.

Larger acoustic tumors often are irregular and nodular, compressing the lateral aspect of the pons and upper medulla and the brachium pontis and the adjacent cerebellum, producing a deformity of these structures proportional to the size of the tumor. Branches of the basilar artery which supply the cerebellum may run over the surface of the tumor. Similarly, large veins are scattered about, apparently with no definite pattern. Very large tumors may extend from the tentorial incisura where the upper pole of the tumor insinuates, compressing and displacing the brainstem toward the opposite side to the foramen magnum. The cerebellum is thrust downward through the foramen magnum by the

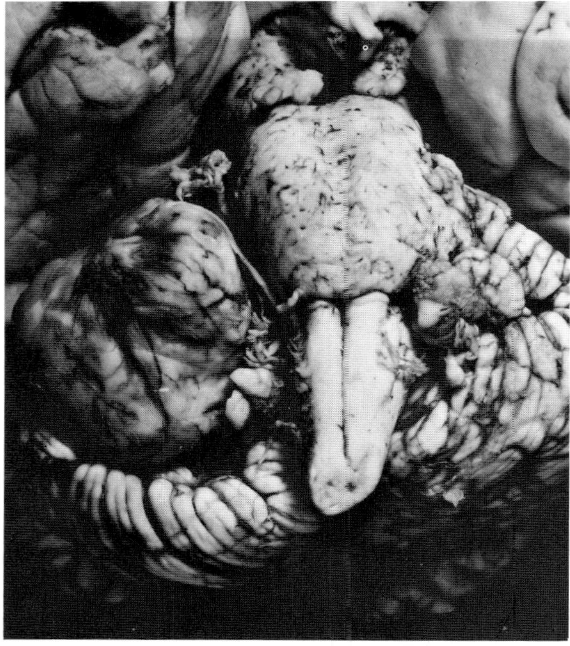

Figure 8. A large acoustic tumor in the right CPA and a small one in the left CPA in a 32-year-old man with von Recklinghausen's neurofibromatosis.

increased pressure above; the imprint of the latter is clearly visible as the tonsils are herniated downward (pressure cone).

The whole tumor is surrounded by a "capsule" of arachnoid membrane clearly visible at operation but difficult to demonstrate at autopsy. The capsule contains a variable amount of CSF, often sufficient to form a "cyst" of variable size over the posterior surface of the tumor. This "cyst" is formed by accumulation of CSF in the lateral cistern of the subarachnoid space. The choroid plexus at this point is greatly displaced and compressed by the tumor. As noted, variations in size of this "cyst" may account for the fluctuations of symptomatology in some cases of CPA tumors.

THE VASCULAR SUPPLY TO THE TUMOR AND BRAINSTEM

The vascular supply to the tumor is of great importance during surgery. The capsule of the tumor contains a large number of arteries and veins.

Branches of the basilar and vertebral arteries also course over the surface of the tumor and are, at times, very numerous. They may surround the neoplasm to present a serious risk of hemorrhage during the operation.

The blood supply to the tumor comes from the posterior-inferior cerebellar artery (PICA) and the anterior-inferior cerebellar artery (AICA). At surgery identification of the origin of the vessels supplying the tumor is often difficult, and great care must be exercised to avoid damage to the blood vessels.

The brainstem and the cerebellum receive arterial blood exclusively from the vertebro-basilar system. The basilar artery is a single vessel that supplies both sides of the neural tube. The pons receives its blood supply from the basilar artery through six to eight branches on each side. The largest vessels—the superior, the anterior-inferior, and the posterior-inferior cerebellar arteries—give off small branches that enter the brainstem before continuing over the cerebellum.

The Anterior-Inferior Cerebellar Artery

The AICA is one of the largest branches of the basilar artery to reach the cerebellum. Its size, course, and level of origin from the basilar artery are variable, even on the two sides. The variation in the caliber of this vessel depends largely upon the size and distribution of the PICA, which are usually in inverse proportion; that is, they are of reciprocal size (38–41). The AICA of both sides were equal in 15%, the right was larger in 48%, and the left in 37%. In 85% the two arteries arose at the same level; of these, 78% arose from the lowest third of the basilar artery, 17% from the middle, and 5% from the lower limit of the basilar artery.

From its origin the AICA courses over the ventral surface of the pons toward the anterior surface of the cerebellar hemisphere of its own side, where it anastomoses extensively with the PICA and SPA. The AICA has important relationships with the sixth nerve. According to Sunderland (42), the artery is anterior to the sixth nerve in 84% of cases on the right and 73% on the left. Immediately before or just after crossing the eighth nerve, the AICA divides into two branches (40). One passes laterally and downward on the medial anterior border of the cerebellar hemisphere. After a short tortuous course, it produces, in most cases, a branch of variable size along the medial surface of the hemisphere that anastomoses with a cerebellar branch of the PICA. The other branch passes laterally and curls around the upper edge of the flocculus, where it lies on the surface of the brachium pontis, and then passes on to the cerebellar hemisphere and anastomoses with the other two main cerebellar arteries (Figures 9–11).

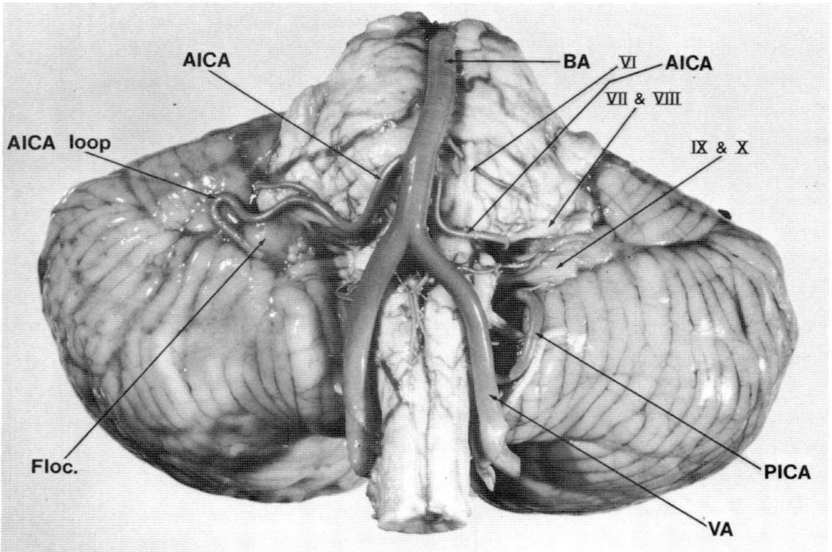

Figure 9. The anterior inferior cerebellar artery (AICA). Its course and relationships.

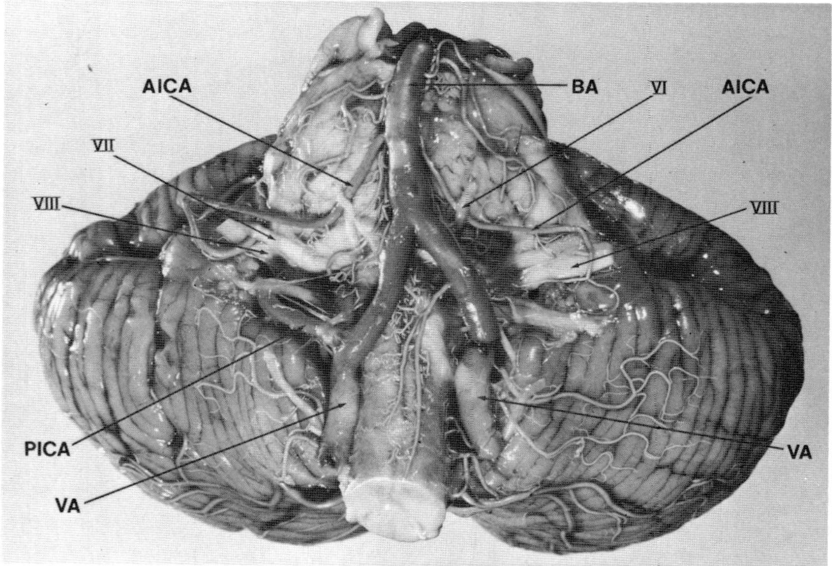

Figure 10. Neurovascular relationships between the cerebellar arteries and cranial nerves. On the right, note the loop of AICA into the IAM before it passes to supply the cerebellar hemisphere.

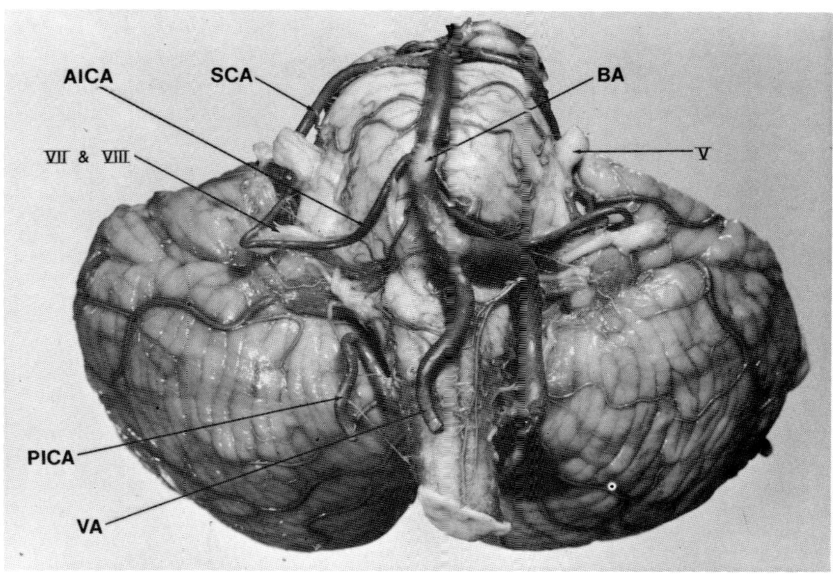

Figure 11. The cerebellar arteries: AICA, PICA, and SCA. Note the course of the AICA and its relationships with the VIII nerve.

During its course the AICA also gives a series of small arteries, variable in number and size and often inconstant, to the region of the pontomedullary sulcus, the lateral medullary fossa, and the brachium pontis. In many specimens these small, unnamed arteries arise directly from the lower portion of the basilar artery. The AICA has two regions of distribution (40). The proximal portion of this vessel supplies the lateral region of the lower pons, and the lateral branches, after crossing the eighth nerve, supply the brachium pontis and an area of variable size in the lateral tegmental region of the lower two-thirds of the pons. According to Atkinson (40), ligation of the artery (AICA) as it crosses the eighth nerve will immediately deprive the lateral pontine tegmentum of blood supply if no anastomosis exists between the PICA or SCA. Alexander and Suh (43) extend the territory of the AICA to the uppermost third of the lateral medullary region.

The AICA gives origin to several small penetrating branches that enter the pons with the rootlets of the seventh nerve and supply the upper third of the medulla and lower pons. This territory includes the facial nucleus, the rostral portion of the medial and lateral vestibular nuclei, the superior vestibular nucleus, the spinal nucleus and tract of the fifth nerve, the lateral portion of the medial lemniscus, and a considerable portion of the inferior and middle cerebellar peduncles. This part of the brainstem does not include the motor and chief sensory nucleus of the fifth nerve, which are supplied by the trigeminal artery (44). As the seventh and eighth nerves pass laterally from the brainstem toward the internal auditory meatus (IAM), they come close to the AICA. These intimate relationships between the arteries and nerves, in such confined spaces as the CPA and the IAM, are anatomical features of considerable practical significance in surgical exploration of the CPA, and, in particular, in the surgical treatment of acoustic tumors.

According to Sunderland (42), who studied these relationships in 132 subjects, the AICA in 39% passed outward, anterior to the facial and acoustic nerves, to enter the IAM, where it looped a variable distance. Stopford (38) found the artery lying more commonly ventral to the nerves, between them and the pons. Before passing to the cerebellum, the recurrent loop of the AICA courses between, above, or below the nerves, either in the meatus or soon after leaving it. In 25% of the specimens, the loop of the AICA just reached the entrance of the meatus ventral to the nerves, then the distal limb of the loop passed to the cerebellum below or between the nerves. In 13% of specimens, the AICA did not extend as far as the IAM, but passed above in 1%, between in 15%, or below the facial and acoustic nerves. In 23% of the specimens, the artery was not related significantly to these nerves (Figure 12).

Internal Auditory Artery

The facial and acoustic nerves in the internal auditory canal are accompanied by the internal auditory artery (IAA), which frequently lies between them. The IAA is often considered a branch of the basilar artery, but most often the evidence favors an origin from the AICA.

The internal auditory (labyrinthine) artery takes origin from a variable site in the AICA; usually the point where this vessel leaves the brachium pontis and continues in close relationship with the seventh and eighth nerves, accompanying these nerves into the internal auditory canal. When the AICA loops into the IAM or well down into the internal auditory canal, the IAA arises from the apex of the loop, and occasionally from the proximal limb at points between the porus and the apex. The reported frequency of such origin varies. Stopford found that the IAA arises from the AICA in 63% of cases. Sunderland reported a similar origin in 83% of 264 sides examined. The IAA arises from the basilar artery in 17% of cases (42). Mazzoni (45), in a study of 100 human specimens, found that the IAA arises from the loop of the AICA in 80% of cases, from the accessory AICA in 17%, and from a branch of

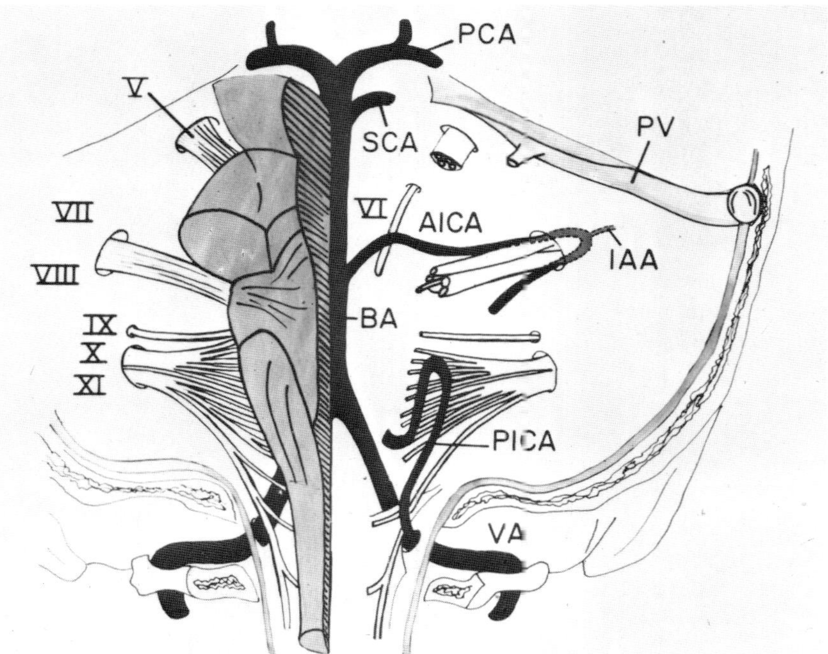

Figure 12. Diagram illustrating the relationships between the AICA and the VII and VIII nerves. A posterior view. (Redrawn from F. W. Bock et al. In Clinical Microneurosurgery. Thieme-Publishing Sciences Group. Stuttgart, 1976).

the PICA in 3%. The loop of the AICA lies inside the internal auditory canal in 40% of cases, at the IAM in 27%, and in the CPA in 33%. Mazzoni considers an independent origin of the IAA from the basilar artery to be rare.

The IAA supplies the dura and nerves in the internal auditory canal, the adjacent bone, and the medial aspect of the inner ear before dividing into its terminal branches, the cochlear, the anterior vestibular, and the vestibular artery (46). The anterior vestibular and cochlear arteries enter the middle ear accompanying the respective nerves. The vestibulocochlear artery penetrates at the median point of the lower quadrant in the depths of the meatus and reaches the middle ear. The cochlear artery divides into cochlear and vestibulocochlear branches. The vestibulocochlear artery gives off the posterior vestibular artery and cochlear branches.

The anterior vestibular artery gives origin to several small branches that supply with blood the macula and utricle, while the macula of the saccule is supplied mainly from the posterior vestibular artery, with minor contribution from the anterior vestibular artery. The osseous branches of the IAA arise either from its intrameatal segment or from its intraosseous portion. A relatively large branch, the artery of the vestibular ganglion, supplies the inferior and superior vestibular ganglia. The subarcuate artery (SA) arises also from the AICA, often from its cerebellar loop outside of the IAM, and rarely from the IAA. The SA enters the dura at the subarcuate fossa.

In summary, the IAA distributes not only to the inner ear, to the dura, and to nerves within the internal auditory canal, but also to the bony structures around it.

In the case of the AICA that is so intimately entwined in a CPA tumor that it requires surgical occlusion of the vessel for the removal of the tumor, it should be remembered that the AICA is a vessel of variable origin, size, and distribution, that it has extensive anastomoses with the distal branches of the SCA and PICA, and that not infrequently it has a direct large anastomosis with the proximal portion of the PICA in the lateral aspect of the medulla. Any surgical occlusion of the vessel (AICA) ought to be made as far lateral as possible from its origin. The circuitous course of the AICA in the CPA angle and the presence of numerous other arteries in this region dictate an extremely cautious dissection of this vessel or, indeed, of any other vessel in this region before occluding it. The IAA arising from the AICA, when occluded during the removal of an acoustic tumor, poses no problem when total hearing loss has already occurred. The acoustic tumors that grow out of the internal auditory meatus into the cerebellopontine angle push the lateral branch of the AICA upward and, as the artery continues over the flocculus and brachium pontis, it lies posteriorly and inferiorly on the surface of the tumor. However, because of the variable course of the artery, it may end up lying over the ventral aspect of the tumor, as some of the illustrations of Cushing (30) and Dandy (47) demonstrate.

In an angiographic study of 30 acoustic tumors (48), elevation of the AICA was noted in 10 patients. In 2 patients the artery was displaced backward. In 18 patients the artery could not be visualized. A faint tumor stain was seen in 8 cases.

The veins of the brainstem develop from a venous plexus. This explains their variable distribution. In general, the veins of the brainstem do not reach the dural sinuses directly. They empty into veins reaching the dorsal aspect of the brainstem and cerebellum before reaching the venous sinuses.

The pattern for the venous drainage of the posterior fossa has been divided according to the direction of flow into 3 groups (49): the superior or galenic group, the anterior or petrosal group, and the posterior or tentorial group.

The superior or galenic group includes the superior cerebellar group, with the precentral cerebellar vein, superior vermis veins, and superior hemisphere veins, and the mesencephalic tributaries of the posterior mesencephalic vein, anterior pontomesencephalic veins, lateral mesencephalic vein, and quadrigeminal veins.

The anterior petrosal group includes the veins related to the anterior aspect of the brainstem, longitudinal running veins, such as the anterior pontomesencephalic vein, the lateral pontomesencephalic vein, the anterior medullary vein, the lateral pontine vein, the numerous transverse running veins, the vein of the pontomedullary sulcus, and the pontomesencephalic vein. This group includes the hemispheric cerebellar veins and its tributaries.

The posterior or tentorial group includes the superior vermian vein and veins related to hemispheric cerebellar veins.

In the pons and medulla, the anterior median vein with the lateral veins form an anastomosing network. The veins of the lower pons empty into the cerebellar veins and with them into the petrosal sinuses. An important vein is the radicular vein associated with the fifth nerve (Dandy's vein), which reaches the superior petrosal sinus.

In the CPA tumors, the most striking feature is the stretching of the petrosal vein over the upper pole of the tumor. The veins converging toward the petrosal veins (tributaries of the petrosal sinuses) are displaced backward in an arcuate fashion. In large tumors growing upward, the peduncular and lateral mesencephalic veins are elevated and displaced medially. Dandy's vein runs in the dorsal aspect of the tumor, beneath the tentorium. This vein is easily torn when trying to dislodge the tumor (31).

The venous drainage system of the cochlea is the posterior spiral veins (spiral ganglion and scala tympani) and the anterior spiral veins (spiral lamina and scala vestibuli), which jointly form the common modiolar vein. This vein is joined by the vestibular cochlear veins (which drain the utricle, saccule, and ampules of the vestibular canals) to empty into the inferior petrosal sinus. The semicircular canals are drained into the lateral sinus.

EFFECTS OF THE TUMOR

The cranial nerves, from the fifth to the twelfth, have close relationships with acoustic tumors occupying the CPA. Anatomically, the eighth nerve occupies a median position among them. Only in the small acoustic tumors will the eighth nerve be found entering the medial surface of the tumor; in the large tumors, it may be impossible to identify it. The peripheral part of this nerve is not visible. Large acoustic tumors can produce considerable stretching of the cranial nerves in the region of the CPA, especially of the trigeminal and facial nerves, without impairing their function. Cushing, in his book *Tumors of the Nervus Acusticus* (30), illustrated dramatically the degree of elongation of these nerves that may occur in large acoustic tumors (see Figure 14). In some examples, the facial nerve appears stretched tightly over the upper pole of the tumor and flattened into a narrow ribbon. In some instances, according to Olivecrona, the facial nerve may be seen on the anterior surface of the tumor. The trigeminal nerve may also be elongated by the superior pole of the tumor, producing a unilateral sensory defect (corneal hypoesthesia, loss of corneal reflex, facial paresthesia, or anesthesia). The abducens nerve usually lies free. Paresis or paralysis of the lateral rectus muscle innervated by this nerve is observed when there is increase of intracranial pressure causing a downward displacement of the brainstem and the compression of the sixth nerve by the AICA, which usually overlies the nerve (30). The ninth, tenth, and eleventh cranial nerves enter in contact with the tumor in the CPA and may be compressed by it, with the corresponding symptomatology (loss of pharyngeal reflex, dysphagia, and dysphonia). Hypesthesia may occur in the posterior aspect of the external auditory canal innervated by the seventh nerve (50), but without corresponding symptomatology. Only during surgical removal of the tumor have autonomic changes (hypotension, respiratory irregularities, and even respiratory arrest) occurred. This is possibly related to mechanical stretching of these nerves.

Compression and deformity of the brainstem and cerebellum are apparent in large tumors of the CPA, as illustrated in the papers of Cushing, Dandy, Olivecrona, and others. The deformity and compression of the pons and the cerebellum are proportional to the size of the neoplasm. Large tumors displace the pons and the medulla toward the opposite side and make a deep indentation in these structures. The cerebellum is also deeply indented; the flocculus and the brachium pontis are especially affected (Figure 13).

The distant effects of the tumor are related to the tumor size and to disturbances of CSF circulation. These are usually related to a deformity and compression of the cerebral aqueduct or of the fourth ventricle and its outlets, resulting in dilation of the lateral and third ventricles, increased intracranial pressure, and papilledema. In addition, cerebral herniations (pressure cones) of variable degrees occur through all possible

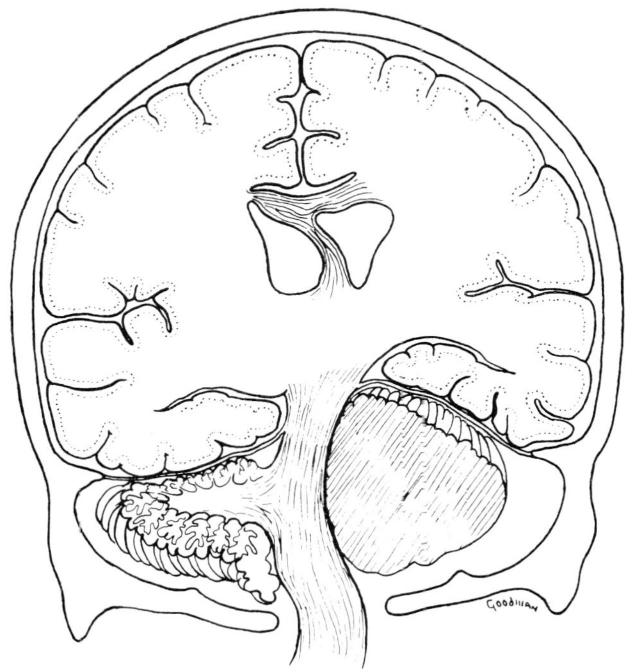

Figure 13. Diagrammatic illustration of the deformity and compression of the brainstem and the cerebellum with production of hydrocephalus and tonsilar herniation.

openings. The most common is the herniation of the cerebellar tonsils at the foramen magnum, where the tonsils are forced down around the medulla into the spinal canal, producing symptoms of medullary compression with notable vasomotor and respiratory dysfunction, which in severe forms result in cardiorespiratory arrest.

In summary, the acoustic tumors are capable of producing three types of gross intracranial changes: changes related to the site of origin of the tumor in the internal auditory meatus that produce enlargement and erosion of the porus acusticus internus; changes related to the compression of nervous structures, brainstem, cerebellum, and cranial nerves in the CPA; and distant effects attributed to internal hydrocephalus, increased intracranial pressure, and associated brain herniation.

Changes in the middle ear produced by acoustic tumors were studied as early as 1871 by Boettcher (51). They have since been fully described by others. Experiments show that division of the eighth nerve leads to a degeneration in the vestibular branch as far as the vestibular ganglion but not beyond, whereas the cochlear branch degenerates beyond the spiral ganglion to its peripheral cells.

In human pathological material, other factors, such as pressure disturbances, vascular stasis, and compression, and changes due to pressure by the tumor modify the experimental results. The changes observed in human material also depend on the size of the neoplasm, its duration, and the extent of its penetration into the internal auditory canal, etc.

SYMPTOMATOLOGY

The symptoms of acoustic tumors (summarized in Table 1) are fairly constant. Considering that almost all known acoustic tumors arise in the vestibular nerve, it is surprising that vestibular symptoms do not figure prominently in the early history of these patients and that, in most instances, the symptoms noted are from the cochlear division. In only a few cases has the history begun with an attack of vertigo and dizziness. The vestibular symptoms include a sensation of unsteadiness and instability of gait, usually present late in the course of the disease. At this time it is difficult to distinguish the role of the labyrinth from that of the cerebellum. Vertigo may occasionally be associated with nausea, and appears as a vague sensation, generally described as "giddiness." It is

Table 1. Frequency of auditory and vestibular symptoms and signs

Investigator	Number of cases	Deafness and tinnitus	Unsteadiness	Nystagmus and impaired caloric response
Cushing (30)	30	100%		63%
Dandy (47)[a]	145	99%	41%	87%
Pool and Pava (52)	122	92%	58%	74.5%
Olivecrona (32)	415	95%	83%	85.3%
House (53)	200	92%		82%[b]
House et al.[c]	500	98.6%	65.6%	82.1%[d]

[a] Reported by Gonzales Revilla (Bull. Johns Hopkins Hosp. 80:254, 1947).

[b] Vestibular tests by Linthicum and Churchill (54).

[c] Personal communication, 1977.

[d] 446 of 500, with adjusted percentages. Reduced vestibular responses greater than 30 degrees per sec. ENG.

not abrupt, as in Meniere's disease. Meniere's disease and an acoustic tumor may occur coincidentally in the same patient (8). In rare cases, the first symptom is a sudden attack of vertigo, with recovery taking a period of weeks (55). When destruction of the vestibular nerve has developed, it is possible that no symptoms will occur, a possibility that attests to the great adaptability of the vestibular system (12). In the majority of cases the first symptoms are auditory. Tinnitus and deafness (92–99% of cases) may precede other symptoms by months or years. Tinnitus often precedes the hearing loss. The loss usually progresses steadily to complete deafness, but occasionally a sudden deafness may appear in the course of the disease. Rarely is there no deafness on the side of the tumor.

Cranial nerves are elongated and compressed by the tumor. As expected, symptoms referable to these nerves appear later, when the tumor reaches considerable size.

Symptoms of irritation of the facial nerve are spasms or twitchings that are constant or intermittent. The slight facial weakness frequently present is usually overlooked by the patient; hypesthesia of the posterior aspect of the external auditory canal, which is innervated by the facial nerve, occurs in 95% of cases (50), probably from pressure on this nerve by a small intracanalicular tumor. Involvement of the trigeminal nerve is the second most common source (acoustic nerve is first) of patients' complaints. Paresthesias are variously described as numbness, tingling in the face, etc.; pain is common and, rarely, paroxysmal.

Symptoms of involvement of the ninth, tenth, and eleventh cranial nerves appear later. Prominent among these are difficulty in swallowing, loss of pharyngeal reflexes, dysphagia, laryngeal paralysis, and dysphonia.

A tumor emerging from the internal auditory meatus may grow in different directions (56). If it grows anteriorly, the fifth and sixth cranial nerves become involved earlier. If the tumor grows predominantly posteriorly and inferiorly, the ninth, tenth, and eleventh cranial nerves are more affected. When the vestibular, cochlear, and facial nerves are the only ones involved by the tumor, Nager (56) terms this the "CPA syndrome."

Preceding the involvement of the cranial nerves, concomitant with it, or, more rarely, much later, symptoms of derangement of the cerebellum appear. The incoordination usually affects the lower more than the upper extremities. The gait becomes unsteady and reeling, with a tendency to deviate or fall to the side of the tumor. The involvement of the cerebellum and its peduncles is manifested by the asynergia, hypotonia, and dysmetria of the extremities on the side of the tumor. The tumor pressing

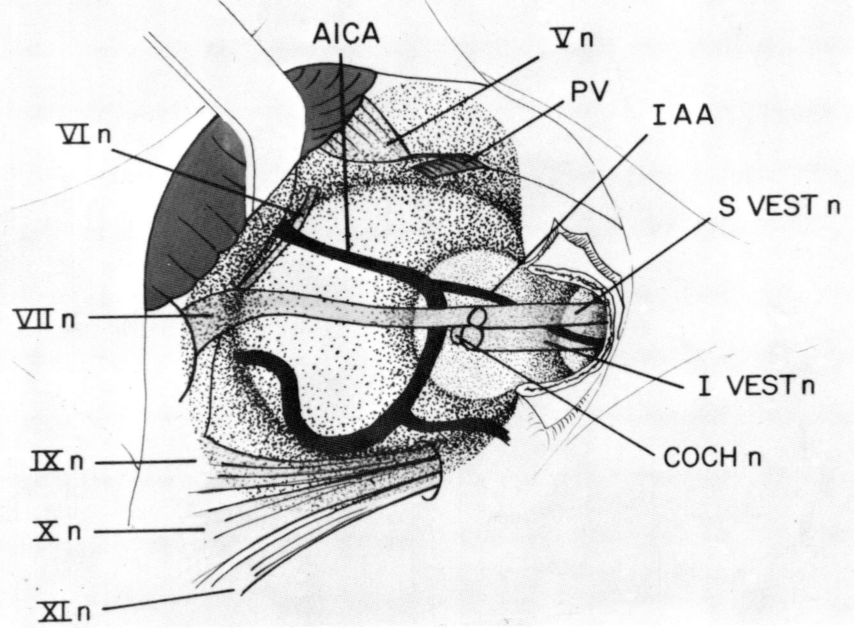

Figure 14. Diagrammatic illustration of the progressive growth of an acoustic tumor into the CPA from a small, intrameatal neoplasm enlarging the IAM, to a large tumor compressing the brainstem, the cerebellum, and adjacent structures. (Redrawn from Koos et al. In *Clinical Microneurosurgery*. Thieme-Publishing Sciences Group. Stuttgart, 1976).

on the brainstem may compress the sensory and motor tracts, giving rise to exaggerated reflexes and numbness in the arms and legs. Usually these symptoms are contralateral, but they may be bilateral. Horizontal nystagmus may be present with the slow component toward the side of the lesion. Rarely, the nystagmus is vertical (Figure 14).

All the signs of involvement of the cranial nerves are usually in the deaf side. The analysis of a large series of cases (Table 1) revealed that the symptoms usually occur in the following order: auditory and labyrinthine symptoms; suboccipital discomfort; incoordination and staggering gait; involvement of other cranial nerves; headaches, vomiting, and papilledema; and dysarthria, dysphagia, and respiratory difficulties. This order usually reflects the anatomic progression of the process.

The mechanisms responsible for auditory and vestibular dysfunction are: 1) destruction of cochlear and vestibular nerve fibers, 2) destruction of sense organs, and 3) biochemical disturbances of the fluids of the inner ear (57).

Destruction of Cochlear and Vestibular Nerve Fibers

The first sign of involvement of the cochlear nerve is a loss of speech discrimination that is disproportionate to the pure tone threshold in the involved ear. The patient may discover the loss when using the telephone. He may say, "I can hear, but I cannot understand what is being said in that ear." In the small acoustic tumors, function is disturbed first by compression and later by destruction of the nerve fibers. The result is a progressive loss of speech discrimination, with minimal or moderate threshold alteration for pure tones. The earliest deficit affects the low frequencies (57). Other auditory signs related to partial loss of nerve fibers are the absence of loudness recruitment and auditory fatigue. These findings correlate well with the results from animal experiments. Schuknecht and Woellner (58) demonstrated that 75% of nerve fibers may be destroyed without producing pure tone threshold losses if the organ of Corti is intact. The implication is that 25% of nerve fibers are sufficient to transmit the threshold response, while many more nerve fibers are needed to ensure speech discrimination. The sudden onset of partial or total deafness, rarely an initial symptom of acoustic tumors, may result from a hemorrhage within the tumor or from sudden occlusion of the IAA.

Vestibular symptoms are often minimal or absent, because the vestibular system readily compensates for vestibular deficits. Sudden attacks of vertigo result from functional derangement of the vestibular nerve followed by compensatory recovery. The loss of vestibular nerve fibers is manifested as a decrease or absence of response to vestibular stimulation, i.e., caloric tests. The correlation between nerve fiber loss and test responses has not been established for this system (59).

Destruction of Sense Organs

The tumors of the eighth nerve, in addition to destroying the nerve fibers in the internal auditory canal, may produce varying degrees of structural damage to the membranous labyrinth (8,9), leading to atrophy or complete destruction of the organ of Corti. The degenerative changes are more severe in the basal turn of the cochlea, and less severe in the maculae and cristae. In rare cases, the tumors of the acoustic nerve may first produce disturbances of sensory function rather than neural involvement.

De Moura suggests that the shrinkage of the sense organs or the loss of sensory and supporting cells was secondary to impairment of the blood supply by tumor compression of the IAA in the internal auditory canal.

Such alterations occur in areas of the cochlea that have little or no loss of nerve cells. Because early acoustic tumors can permanently injure the cochlear nerve fibers, the sensory organ, or both, the audiometric findings are varied, with no consistent patterns of dysfunction.

The audiometrics in 500 patients with acoustic tumors treated by the Otologic Medical Group, Inc., in Los Angeles (60) revealed the pure tone loss patterns in 497 cases as follows: no hearing, 15.3%; high tone loss, 55.3%; through type loss, 4.4%; low tone loss, 6.4%; and flat loss, 18.5%. These data indicate that the most common hearing deficit is in the high frequencies.

Perlman and Kimura (61), by temporarily interrupting the blood supply to the inner ear by pressure in the IAA, demonstrated that an arrest of blood flow of more than 30 min produced a permanent loss of electrical responses to auditory stimuli. The histological alterations present were directly proportional to the duration of the arterial occlusion. Interruption of blood supply for 5 minutes or more resulted in scattered degeneration in the cochlear and vestibular labyrinth. In the cochlea, the external hair cells are more sensitive to injury than the internal hair cells and supporting cells. Arterial obstruction for one hour produced additional degeneration in the vestibular sense organs.

Dandy (62) partially sectioned the eighth nerve in patients with Meniere's disease. These patients frequently show no change in auditory thresholds, and the hearing losses that occurred were in high frequencies. Observation of humans seems to indicate that the earliest manifestation of pure nerve degeneration is loss of speech discrimination (12). A loss of 75% of cochlear neurons is not associated with threshold losses. More than 90% of ganglion cells may be lost in a particular cochlear region without influencing pitch discrimination for frequencies with displacement patterns in that region. Loudness recruitment characteristic of sensory lesions does not occur with pure cochlear nerve lesions (12). Experimental interruption of venous drainage by blocking the inferior cochlear vein and tributaries (63) for 24 hr resulted in loss of external hair cells. After 48 hr there were scattered areas of degeneration. Coagulation of the IAA produced rapid and profound changes in the labyrinth. The external hair cells began to degenerate within 30 min, and a few hours later similar changes were seen in the internal hair cells and supporting cells, resulting in severe degeneration of the organ of Corti and stria vascularis. The changes in the vestibular labyrinth parallel those of the cochlea. Kimura (quoted by Schuknecht, 12) ligated the AICA in four cats, producing total destruction of the inner ear in three. The changes were more severe in the apical region in one cat. The ligation of the basilar artery produced no pathological changes in the inner ear. Bernstein and Silverstein (63) ligated the AICA and its branches in 21 cats. Three animals showed sensory lesion restricted to the cochlear apex. The damage of the apical cochlear region following vascular lesions is well known and well documented, but its pathophysiological mechanisms remain obscure (12). Surgical removal of acoustic tumors usually interferes with the blood supply to the inner ear, resulting in necrosis of the membranous labyrinth. After surgery, the bone of the modiolus and osseous spiral lamina is partially reabsorbed. Later a pink granular precipitate becomes organized into a thick fibrous tissue with necrosis of the scala. As a rule, the macula is well preserved, but in advanced cases it shows atrophy. An exception to this process would be a small tumor removed by the middle fossa approach without affecting the vascular supply to the middle ear.

Biochemical Disturbances of Fluids of the Inner Ear

Biochemical disturbances in the fluids in the staining characteristics of the perilymph, which appears deeply eosinophilic and finely granular, indicate a possible increase of protein (64). Silverstein and Schuknecht (65) confirmed this finding in seven patients with acoustic tumors. The perilymph of these patients contained elevated protein values (average 2,444.3 mg/100 ml).

POSTOPERATIVE DEATHS

In 1967 Olivecrona (32) published an analysis of 415 cases treated by him. In this series, there were 67 deaths. In the cases with complete removal of the tumor, pulmonary embolism caused one death; meningitis, one; cardiac failure, one; postoperative hematomas, seven; shock and hemorrhage, six. In all remaining 51 cases, death was caused by "postoperative clot" in the tumor bed or hemorrhagic softening of the pons. In these cases the brainstem injury was considered the dominant factor. The hemorrhagic softening of the pons was attributed to occlusion of the AICA and to electro-coagulation of the petrous and other veins on the lateral surface of the pons. This could be seen in cases known to have minimal injury to the brainstem at the operation.

Atkinson (40) wrote an important paper on the significance of the AICA in surgery of cerebellopontine angle tumor. At Queen Square in London he did postmortem studies of seven patients with acoustic tumors (Table 2). At necropsy, he found infarction of the lateral tegmental

Table 2. Findings in 7 deaths following removal of acoustic tumors (Atkinson's series)

Cases			Consciousness		Pulse	Resp.	Blood	Death and
No.	Age	Sex	PO	Temp.	(beats per min)	(per min)	pressure	postmortem findings
1	45	F	Coma 4 h.	104°F	150	N	?	10 d., inf. lat. pons, AICA ?
2	?	F	Coma	102.4°F 104°F	140 176 200	28 40	150/95	48 h., ext. hem. inf., r. lat. pons & med., cereb., AICA clipp.
3	47	F	Awake, coma	?	120 110 140		120/90 160/110 110/85, 80/60	24 h., ext. hem. inf. r. pons, AICA clipp.
4	57	M	Coma	102°F	72 150	N 30	150/80	23 h., pontine inf., AICA ?
5	58	F	Coma		120	22	100/60	24 h., l. hem. inf. pons & upper med., AICA clipp.
6	56	F	Coma 4h., drowsy	102°F	78		94/70, 110/72, 120/78, 98/70, 130/100	24 h., l. pons hem. inf., AICA clipp.
7	62	F	Drowsy 3d., coma				160/100	7 d., l. pons teg. isch. inf., AICA thromb.

region of the pons, in the area corresponding to the distribution of the AICA.

In four cases (2,3,5, and 6) the AICA was clipped during the operations; in two cases (1 and 4) the condition of the vessels is not stated; and in one case (7) the artery thrombosed without being clipped at the operation. The operative and postoperative records of these cases revealed a series of autonomic disturbances in the pulse rate, respiration, temperature, and blood pressure, and alterations in the level of consciousness. Most of the patients were in coma in the postoperative period and did not regain consciousness. In many of these patients, these signs indicated increased intracranial pressure. Atkinson considered that clipping or injury of the AICA during surgery may be associated with many of these disturbances. He stated that the area of infarction in these cases "coincides almost exactly" with the distribution of the AICA, and the region of primary importance, as far as the patient's life is concerned, is the tegmental area.

The autopsy series of Olivecrona (32), Pool (52), Pertuiset (66), and those of House listed in Table 3 seem to indicate that the cause of death following total removal of acoustic tumors in the CPA is nearly always a pontine hemorrhagic infarction. The site of the lesion was the same in all the autopsied cases. It usually included the lateral half of the lower pons and seldom extended into the upper medulla or the upper pons and mesencephalon. The damaged territory included portions of the pyramids, lateral tegmentum, proximal middle cerebellar peduncle, and often reached the wall of the fourth ventricle. Atkinson gave a detailed

Table 3. Causes of death

	Investigators				
	Olivecrona	Pool	Pertuiset	House et al.	
Number of cases	415	96	60	200[a]	500[b]
Number of autopsies	67	22	12	8	
Pontine infarction	51		5	3	4
Hematoma PO	7	7	2	4	3
Shock	6				
Brain edema		4	1	3	
Cardiac failure	1	5			1
Pulmonary embolism/infarction	1	6	1	2	1
Meningitis	1	1	1		1
Other		1	2		3

[a] First series 1968.
[b] Second series 1977.

anatomical description of the autopsy findings in cases 3 and 5 and briefly described the extension of the lesion in the others. From these, and from the examination of the illustrations in papers by Atkinson (40), Pertuiset (66), and others, one must conclude that the lesions extend beyond the confines of distribution of the AICA and include adjacent and even distant territories, depending on their blood supply from other arteries. These require participation of other blood vessels (arteries and veins) and/or the presence of "other factors" in the causality of these extensive lesions. Nevertheless, an extensive involvement of the pontine tegmental region is a constant feature in the postmortem findings.

The vascular supply to the tumor and to this region is of great significance for the understanding of the lesion. The capsule of the tumor possesses a good number of small blood vessels, arteries, and veins, and the tumor itself is also supplied with many blood vessels of variable size.

The AICA and PICA supply branches to the tumor. Other nutrient arterial branches arise directly from the basilar and vertebral arteries. Olivecrona (31) remarks that, at operation, it is rarely possible to identify the origin of all vessels supplying the tumor. In case of bleeding, the only course is to clip the arteries as close to the tumor as possible, to avoid damage to branches that supply the brainstem. Pertuiset believes that most of the vessels to the tumor are behind it and mingling with vessels directed to the pons. At this site the surgeon must exercise caution to avoid injury to vessels distributed to the brainstem.

SIGNIFICANCE OF THE PONTINE LESION

A hemorrhagic infarction in the pons and a blood clot in the tumor bed at the CPA have similar symptomatology, making clinical distinction difficult. Moreover, the two conditions may occur simultaneously. An early symptom is restlessness, followed by unconsciousness, inability to swallow, and temperature elevation. These symptoms gradually worsen over the next few days. The patient usually dies by the end of the first week. In large pontine infarcts, consciousness is lost and never regained. Death occurs a day or two after the operation. In less severe lesions the patient becomes semicomatose on the second postoperative day and gradually lapses into coma. The temperature rises and death usually occurs within a week. In small infarcts, the patient may survive with a serious cerebellar deficit.

Hitselberger and House (68), discussing the surgery of acoustic tumors, considered that some of the difficulties at surgery were related to vascular and respiratory disturbances secondary to interruption of the vascular supply to centers in the brainstem. They observed that 34 of 114 patients with acoustic tumors operated by the Otologic Medical Group, Inc., had changes in vital signs during surgery. The most frequent was a rise of blood pressure. Pulse alterations were variable; irregularities and increment or decrement of pulse rate paralleled changes in blood pressure. The respiratory alterations were inconstant and consisted of apnea of variable duration. In many instances these changes heralded more serious complications dictating a modification of the intended operative procedure. In only 12 of these cases was the planned total excision of the tumor completed.

Of 251 cases out of 500 patients treated by the OMB (House et al., 60), 72.5% had no changes in vital signs during surgery; 13.5% had changes due to the surgical procedure; 8.4% due to the anesthesia; 1.6% due to the anesthesia and operation; and 4% for unexplained reasons. Significant alterations of blood pressure occurred in 18% of patients. It increased in 9%, decreased in 8%, and was uncertain in 1%. The pulse stopped in two patients; various forms of arrhythmia occurred in 8 patients. Respiratory changes were observed in 5% of cases; one-half of these exhibited acceleration and the other half slowness of the respiratory frequency. Two patients became apneic and one of them arrested.

Many implications arise from these observations. Significant autonomic changes have been recorded by surgeons during operations on acoustic tumors. They are a rise in blood pressure, and respiratory and vasopressor disturbances, often transient but sometimes persistent and progressive. Occasionally, these are followed by disturbances of consciousness, and in a few instances by coma and death. These changes have been attributed to spasm or occlusion of the AICA impairing the blood supply to the brainstem tegmentum and the structures and pathways subserving these functions. This theory is supported by the postmortem findings of the cases studied by Atkinson (40), Olivecrona (32), Pertuiset (66), House et al. (53), and others.

Analysis of these cases reveals that the most frequent lesion responsible for death occurred in the brainstem. This is described as a pontine infarction, hematoma, or brainstem edema. However, these findings have not been present in all the cases examined anatomically. Moreover, in the majority, the functional disturbances and the structural damage in the brainstem disclosed in neuropathological examination surpass the territory supplied by a single artery. This fact would suggest that an additional factor or factors, such as injury to the brainstem, hemorrhage, increased intracranial pressure, anesthesia, and others unknown, play a role in the casuality of the events observed during and after surgery. A prominent role seems to be played by the sudden rise of intracranial pressure, which, when excessive, cannot be compensated. A further consequence is the development of cerebral edema with compression of the ventricles, reduction of the cisterns, and mass displacement of brain tissue (herniation). This results in distortion and compression of the brainstem and circulatory disturbances (capillary and venule compression). The compression of large arteries may be so severe as to result in ischemia in the areas they supply. Thus, all these events create the conditions for the development of vascular and respiratory disturbances that lead to hypoxia, anoxia, cerebral edema, and increased intracranial pressure. In this way a vicious circle is perpetuated that terminates only in death.

REFERENCES

1. Henschen, F. 1910. Om acusticustomoren. Hygeia (Stockh.) 10:31.
2. Henschen, F. 1915. Uber Geschwulste der hinteren Schadelgrube, insbesondere der Kleinhirnbruckenwinkeltumoren. Arch Psychiatr. 56:20–122.
3. Henschen, F. 1955. Tumoren des Zentralnervensystems und Seiner Hullen. In: Handbuch der Speziellen Pathologischen Anatomie und Histology, Vol. 13. Erkan-Kungen des Zentral Nervensystems. Springer-Verlag, Berlin.
4. Skinner, H. A. 1929. The Origin of Acoustic Tumors. Brit. J. Surg. 16:440–463.
5. Maxwell, D. S., Kruger, L., and Pineda, A. 1969. The trigeminal nerve root with special reference to the central peripheral transition zone: An electron microscope study in the macaque. Anat. Rec. 164:113–126.
6. Nager, G. 1964. Association of bilateral VIII nerve tumor with meningiomas in von Recklinghausen's disease. Laryngoscope 74:1220–1261.
7. Jorgensen, M. B. 1962. Intracochlear neurinoma. Acta Otolaryngol. 54:227–232.
8. De Moura, L. 1967. Inner ear pathology in acoustic neurinoma. Arch. Otolaryngol. 85:125–134.
9. De Moura, L., Hayden, R., and Conner, G. 1969. Further observations on acoustic neurinoma. Trans. Amer. Acad. Ophthal. Otolaryngol. 73:60–70.
10. Hardy, M., and Crowe, S. J. 1936. Early asymptomatic acoustic tumors. Arch. Surg. 32:292–301.
11. Leonard, J., and Talbbott, M. 1970. Asymptomatic acoustic neurilemoma. Arch. Otolaryngol. 91:117–124.
12. Schuknecht, H. F. 1974. Pathology of the ear. Harvard University Press, Cambridge, Mass.
13. Pirsig, W., Eckermeier, L., and Mueller, D. 1978. As to the origin of vestibular Schwannomas. Seminar on diagnosis and management of acoustic tumors and skull base tumors. Ear Research Institute, Los Angeles, Cal. (Feb. 28–March 3, 1978).
14. Willis, R. A. 1960. Pathology of Tumors, 3rd Ed. Butterworths, London.

15. Verocay, J. 1910. Zur Kenntniss der Neurofibrome. Beitr. Path. Anat. 48:1–68.
16. Masson, P. 1932. Experimental and spontaneous Schwannomas (peripheral gliomas). Am. J. Pathol. 8:369–416.
17. Stout, A. P. 1949. Tumors of the Peripheral Nervous System. Atlas of tumor pathology. Armed Forces Institute of Pathology, Section II, Fasc. 6, Washington.
18. Rio-Hortega, P. del. 1943. Estudio citologico de los Neurofibromas de Recklinghausen (lemmocitomas). Ach. Hist. (BsAs). 1:373–414.
19. Russell, D. S., and Rubinstein, L. J. 1971. Pathology of Tumors of the Nervous System, 3rd Ed. Edward Arnold, London.
20. Mallory, T. 1920. The type of the so-called dural endothelioma. J. Med. Res. 41:349–364.
21. Penfield, W. 1932. Tumors of the sheaths of the nervous system. In: Cytology and Cellular Pathology of the Nervous System, Vol. 3. Hoeber, New York.
22. Tarlov, I. M. 1940. Origin of the perineural fibroblastoma. Am. J. Pathol. 16:33–40.
23. Murray, M. R., and Stout, A. P. 1940. Schwann cell versus fibroblast as origin of specific nerve sheath tumor; observations upon normal nerve sheaths and neurilemomas in vitro. Am. J. Pathol. 16:41–60.
24. Luse, S. A. 1960. Electron microscopic studies of brain tumors. Neurology 10:881–905.
25. Pineda, A. 1964. Submicroscopic structure of acoustic tumors. Neurology 14:171–184.
26. Poirier, J., Escourolle, R., and Castaigne, P. 1968. Les neurofibromes de la maladie de Recklinghausen. Acta Neuropathol. 10:279–294.
27. Cravioto, H. 1969. The ultrastructure of acoustic nerve tumors. Acta Neuropathol. 12:116–140.
28. Raimondi, A. J., and Beckman, F. 1967. Perineural fibroblastomas. Their fine structure and biology. Acta Neuropathol. 8:1–23.
29. Henneberg and Koch 1902. Uber centrale Neurofibromatose und die Gaschwulste des Kleinhirnbruckenwinkels (Acusticus neurome). Arch Psychiat. 36:251–304.
30. Cushing, H. 1917. Tumors of the Nervus Acusticus and the Syndrome of the Cerebellopontile Angle. W. B. Saunders Co., Philadelphia.
31. Olivecrona, H. 1967. The surgical treatment of intracranial tumors. In: Handbuch der Neurochirurgie, Vol. IV. Springer-Verlag, Berlin.
32. Olivecrona, H. 1967. Acoustic tumors. J. Neursurg. 26:6–13.
33. Toynbee, J. 1853. Neuroma of the auditory nerve. Trans. Pathol. Soc. Lond. 4:259–260.
34. Panse, R. 1904. Ein Gliom des Akusticus. Arch F. Ohrenh. 41:251–255.
35. House, W., and Hitselberger, W. E. 1968. Surgical complications acoustic tumor surgery. Arch. Otolaryngol. 88:659–667.
36. Fischgold, H., Metzger, J., and Salamon, G. 1961. Les Neurinomes du VIII, Vol. I. Garnier, Paris.
37. Cruveilhier, J. 1829–1842. Anatomie Pathologique du Corps Humain, Part 26:1–8. J. B. Bailliere, Paris.

38. Stopford, J. S. B. 1915. The arteries of the pons and medulla oblongata. Part I. J. Anat. Physiol. 50:131–164.
39. Stopford, J. S. B. 1916. The arteries of the pons and medulla oblongata. Part II. J. Anat. Physiol. 50:255–280.
40. Atkinson, W. J. 1949. The anterior inferior cerebellar artery; its variations, pontine distribution and significance in the surgery of the cerebellopontine angle tumors. J. Neurol. Neurosurg. Psychiat. 12:137–151.
41. Bebin, J. 1968. The cerebellopontine angle. The blood supply of the brain stem and the reticular formation. Anatomical and functional correlations relevant to surgery of acoustic tumors. Henry Ford Hosp. Med. J. 16:61–83 and 163–183.
42. Sunderland, S. 1945. The arterial relations in the internal auditory meatus. Brain 68:23–27.
43. Alexander, L., and Suh, T. H. 1937. Arterial supply of lateral paraolivary area of the medulla oblongata in man. Arch. Neurol. Psychiat. 38:1243–1260.
44. Gillilan, L. A. 1964. The correlation of the blood supply to the human brain stem with clinical brain stem lesions. J. Neuropath Exp. Neurol. 23:78–108.
45. Mazzoni, A. 1969. Internal auditory canal. Arterial relations at the porus acusticus. Ann. Otol. Rhinol. Laryngol. 78:797–814.
46. Mazzoni, A. 1972. Internal auditory artery supply to the petrous bone. Ann. Otol. Rhinol. Laryngol. 81:13–21.
47. Dandy, W. E. 1955. The Brain. In: Lewis and Walters (eds.), Practice of Surgery, Vol. 12, W. F. Prior Company, Hagerstown, Maryland.
48. Takahasi, M., Okudera, T., Tomonaga, M., and Kitamura, K. 1971. Angiographic diagnosis of acoustic neurinomas. Analysis of 30 cases. Neuroradiology 89:834–840.
49. Huang, Y. P., and Wolf, W. S. 1974. Veins of posterior fossa. In: T. H. Newton and D. G. Potts (eds.), Radiology of Skull and Brain, Vol. II. Book 3, pp. 2155. The C. V. Mosby Company, St. Louis.
50. Hitselberger, W. E. 1966. External auditory canal hypesthesia. An early sign of acoustic neurinoma. Am. Surgeon 32:741–743.
51. Boettcher, A. 1876. Uber die Veranderungen der Netzhaut und des Labyrinths in einem Fall von Fibrosarcom der N. acusticus. Arch. Augen. Ohrenheilk. 2:87–115.
52. Pool, J. L., and Pava, A. A. 1957. Early Diagnosis and Treatment of Acoustic Nerve Tumors. Charles C Thomas, Springfield, Illinois.
53. House, W. F. 1968. Case summaries. Arch. Otolaryngol. 88:586–591.
54. Linthicum, F. H., Jr., and Churchill, D. 1968. Vestibular test results in acoustic tumor cases. Arch. otolaryngol. 88:604–607.
55. Hallberg, O., Uihlein, A., and Siekert, R. 1959. Sudden deafness due to cerebellopontine angle tumor. Arch. Otolaryngol. 69:160–169.
56. Nager, G. 1969. Acoustic neurinomas. Pathology and differential diagnosis. Arch. Otolaryngol. 89:252–279.
57. Schuknecht, H. F. 1966. The pathophysiology of angle tumors. In: R. J. Wolfson (ed.), The Vestibular System and Its Diseases. University of Pennsylvania Press.
58. Schuknecht, H. F., and Woellner, R. 1955. An experimental and clinical study of deafness for lesions of the cochlear nerve. J. Laryngol. 69:75–97.

59. Litton, W., and McCabe, B. 1966. Neural vs sensory lesions: Vestibular signs. Laryngoscope 76:1113–1127.
60. House, W. Personal communication.
61. Perlman, H., and Kimura, R. 1955. Observations of the living blood vessels of the cochlea. Ann. Otol. Rhinol. Laryngol. 64:1176–1192.
62. Dandy, W. E. 1934. Effects on hearing after subtotal section of cochlear branch of auditory nerve. Bull. Johns Hopkins Hosp. 55:240–243.
63. Bernstein, J., and Silverstein, H. 1966. Anterior cerebellar and labyrinthine arteries, a study in the cat. Arch. Otolaryngol. 83:422–435.
64. Dix, M., and Hallpike, C. 1950. Observations on the pathological mechanisms of conductive deafness in certain cases of neuroma of the VIII nerve. J. Laryngol. 64:658.
65. Silverstein, H., and Schuknecht, H. F. 1966. Biochemical studies of inner ear fluid in man. Arch. Otolaryngol. 84:395–402.
66. Pertuiset, B. 1970. Les Neurinomes de L'Acoustique developpes dans l'angle ponto-cerebelleux Neuro-Chirurgie. Supp. 16.
67. House, W. 1968. Fatalities in acoustic tumor surgery. Arch. Otolaryngol. 88:687–699.
68. Hitselberger, W. E., and House, W. F. 1966. Acoustic tumor surgery. The significance of vital sign changes. Arch. Otolaryngol. 84:255–260.

Acoustic Tumors
Volume I, *Diagnosis*
Edited by W. F. House and C. M. Luetje

Chapter 6

Pathology of Acoustic Tumors

Philip Gruskin, M.D., F.C.A.P.*

Assistant Clinical Professor of Pathology, University of Southern California School of Medicine, Los Angeles; Associate Director of Pathology, St. Vincent Medical Center, Los Angeles; Pathologist, Clinical Laboratory Medical Group, Los Angeles

Joseph N. Carberry, M.D., F.C.A.P.*

Associate Clinical Professor of Pathology, University of Southern California School of Medicine, Los Angeles; Director of Pathology, St. Vincent Medical Center, Los Angeles; Pathologist, Clinical Laboratory Medical Group, Los Angeles

---

The acoustic tumor is one of the more common intracranial tumors, after the various gliomas and meningiomas. Multiple studies have shown

* Mailing addresses: Department of Pathology, St. Vincent Medical Center, 2131 West Third Street, Los Angeles, California 90057, and Clinical Laboratory Medical Group, 2222 Ocean View Avenue, Los Angeles, California 90057

approximately similar incidence—acoustic tumors representing 8.7% of over 2,000 intracranial tumors in one series (1) and 11.5% of 642 cases in another (2). "Neurinomas" accounted for 7.6% of 6,000 brain tumors (3) and 8% of 5,250 verified brain tumors in Olivecrona's series (4). The overwhelming majority of intracranial schwannomas originate from the acoustic nerve, particularly the vestibular branch (see "Site of Origin"), while other cranial nerves account for a small fraction. "Neurinomas" are approximately 78% of tumors in the cerebellopontine angle (5). About 5% of acoustic tumors are bilateral (6).

Sandifort (Leyden, Germany, 1777) (7) is credited with the original postmortem description of what was presumably an acoustic tumor. Later (1810) Leveque-Lasource (8) correlated postmortem findings of a probable acoustic tumor with clinical findings. [Cushing (9) believed, however, that these two cases may have been meningiomas rather than acoustic tumors.] In Charles Bell's 1830 monograph is his sketch of an acoustic tumor showing cystic degeneration (10). Subsequently the acoustic tumor became a more recognized entity both clinically and pathologically.

ANATOMICAL CONSIDERATIONS

The gross anatomy of the eighth cranial nerve is well known. Each of the two components of the eighth nerve, cochlear and vestibular, is approximately 17–20 mm in length (6). The neuroglial-neurolemmal (glial-Schwann cell) junction is 10–13 mm distal to the brainstem in the male and 7–10 mm distal to the brainstem in the female. This junction is frequently more distal in the vestibular branch than it is in the cochlear component (11).

Much of the overall microscopic anatomy is demonstrated in Figures 1–3. As the nerve emerges from the brain it resembles bundle-like extensions of the central nervous system. Initially it does not contain Schwann cells but rather neuroglial cells. The glial-Schwann cell junction is often relatively distinct but not always sharp. Occasionally islands of glial cells are distal to this junction. In most instances the glial-Schwann cell junction is within the region of the acoustic meatus. There is, however, variation in this position; sometimes it is more proximal, and sometimes it is more distal. The more distal part of the nerve lies in the internal auditory canal and is invested by Schwann cells.

SITE OF ORIGIN

In most cases the tumor arises in the region of the internal acoustic meatus. However, the tumor may arise in any area of the nerve covered by

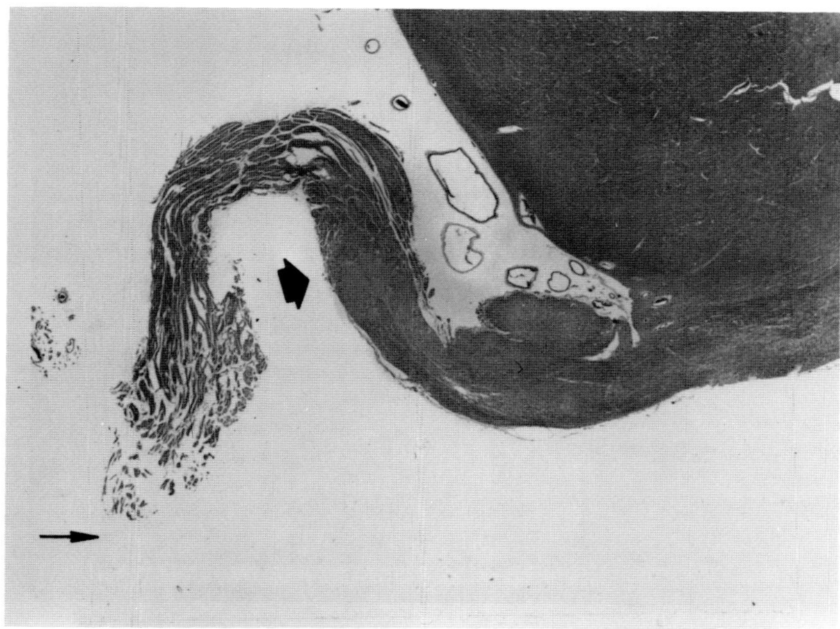

Figure 1. Normal anatomy of the eighth cranial nerve. Glial-Schwann cell junction (broad arrow), nerve entering brain (upper right), and region of Scarpa's ganglion (small arrow). (Ganglion not seen in this section—see Figure 3.) Routine autopsy specimen. (H & E × 9)

Schwann cells, i.e., the more distal part. As stated above, the glial-Schwann cell junction usually lies in the region of the internal acoustic meatus, but it may be more central, outside the temporal bone, or it may be more distal. Schuknecht (11) states there is no evidence to support the contention that schwannomas arise predominantly at the glial-Schwann cell junction; they may arise anywhere between this junction and the cribrose area. There are no reports of primary tumors occurring in the neuroglial portion (12).

Most tumors originate from the vestibular branch, but some can originate from the cochlear nerve. The classic study of Skinner (13) [with reference to Henschen (14)] might explain why these tumors are much more apt to occur in the vestibular division and in the distal segment, and why this tumor, common in this nerve, is most uncommon in other cranial nerves. It was determined that the vestibular ganglion, as opposed to others, has an increased number of cells between the ganglion cells and that these cells have a disordered appearance. This may predispose the vestibular nerve to develop tumors.

Various temporal bone studies have disclosed small asymptomatic schwannomas and have demonstrated their early features, including site of origin. The 1936 Hardy and Crowe study (15) of temporal bones in 250 cases disclosed an acoustic tumor in six. Later, in 1970, Leonard and Talbot (16) reviewed the original Hardy and Crowe series and added additional cases. They accepted only three of the original six cases as being "neurilemmomas" and added one more (total of four cases of early asymptomatic "neurilemmomas" in 883 temporal bones). These four tumors arose from the vestibular nerve or between the vestibular nerve and cochlear nerve. Another series of 893 temporal bones (17) revealed five occult vestibular schwannomas. Gussen (18) described an acoustic tumor limited to the modiolus. There was no evidence of tumor extending into the modiolus from the internal auditory canal, and the tumor appeared to arise from that portion of the nerve peripheral to the spiral ganglion. A tumor apparently arising in the vestibule was presented by Wanamaker (19), who felt that tumors could develop from the nerves to either the saccule or utricle. Naunton and Petasnick (20) encountered six

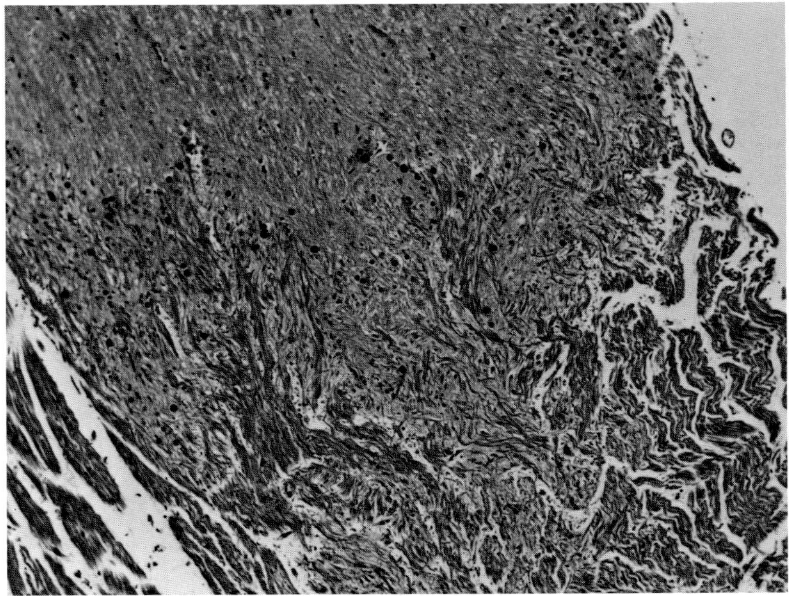

Figure 2. Higher power of Figure 1: glial-Schwann cell junction. Lighter area (top half) glial portion with calcospherites. Myelinated fibers covered by Schwann cells (lower half). (H & E × 90)

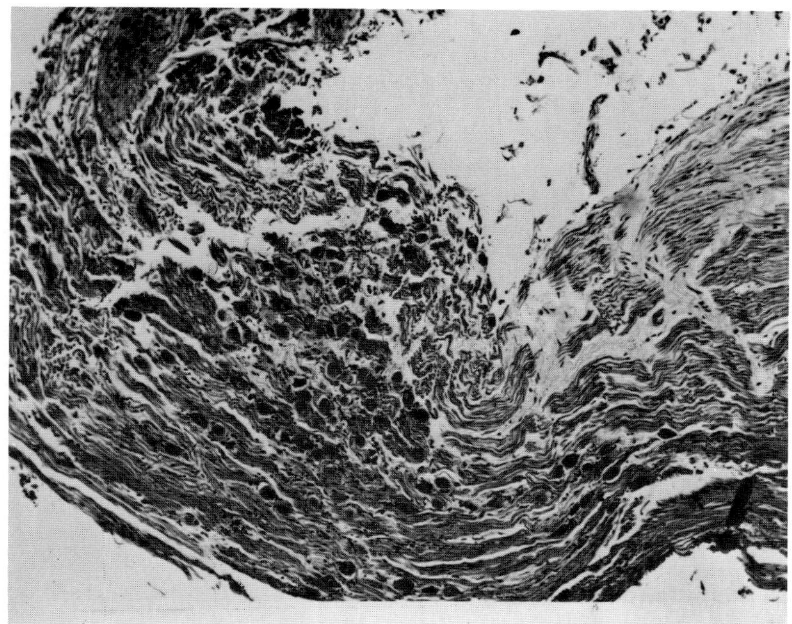

Figure 3. Deeper section of nerve in Figure 1 (in region of small arrow in Figure 1) to show Scarpa's ganglion. (H & E × 90)

acoustic tumors in which the internal auditory meatus were normal or without significant asymmetry, yet the tumors were large and predominantly in the cerebellopontine angle, with extension into the internal auditory meatus. Their impression was that these tumors arose from a portion of the nerve trunk central to the internal auditory meatus.

It is now evident that acoustic tumors may arise from either branch of the eighth nerve and anywhere between the glial-Schwann cell junction and the origin of the nerves in the labyrinth (17).

Multiple schwannomas occurring at almost any site are usually considered part of von Recklinghausen's disease.

TERMINOLOGY AND CELL OF ORIGIN

To date, numerous names (more than 25) have been applied to eighth nerve tumors. The multitude of names stems from the confusion regarding the cell of origin, with the name of the tumor based on the presumed cell of origin. Names for eighth nerve tumors have included acoustic nerve tumor, acoustic neuroma, angioneurofibroma, false neuroma, fibroglioma, fibromyxoma, glioma, myoschwannoma, neurilemoblastoma (Geschickter), neurinoma, neurofibromyxoma, neurilemmoma, neurolemmoma, neuroma fibrillare, peripheral glioma, perineural fibroblastoma, perineural glioma, schwannoglioma, and schwannoma (21). Additional terms have included neurofibroma, fibroma of the eighth nerve, lemmoma, lemmoblastoma, cerebellopontine tumor, acoustic tumor, tumor of the acoustic nerve, and recess tumor (6). Other names have been used.

The neuroectodermal origin from Schwann cells was first suggested in 1908 by Verocay (22), who expressed the opinion that the tumor arose from "nerve fiber cells" which he thought were capable of producing nerve fibers. The term "neurinoma," meaning nerve fiber tumor, was therefore suggested. Mallory (23) believed that the common tumor of the nervus acusticus and other central nerves was a perineurial fibroblastoma, while Antoni (24) maintained that the tumors originated from the cells of Schwann (lemmoblasts) and thus suggested the name "lemmoma" or "lemmoblastoma." It was Masson's thought that the tumors arose from the sheath of Schwann, and thus the tumor was termed a "schwannoma" (25). To Stout (26) the previous terms were not totally acceptable as indicating the cell of origin. Therefore, he took the phrase "nerve sheath tumor," which was descriptive as far as a cellular origin from fibroblast or Schwann cell, and constructed a new term, "neurilemmoma." Friedmann (27) uses the term "Schwann cell tumor of the ear."

Before continuing the discussion of cell of origin and terminology of eighth nerve tumors, a current definition of solitary schwannoma and solitary neurofibroma is appropriate.

A solitary schwannoma is a benign, slowly growing, encapsulated neoplasm that originates in a nerve and is composed of Schwann cells in a collagenous matrix (28). A solitary neurofibroma is a benign, slowly growing, relatively circumscribed but nonencapsulated neoplasm originating in a nerve and composed principally of Schwann cells. The intercellular matrix contains collagen fibrils in a nonorganized mucoid or myxomatous component (28). The neurofibroma has a different appearance and natural history from that of schwannoma. The neurofibroma is formed by a combined proliferation of all the elements of the peripheral nerve—Schwann cells, neurites, fibroblasts, and probably perineurial cells. Schwann cells usually predominate (29).

Peripheral nerves contain axons, Schwann cells, fibroblasts of the endoneurium and epineurium, and perineurial cells. Ordinary fibroblasts, such as those found in the endoneurium, have no basement membrane, and since the tumor cells are surrounded by basement membrane (see "Electron Microscopy"), fibroblasts are not thought to be the cell of origin. Also, nerve fibers themselves do not proliferate in acoustic tumors and therefore are not thought to be the cell of origin. The term "neurinoma" is therefore not correct.

Almost all the current debate regarding the cell of origin revolves around the Schwann cell and perineurial cell. Harkin and Reed (28) felt the two could not be distinguished by any techniques then in use, including histochemistry, electron microscopy, or tissue culture. Since Schwann cells and perineurial cells differ only in their location in the nerve sheath, they thus adhere to the single term of schwannoma, postulating that it may arise from either or both cell types.

There is not, however, general acceptance that the Schwann cell and perineurial cell are identical. Perineurial cells also have a basement membrane like Schwann cells, but unlike them, perineurial cells contain large numbers of micropinocytotic vesicles (30) and terminal bars (31).

Most electron microscopists and others feel today that nerve sheath tumors are derived from Schwann cells, while others still consider that perineurial cells may be the cells of origin (30, 31, 32).

Acoustic tumors contain, in addition to the predominant tumor cell, connective tissue fibers, collagen, and reticulum. Schwann cells may be able to produce collagen (28, 33). Silver reticulum stains on acoustic tumors often show abundant argyrophilic fibers (see "Microscopic Pathology" and Figure 68).

Pineda and Feder (34) discuss the term "acoustic neuroma" and feel it may be misleading. True neuroma should be composed of nerve cells and nerve fibers, while a false neuroma is a tumor of nerve sheath without neoplastic proliferation of genuine nerve cells. Therefore, acoustic nerve neoplasms should more properly be called "false neuromas." The term "neurolemmoma," although it reflects the cell of origin more accurately (sheath of Schwann, or neurolemma), is too often confused with the term neurilemmoma (neurilemma: a thin outer covering, not properly the Schwann or sheath cell). They therefore suggest that neoplasms of the acoustic nerve be called schwannomas.

In conclusion, then, most authorities feel that the Schwann cell is the cell of origin. The term neurofibroma does not seem appropriate. Acoustic tumor, acoustic neuroma, neuroma, neurilemmoma, and neurolemmoma are all terms in general use, but with regard to all of the above discussion, we feel that schwannoma is the most acceptable term at this time.

GROSS PATHOLOGY

The schwannoma is considered one of the few truly encapsulated neoplasms, with the capsule formed by the perineurium. In practice, however, the capsule is difficult to identify in surgical material of acoustic tumors. The nerve of origin may be demonstrated at the periphery, flattened along the edge of the tumor.

The acoustic tumor may vary considerably in size, from a microscopic tumor to one that is quite large. We have received specimens up to 5 or 6 cm in diameter and weighing up to 30 g or more. Some of these have been tumors only partially removed, either in a first-stage operation or for other reasons, and therefore may have been even larger.

The shape of the tumor may depend on its location. Those originating in the internal auditory canal are usually round or oval, as are tumors that originate central to the internal auditory meatus and that are therefore primarily in the cerebellopontine angle. Externally, tumors are relatively smooth and lobulated.

Classically, however, most tumors originate in the region of the internal auditory meatus, and, as they grow, they enlarge the meatus and extend into the cerebellopontine angle. Expansion of the meatus causes the classic funnel-shaped appearance. When they reach the cerebellopontine angle, they may attain considerable size. Many tumors therefore consist of two portions: a stalk within the meatus and a larger extratemporal portion, the overall configuration resembling a mushroom.

An arachnoidal cyst containing xanthochromic or clear fluid often overlies the dorsolateral aspect of the tumor (6).

The color and consistency, in our experience, often depend on the size of the tumor and the degree of degenerative change. Small tumors (less than 15 mm) may be yellow or pink to pink-grey and have a rubbery consistency. On cut section they have a semi-translucent appearance and are solid (Figure 4). Medium size tumors have the gross appearance of schwannomas seen elsewhere in the body, with a pale yellow color. Usually firm to rubbery, they are glistening on cut section and usually solid (Figure 5).

The larger tumors (Figure 6) have a much more varied gross appearance due to degenerative changes. The color is more mottled, with the most consistent finding being a bright yellow (predominantly from histiocytes) to yellow-tan color, which is opaque rather than semi-translucent on section. Areas of acute or recent hemorrhage appear red, while older hemorrhage appears brown. Fibrosis is more grey. The larger tumors may be solid, but often are not, and cystic change can be

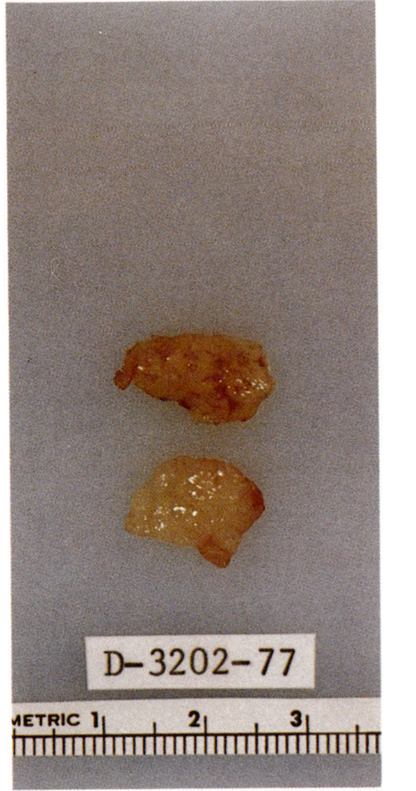

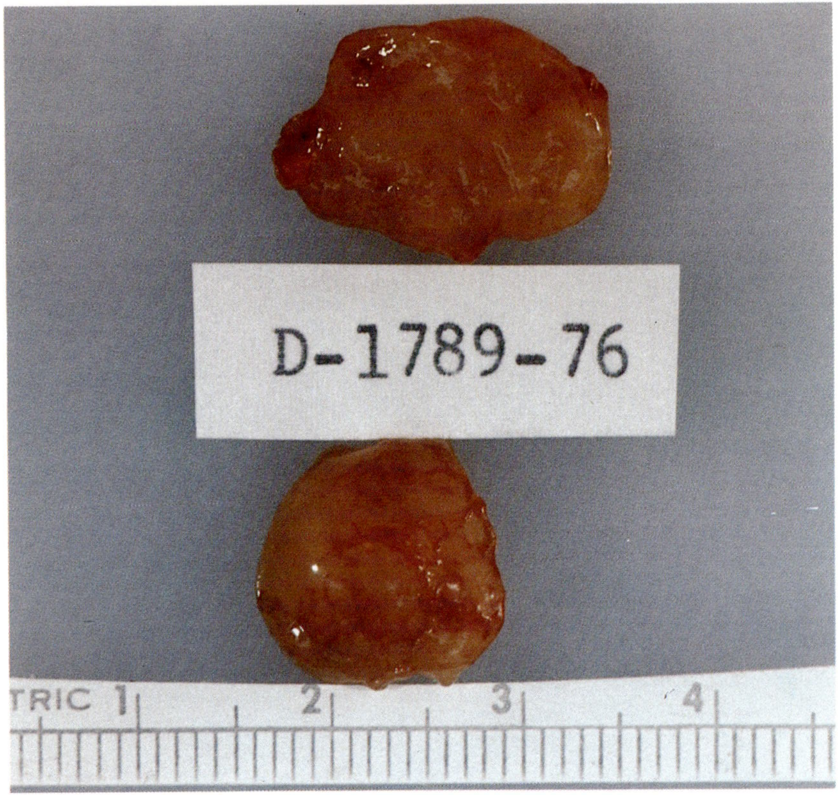

Figure 4. (*left*) Small acoustic schwannoma, bisected. External surface (top) and cut surface (bottom).
Figure 5. (*right*) Medium size acoustic schwannoma, bisected. Cut surface (top) shows solid tumor with focal hemorrhage. External surface (bottom) is lobulated. Note the characteristic pale yellow color.

prominent. The consistency also is quite variable. There may be areas that are rubbery, edematous, soft, or fibrous. Some tumors represent all these characteristics in one part or another, while others are predominantly of one type.

From a practical standpoint regarding the biopsy material received from surgery, the color alone is often a clue to the diagnosis. Yellow tissue (Figure 7), even in small biopsy fragments, usually is indicative of schwannoma, while white or grey fragments are often meningiomas. This is not, however, absolute, as we have encountered a few biopsies of yellow meningiomas (Figure 74) and white or grey schwannomas.

The gross features of acoustic tumors, including the relationship to the surrounding structures, are demonstrated in Figures 8 and 9.

Some of the clinical symptomatology may be explained by changes in the tumor and by involvement of adjacent structures. Hemorrhage may produce enlargement, as may edema. The tumor may again shrink when the edema disappears. Occasionally degenerative change with fibrosis may actually shrink the tumor.

As the lesion grows, it destroys its nerve and ganglia, with a resultant loss of vestibular function and hearing. The facial nerve, which is in proximity to the eighth nerve, may also be affected. The internal auditory and other arteries, e.g., anterior inferior cerebellar, may be compressed, with resultant dysfunction and degenerative changes. When the tumor extends into the cerebellopontine recess, symptoms may be those of a classic mass lesion in this area, and even death may result.

MICROSCOPIC PATHOLOGY

More than 1,000 acoustic tumors have been surgically removed by William F. House, M.D., and associates, at St. Vincent Medical Center, Los Angeles. The authors have reviewed most of the available microscopic sections. Although any tumor may have the "classic" pattern of a schwannoma in a given area, any one may manifest myriad patterns, particularly in a localized area. There is probably more variation in histologic patterns in acoustic tumors than in many other tumors.

Figures 10–13 demonstrate the overall relationship of a typical acoustic tumor to its nerve of origin. Figures 14–19 also show the nerve of origin in relation to the tumor. Often the nerve is compressed at the periphery (Figure 14), or the nerve may be partially split by the tumor (Figures 15 and 16). Ganglion cells may be noted in the nerve. Sometimes fibrous tissue of perineurium is included; this tissue forms the capsule of these tumors, although we often find this difficult to demonstrate. The

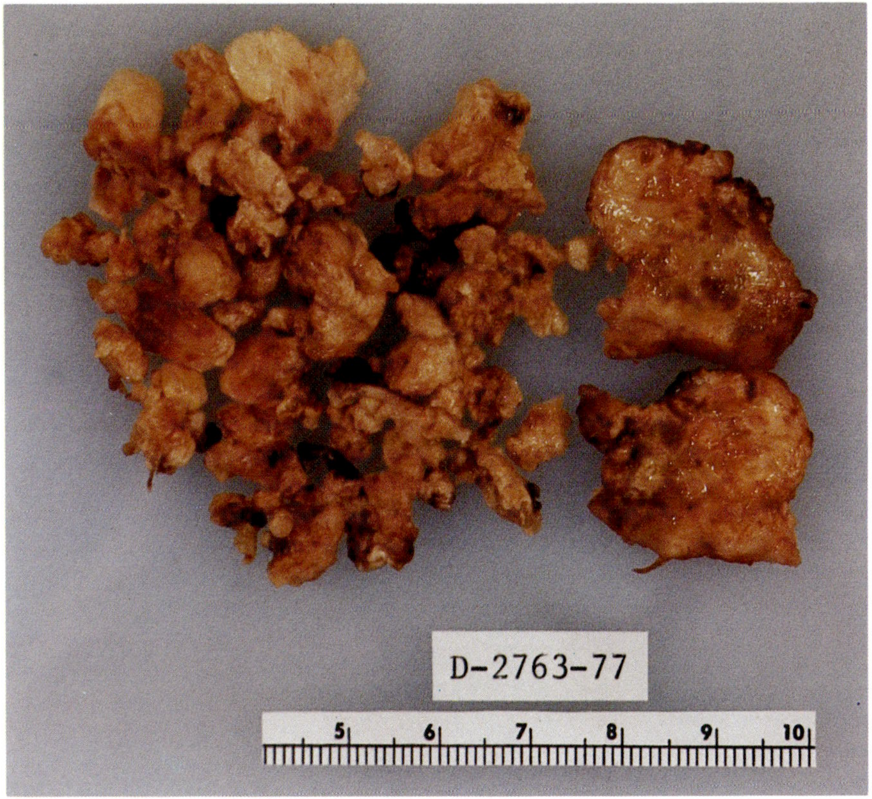

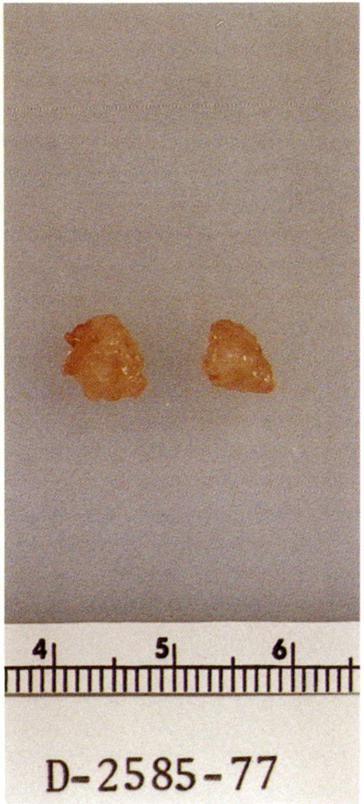

Figure 6. (*left*) Large acoustic schwannoma, as often received in multiple pieces. Variegated appearance with bright yellow areas and hemorrhage.

Figure 7. (*right*) Typical biopsy specimen of acoustic schwannoma. Yellow color and glistening surface arc characteristic.

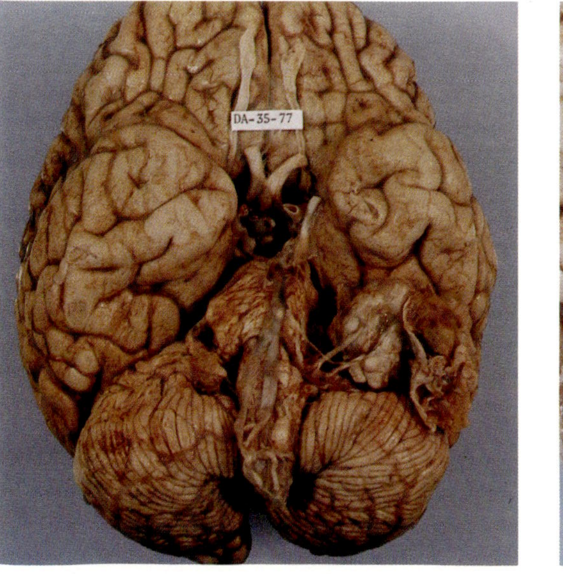

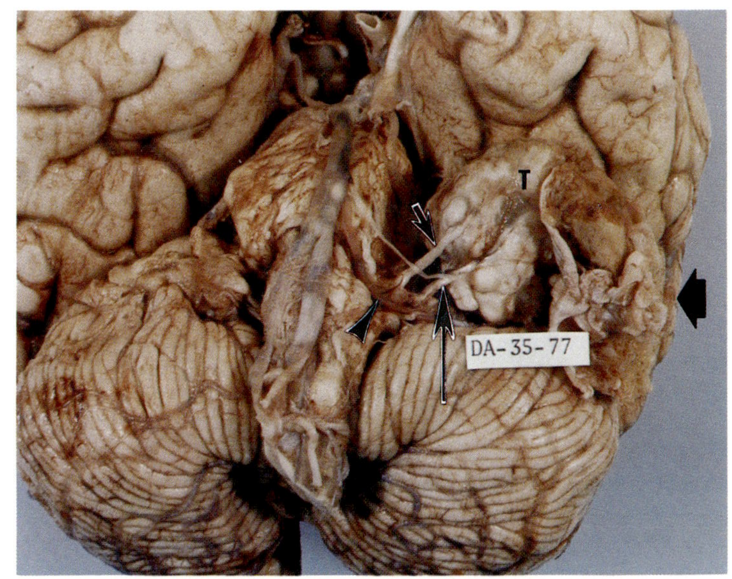

Figure 8. (*left*) Brain from a patient with von Recklinghausen's disease and bilateral acoustic tumors. (Right tumor previously surgically removed.)

Figure 9. (*right*) Same specimen as in Figure 8. The tumor (T) is 3.4 cm in diameter and originates from the eighth cranial nerve (long arrow). The seventh cranial nerve (short arrow) is stretched over the tumor. Crossing these two nerves is the small internal auditory artery arising from the basilar artery. The anterior inferior cerebellar artery (arrowhead) is compressed between tumor and cerebellum. The temporal bone (broad arrow) is removed en bloc with the tumor.

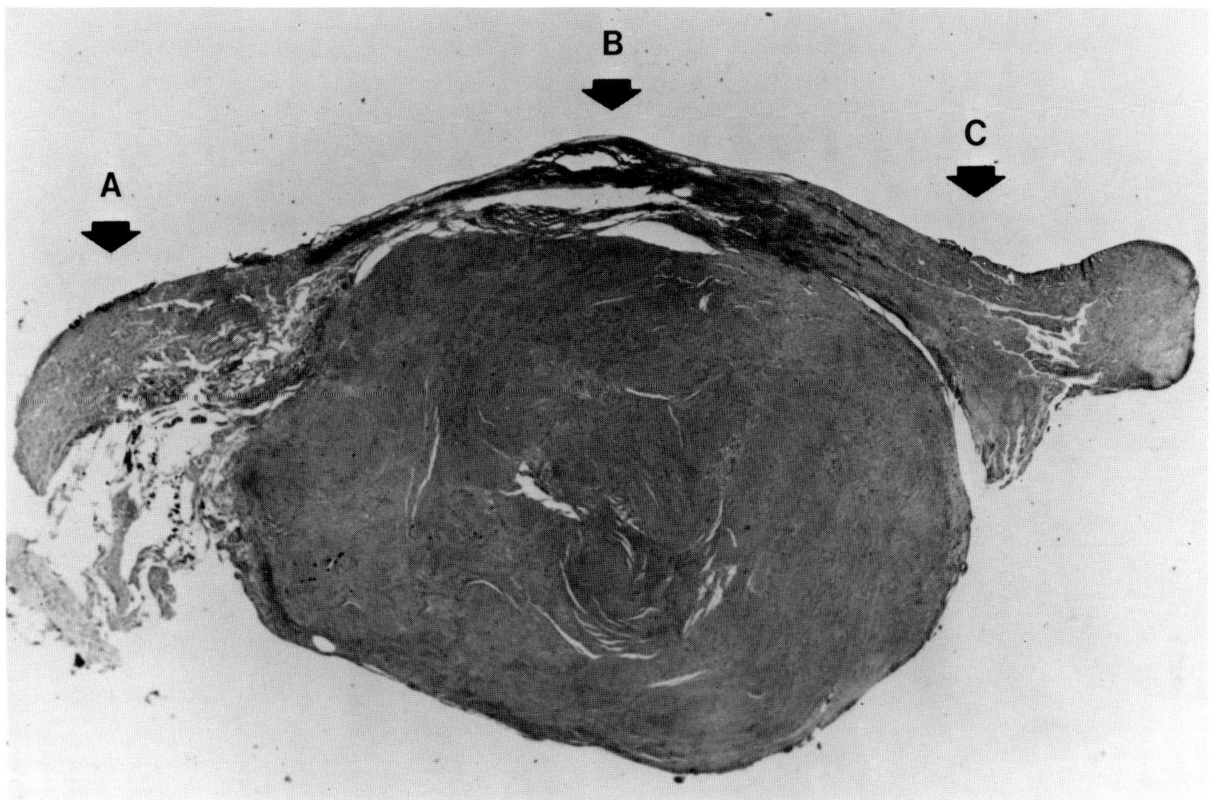

Figure 10. An acoustic schwannoma and its nerve of origin. Scarpa's ganglion (arrow A and Figure 11), compressed nerve with hemorrhage (arrow B and Figure 12) and glial-Schwann cell junction (arrow C and Figure 13). (H & E × 14)

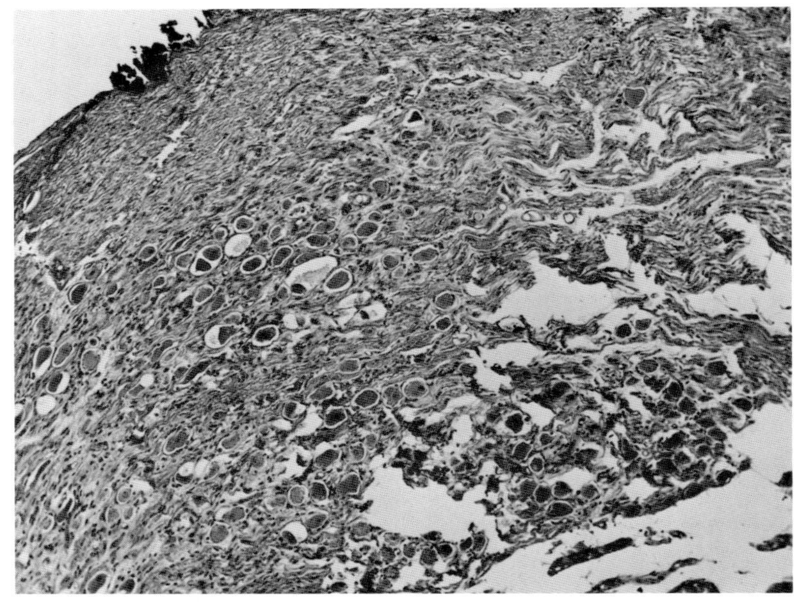

Figure 11. Same specimen as Figure 10 (at arrow A). Scarpa's ganglion. (H & E × 90)

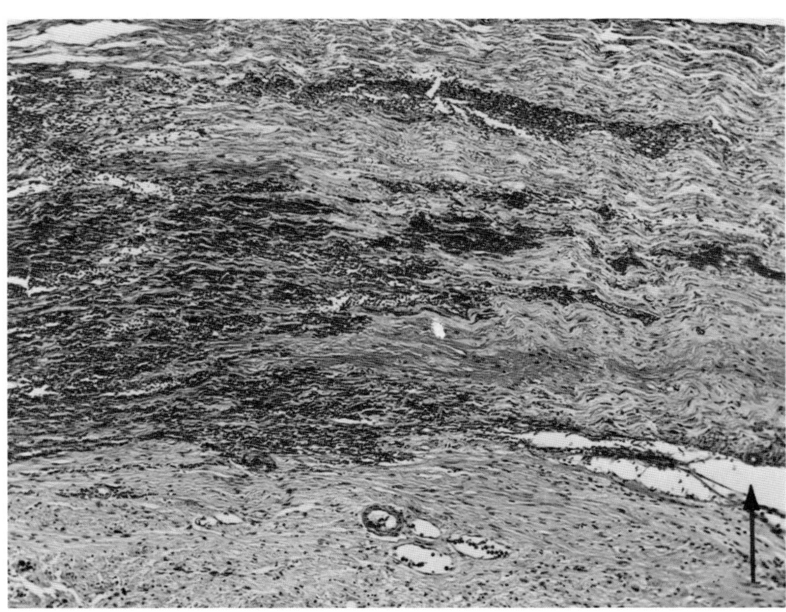

Figure 12. Same specimen as Figure 10 (at arrow B). Compressed nerve with hemorrhage (top) is separated (arrow) from tumor (bottom). (H & E × 90)

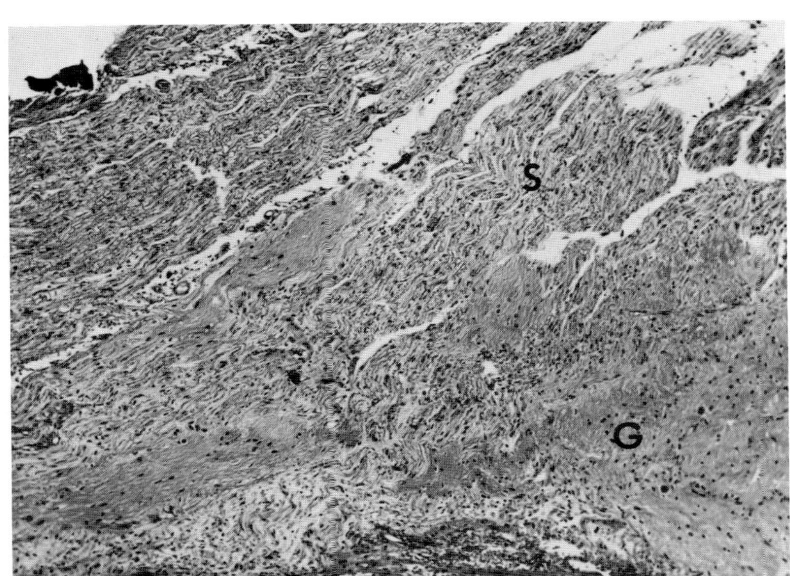

Figure 13. Same specimen as Figure 10 (at arrow C). Glial (G) and Schwann cell (S) junction. (H & E × 90)

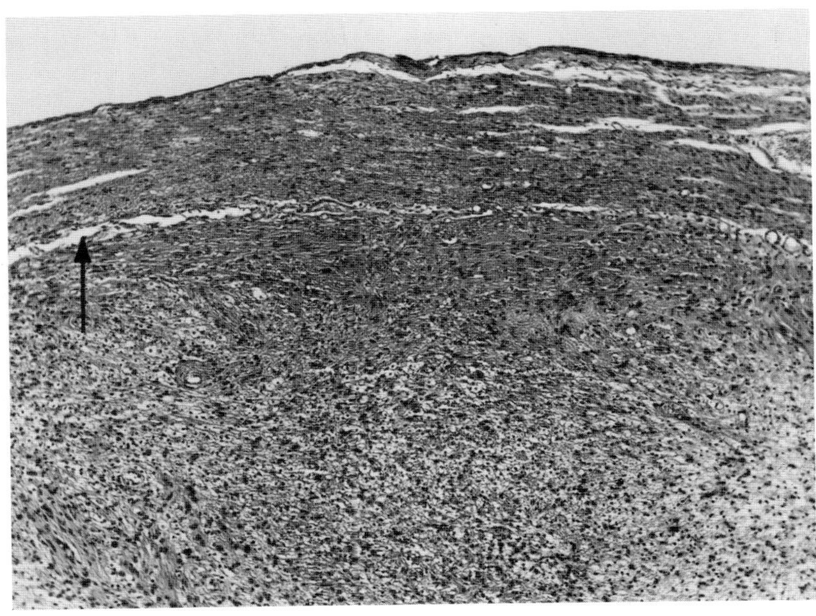

Figure 14. *Relation of acoustic schwannoma to nerve of origin and ganglion cells (Figures 14–19).* Compressed nerve (top) separated (arrow) from tumor (bottom). (H & E × 108)

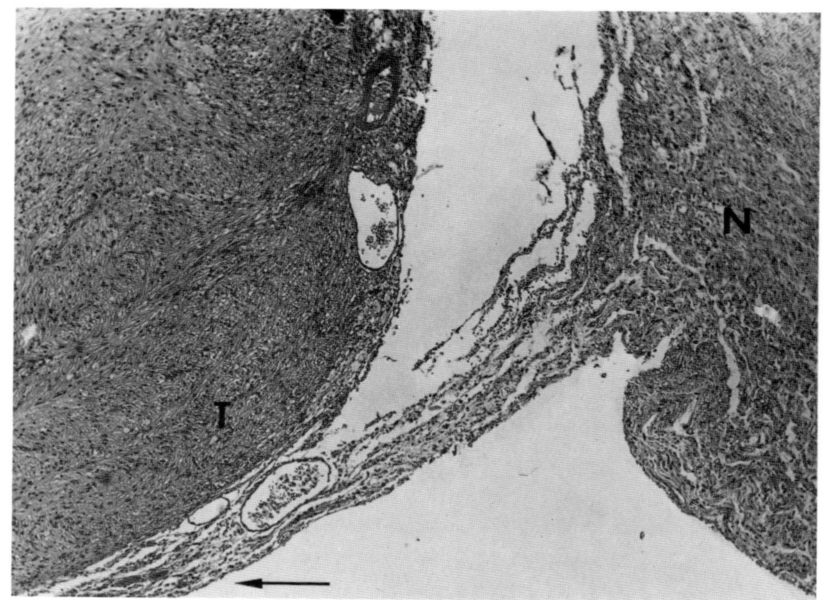

Figure 15. Nerve (N) partially split by tumor (T). Ganglion cells in the nerve (arrow). (H & E × 90)

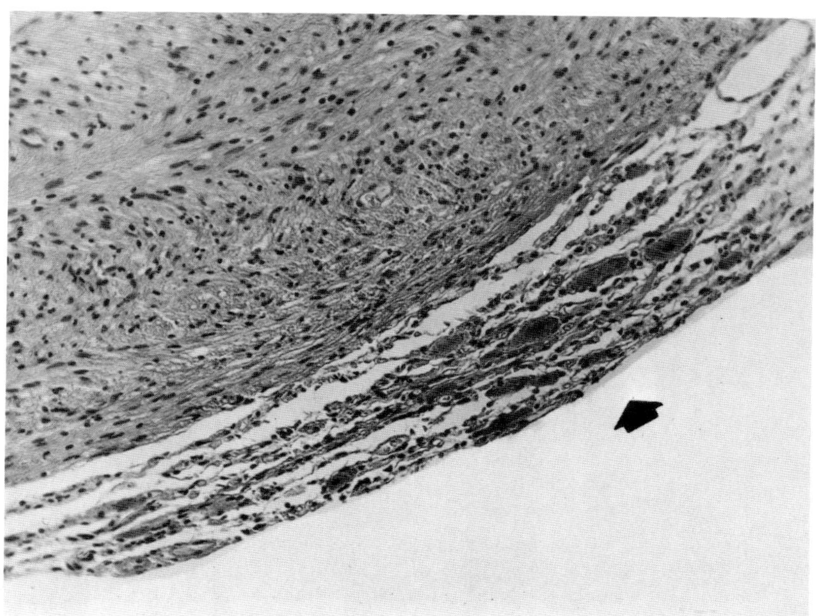

Figure 16. Higher power of Figure 15. Ganglion cells (arrow). (H & E × 216)

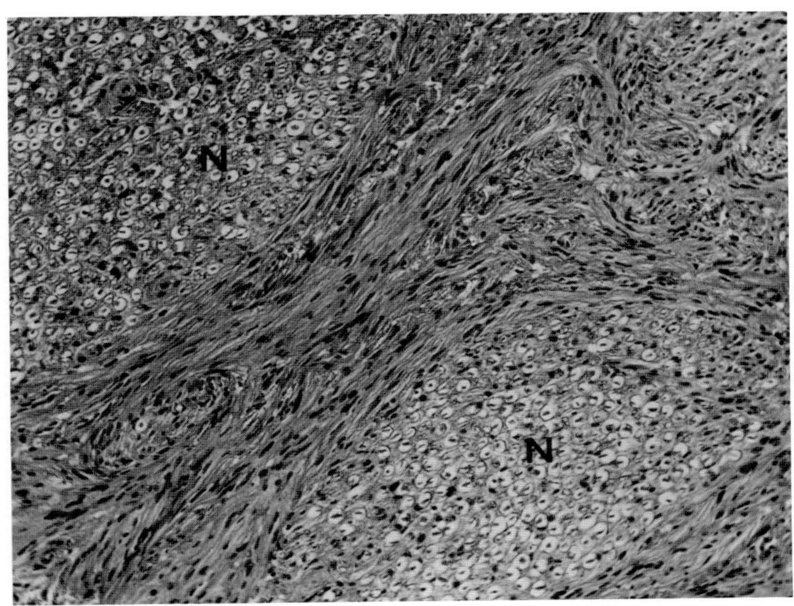

Figure 17. Nerves (N) as seen on end are surrounded by tumor. (H & E × 180)

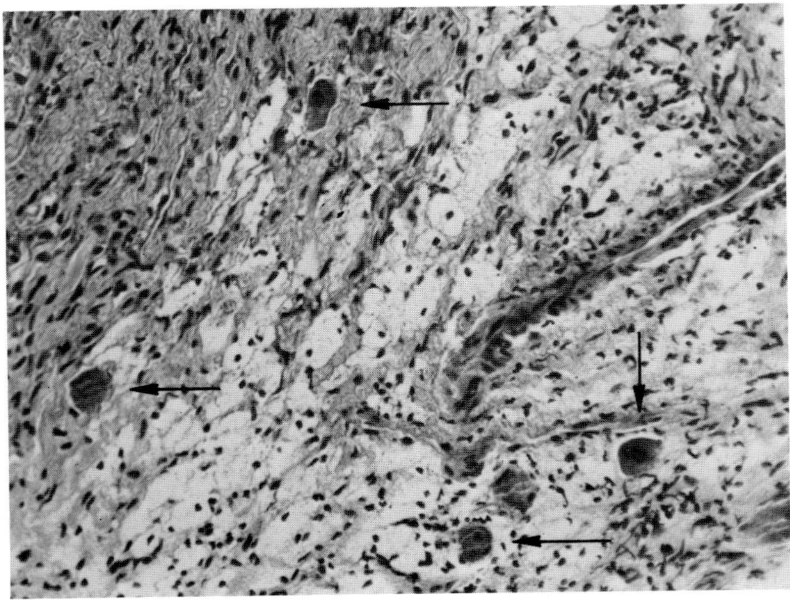

Figure 18. Ganglion cells (arrows) surrounded by tumor, near an Antoni B area with histiocytes. (H & E × 288)

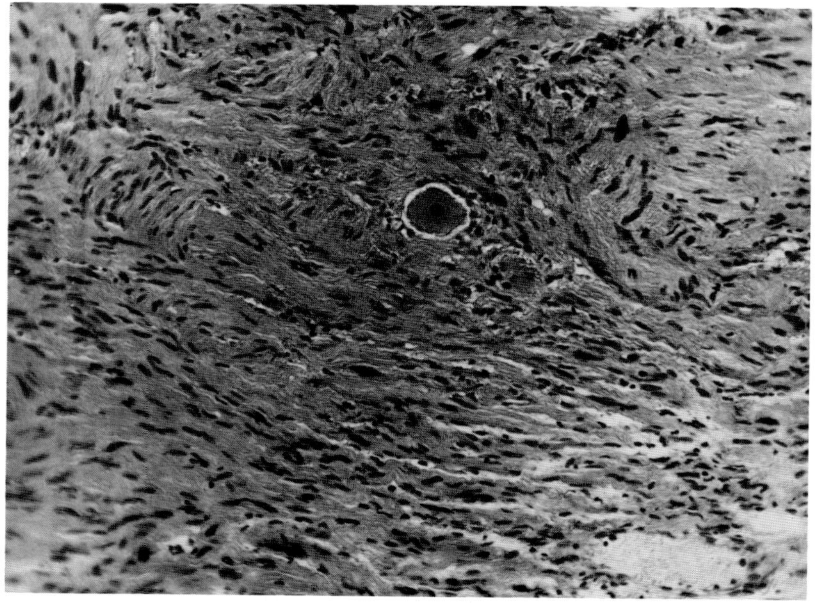

Figure 19. Ganglion cell entrapped in neoplasm (Antoni A area). (H & E × 216)

nerve may be surrounded by the tumor rather than compressed along an edge (Figure 17), and ganglion cells may be intermixed with the tumor cells (Figures 18 and 19).

The classic description of a schwannoma is a tumor composed of Antoni type A and type B tissue. Type A is composed of more compact tissue, with elongated spindle cells, in irregular streams, and with a tendency to palisading. Type B tissue, often intermingled with type A, is characterized by a loose texture, often with sponginess and cyst formation.

Figure 20 and Figures 21–24 show typical acoustic tumors with Antoni A and B areas. Much of the tumor is composed of bundles of interlacing eosinophilic spindle cells with a moderate degree of cellularity. There is mild nuclear pleomorphism. Most acoustic tumors are predominately type A tissue.

The various patterns found in acoustic schwannomas may be either focal or diffuse. The following descriptions cover the vast array of patterns. Although patterns may be of more importance to the pathologist, the surgeon should be aware of these possibilities, particularly as they relate to diagnosis of small biopsies and frozen sections. If the entire

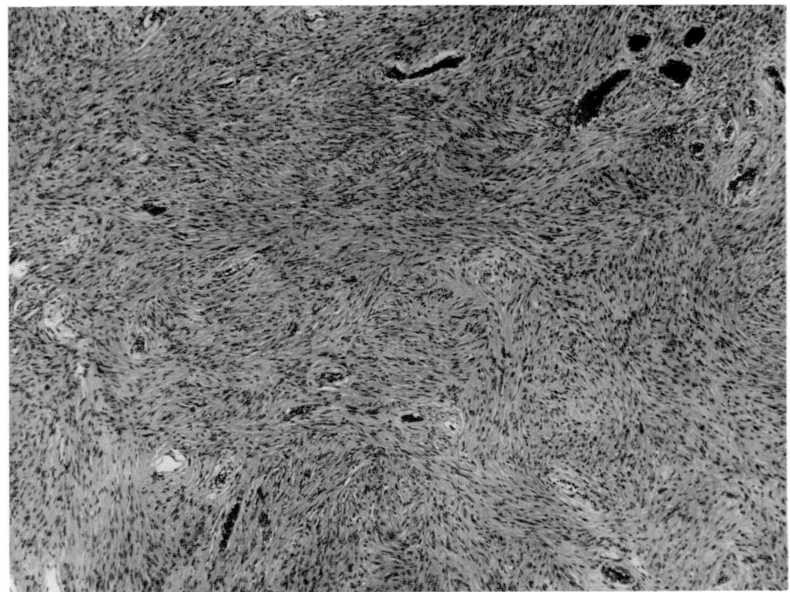

Figure 20. Typical acoustic schwannoma (Antoni A area) composed of irregular interlacing bundles of spindle cells. (H & E × 57.6)

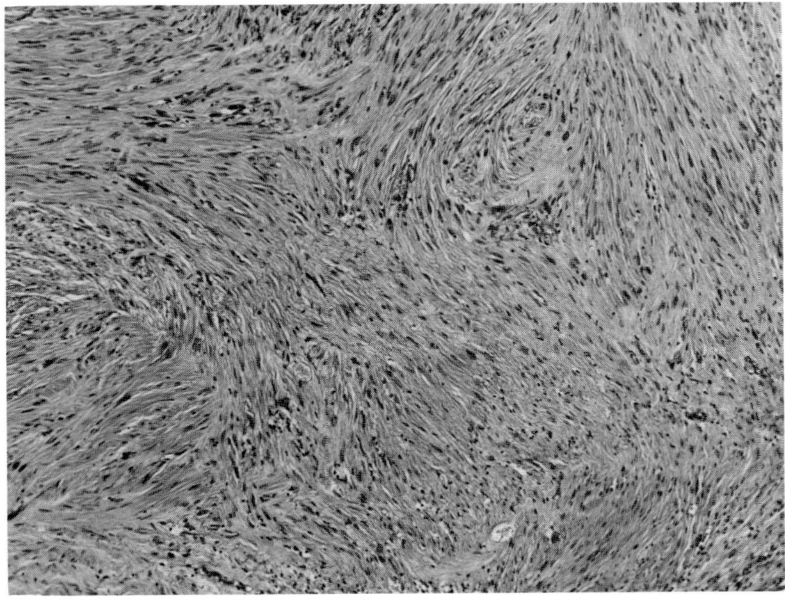

Figure 21. Typical schwannoma with interlacing bundles and lack of palisading. Same case as Figure 10. (H & E × 90)

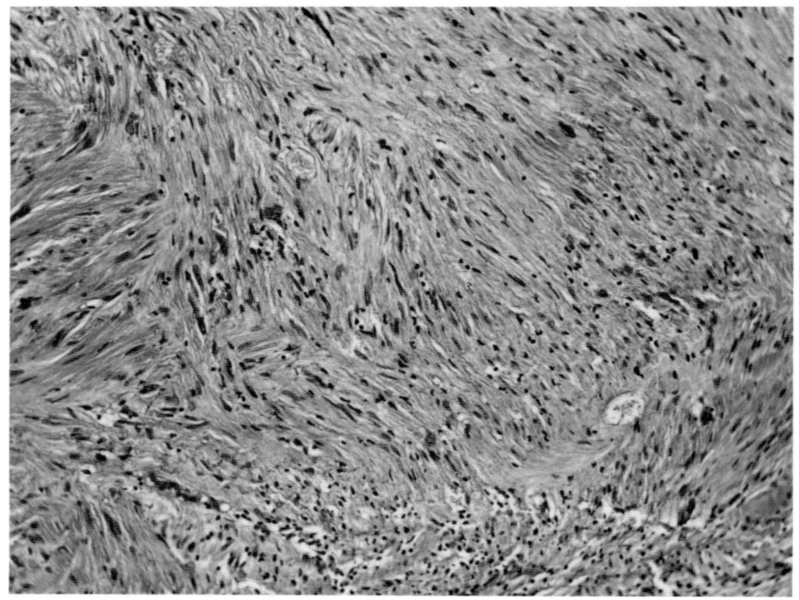

Figure 22. Higher power of Figure 21. Spindle cells with mild nuclear pleomorphism and average degree of cellularity. (H & E × 144)

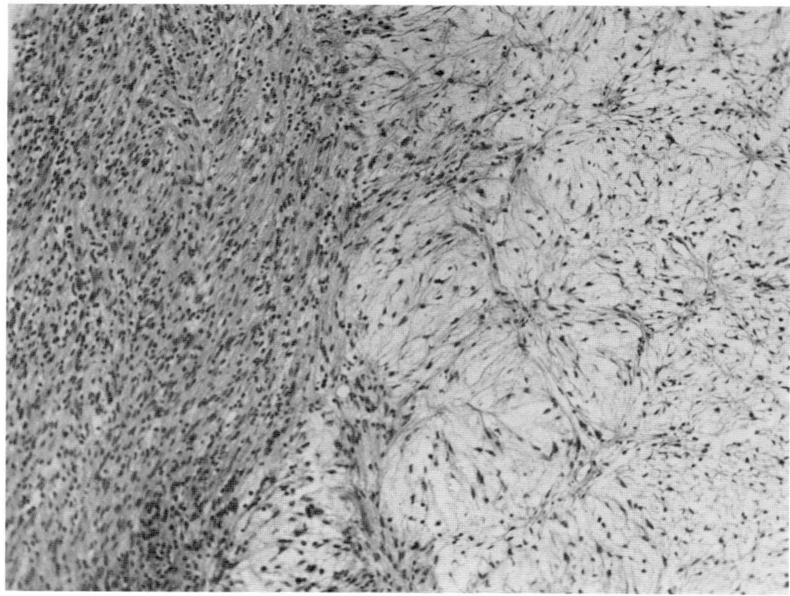

Figure 23. Acoustic schwannoma showing junction of Antoni A tissue (left) and Antoni B tissue (right). (H & E × 144)

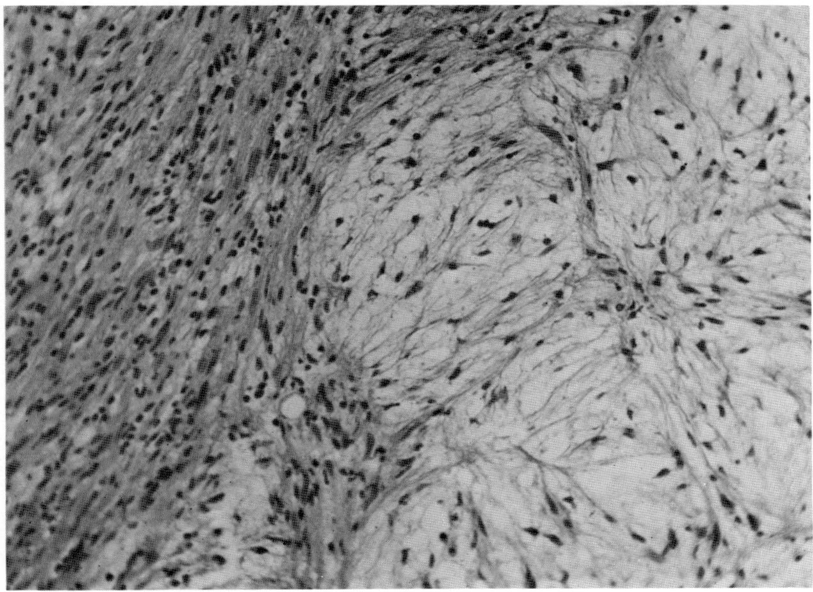

Figure 24. Higher power of Figure 23. Antoni A tissue (left) and Antoni B tissue (right). (H & E × 288)

tumor were submitted, most tumors could be diagnosed by the surgical pathologist. The routine biopsy material of 5 mm or less may, however, create problems in diagnosis, as only a small area is seen. Even when an entire tumor is available, a rare one will be difficult to diagnose.

Various patterns and changes may occur in the tumors because of compression of vessels, compression against bone, degeneration, inherent nature of the tumor, hemorrhage, and other factors.

Spindle cells in more compact areas can vary in arrangement, including typical interlacing bundles (Figure 21), herringbone pattern (Figure 25), whorled bundles resembling meningioma (Figures 26 and 27), parallel fibers (Figure 28), bundles or cords (Figure 29), or small bundles resembling neurofibroma (Figure 30).

Schwannomas are also well noted for their various patterns of palisading. A large part of a tumor may show palisading of cells, such as that in Figure 31. Other patterns (Figure 32) may be seen focally. Sometimes there is palisading of nuclei with more central eosinophilic fibrillar material, as illustrated in Figure 33. Palisading structures resembling tactile corpuscles are called Verocay bodies. However, the term "Verocay body" has been used by many to mean any body-like con-

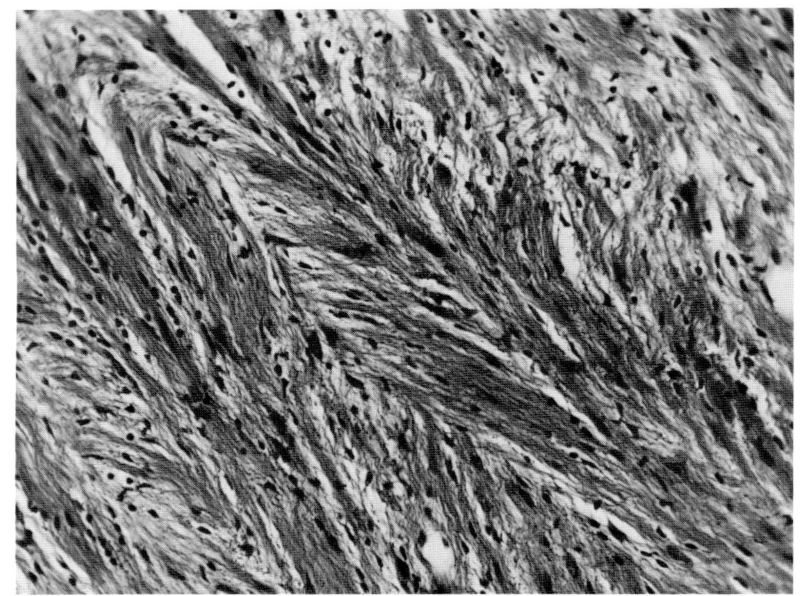

Figure 25. *Spindle cell patterns in acoustic schwannomas* (*Figures 25–30*). Herringbone pattern. (H & E × 225)

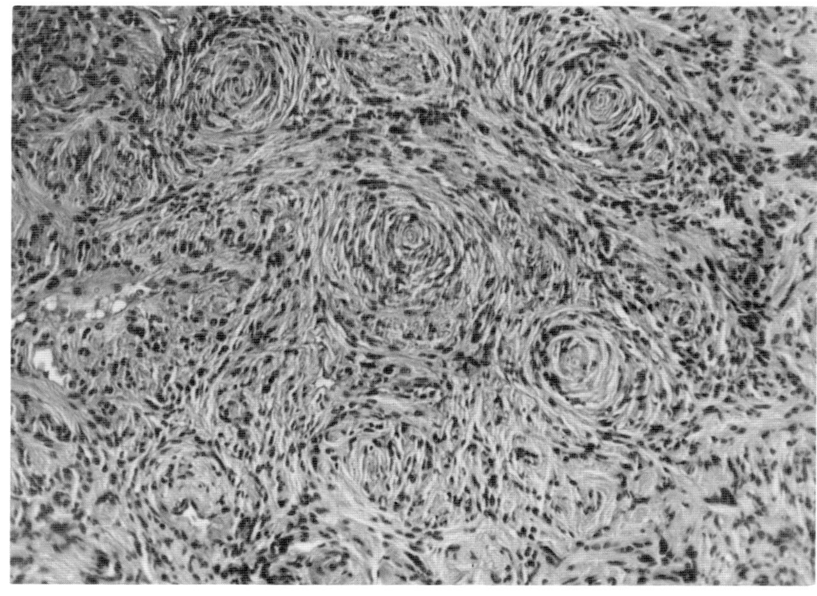

Figure 26. Meningioma-like whorls. (H & E × 216)

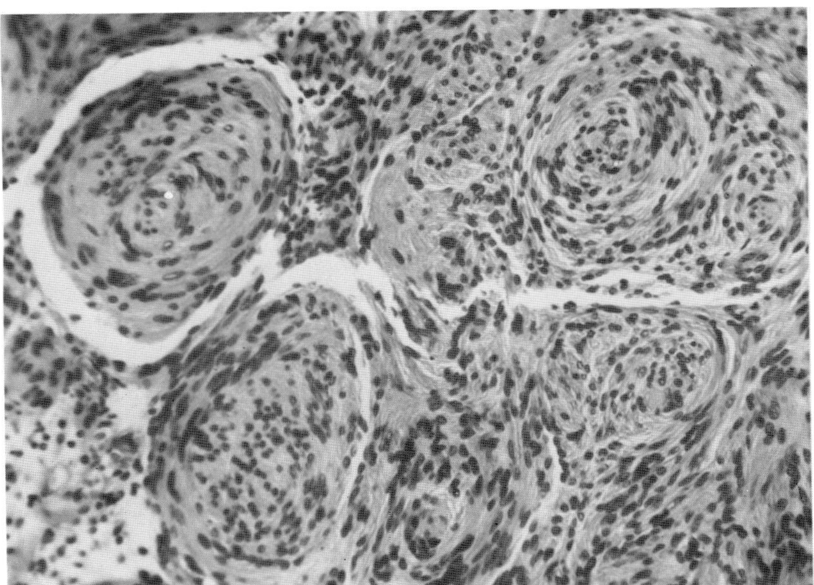

Figure 27. Meningioma-like whorls (different case than Figure 27). (H & E × 252)

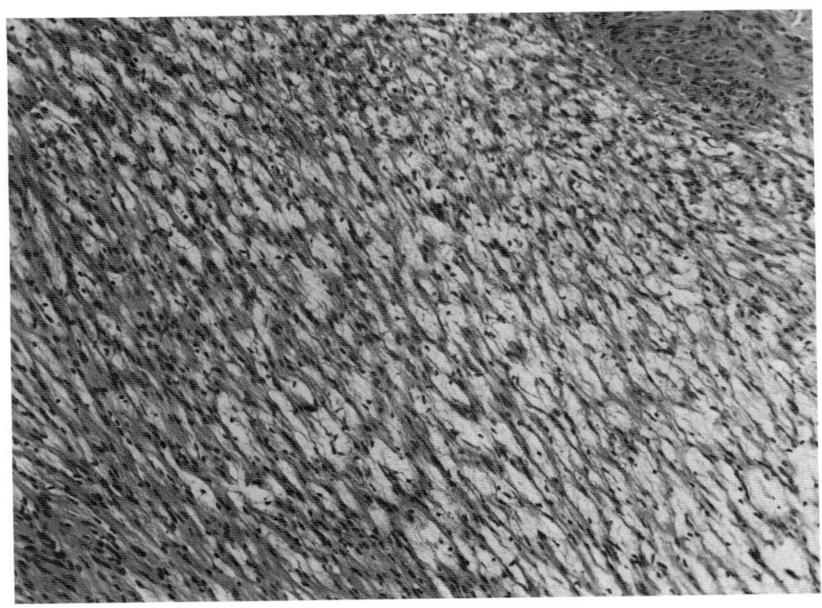

Figure 28. Parallel fibers separated by histiocytes. (H & E × 144)

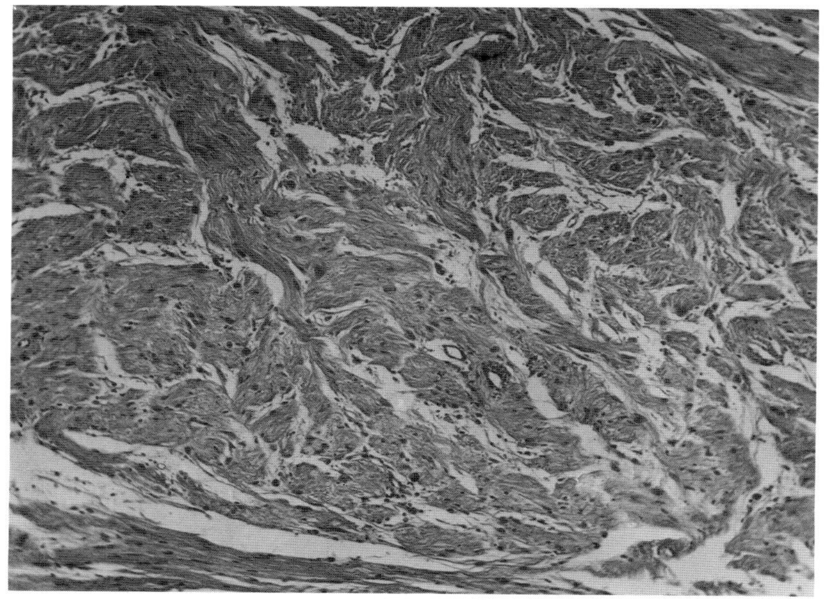

Figure 29. Bundles or cords. (H & E × 144)

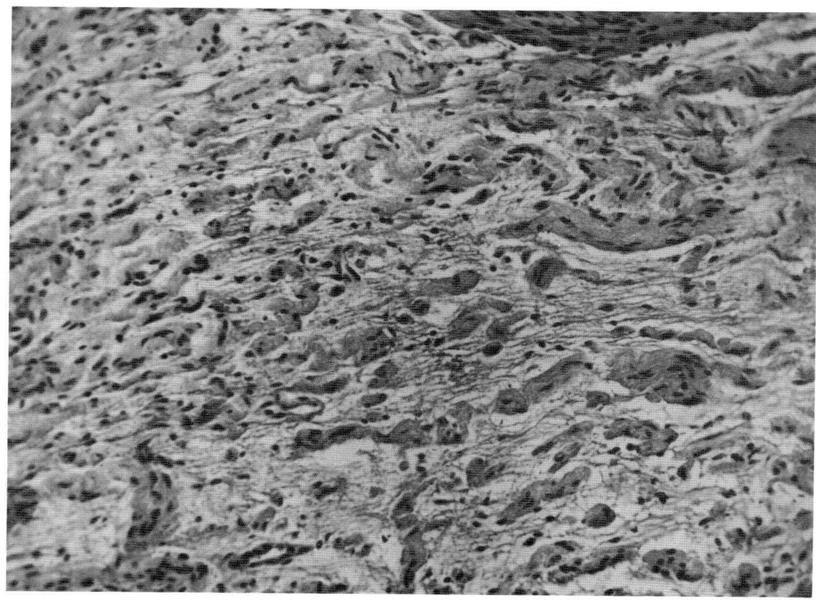

Figure 30. Neurofibroma-like area. (H & E × 216)

figuration of tumor cells. It has been our experience that palisading and Verocay bodies are frequently absent in many acoustic tumors. In addition, palisading is a phenomenon not limited to schwannomas and can be found in other tumors, e.g., leiomyoma, leiomyosarcoma, and those of fibrous tissue origin.

Looser areas may have a myxoid pattern (Figure 34) with acid mucopolysaccharide material in the intercellular space (confirmed by Alcian blue stain).

Foamy histiocytes vary tremendously in number and may be localized or diffuse (Figure 35). These impart the bright yellow color often seen grossly. They may or may not be seen in a region of acute or old hemorrhage. Characteristically they are part of Antoni B areas but they may be present in Antoni A tissue.

The prominent vascular pattern is one of the most consistent histologic findings. Almost all tumors are prominently vascular, both in the Antoni A and Antoni B areas. The blood vessels, however, show considerable variation, not only from tumor to tumor but within any given tumor.

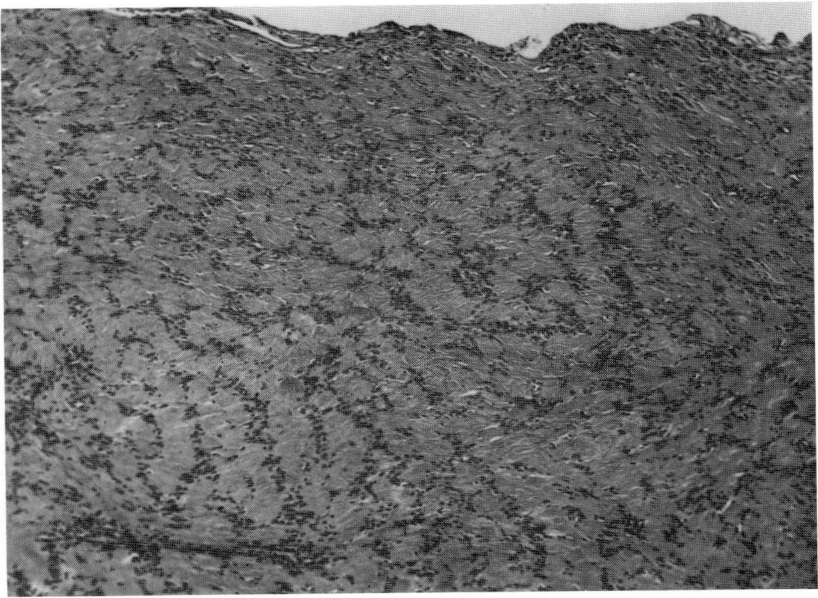

Figure 31. Prominent palisading pattern composes most of this schwannoma. (H & E × 126)

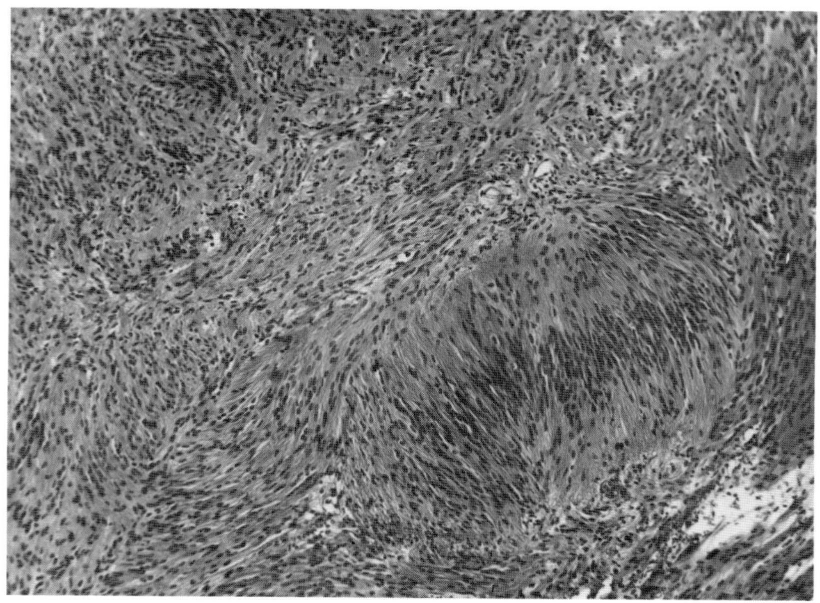

Figure 32. Schwannoma with organoid pattern of palisading (lower right). (H & E × 126)

Vessels can be of relatively small diameter, closely packed, and resemble a capillary hemangioma, glomus tumor, or other vascular tumor (Figures 36 and 37). Occasionally one encounters a localized area with quite dilated thin-walled blood vessels resembling a cavernous hemangioma (Figure 38). Usually vessels are of moderate size (Figure 39), and they may contain thrombi (Figure 40). Other areas may contain irregularly dilated vessels with hyalinized walls (Figure 41). Not infrequently there is bright eosinophilic material, probably fibrin, in the walls of some vessels (Figure 42). Other vessels, individually or in groups, may have intensely hyalinized walls (Figure 43). Hemorrhage and hemosiderin deposits are often found in the region of thrombi (Figure 44). Hemorrhage of varying ages is a fairly consistent finding in larger tumors. Acute hemorrhage can easily be recognized but often cannot be distinguished from surgical artifact. Slightly older hemorrhage with hematoidin pigment can be found, but hemosiderin pigment is the more usual finding.

Necrosis occurs microscopically and in larger areas. Figure 45 shows a microscopic area of necrosis with an associated thrombus in a vessel. Often such a thrombus is not seen.

Cellularity can also vary considerably. Average cellularity is as previously shown (Figure 22), but some areas can be sparsely cellular and some intensely cellular (Figure 46). Fibrosis ranges from focal to broad areas composed almost entirely of hyalinized tissue (Figure 47). Some fibrosis may be old healing from ischemic necrosis. Fibrosis is, however, not always an inherent part of the tumor and may be related to previous operation. Rarely, microscopic islands of hyalinized fibrous tissue, probably not blood vessels, are encountered (Figure 48).

Another feature of acoustic schwannoma, or any schwannoma, is the type and degree of nuclear pleomorphism. An ordinary acoustic tumor (Figure 22) may have mild nuclear pleomorphism. The degree of pleomorphism can be more marked, such as that seen in Figure 49, and multinucleation is possible (Figure 50). Sometimes pleomorphism is seen in areas of necrosis (Figure 51) or adjacent to thrombi (Figure 52). Some feel that pleomorphism is a degenerative change, but often there is no necrosis or obvious degenerative change associated with it. To the unwary, pleomorphism may imply malignancy. In our experience, however, pleomorphism alone should not raise a suspicion of malignancy.

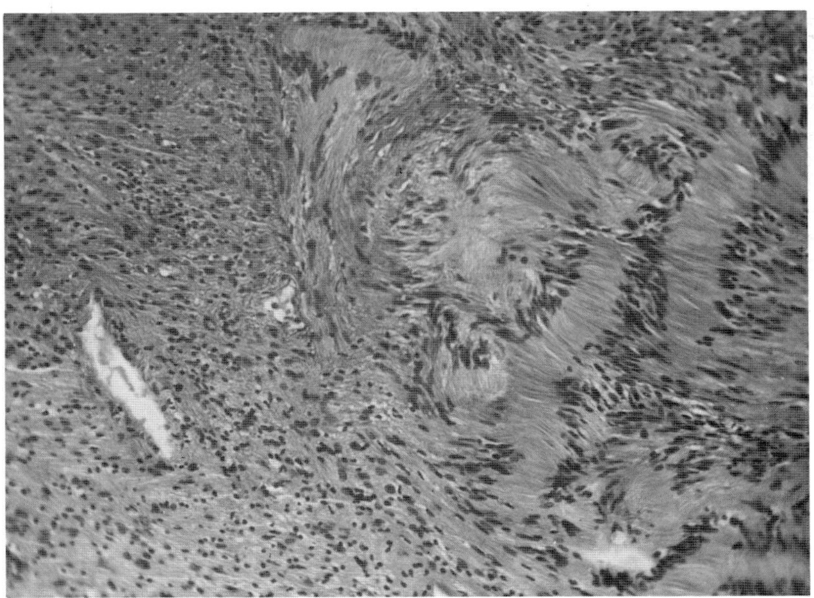

Figure 33. Palisading in acoustic schwannoma—columns of nuclei separated by anucleate eosinophilic fibrillar material. (H & E × 180)

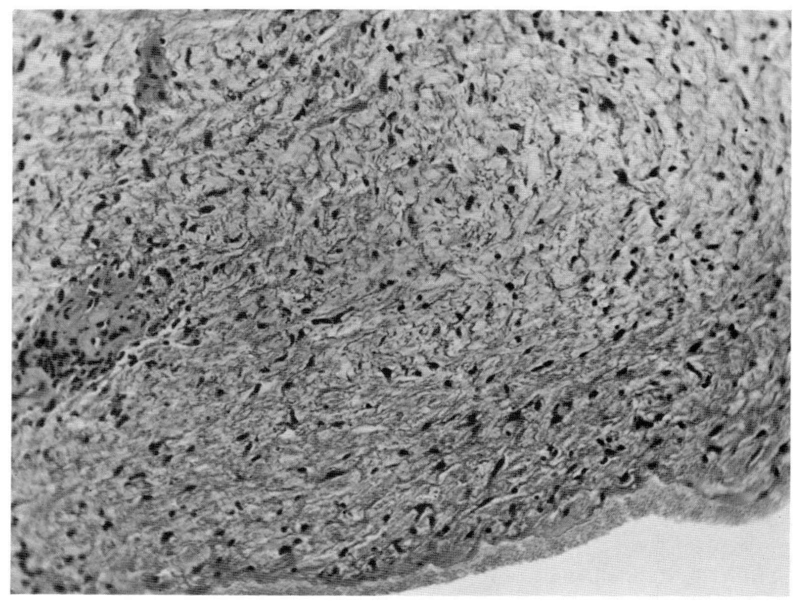

Figure 34. Myxoid area of schwannoma (Antoni B area). (H & E × 252)

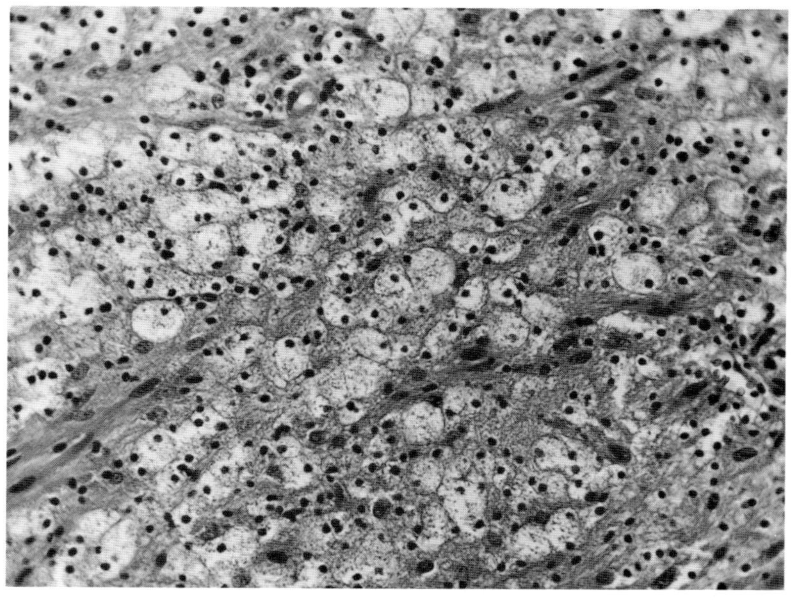

Figure 35. Histiocytes in acoustic schwannoma. (H & E × 288)

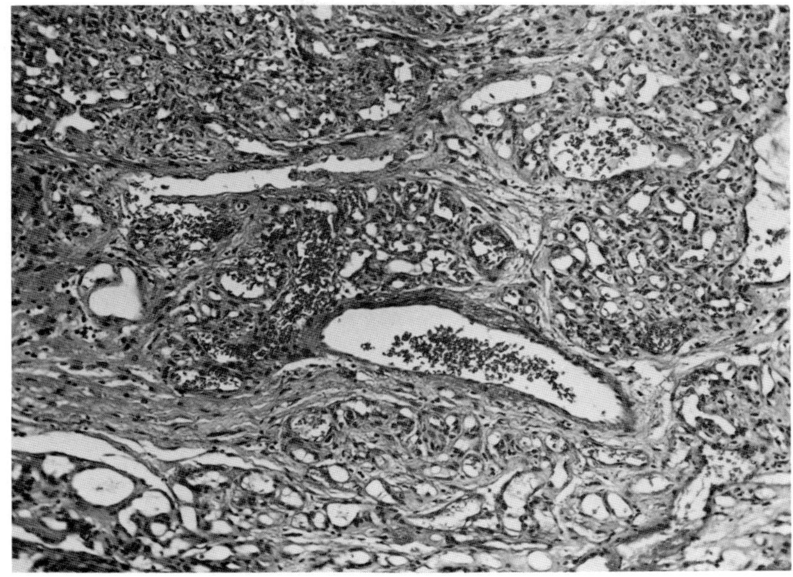

Figure 36. *Vascular patterns in acoustic schwannomas (Figures 36–44).* Small vessel proliferation is so marked it obscures the underlying schwannoma. (H & E × 144)

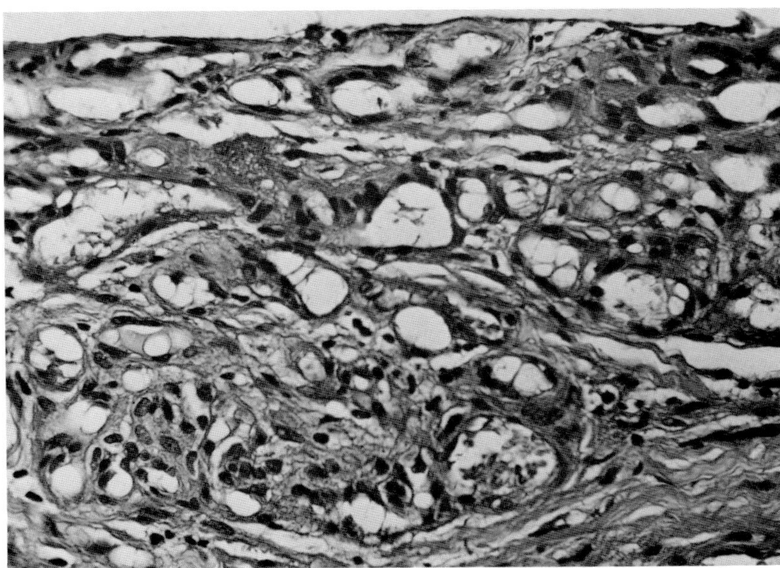

Figure 37. Higher power of Figure 36. The numerous small blood vessels mimic capillary hemangioma. (H & E × 378)

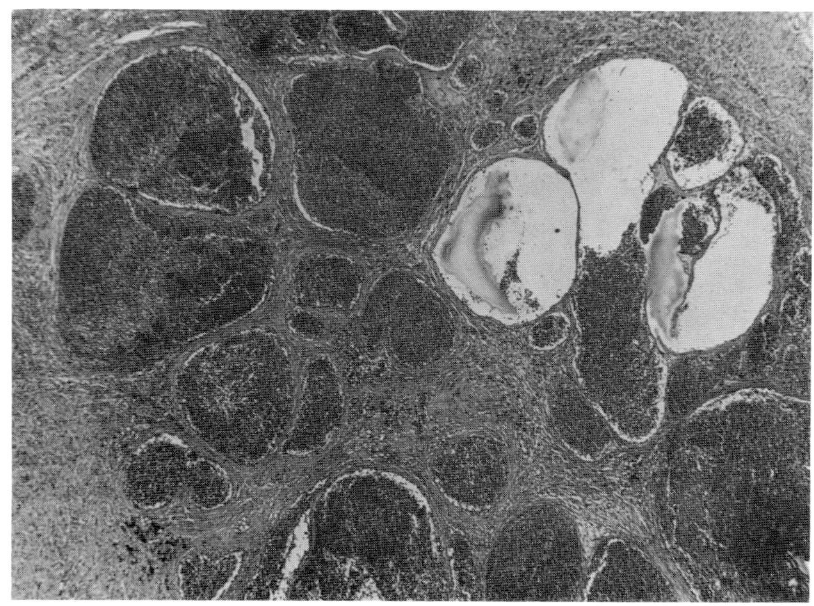

Figure 38. Numerous dilated thin-walled blood vessels resembling cavernous hemangioma. (H & E × 90)

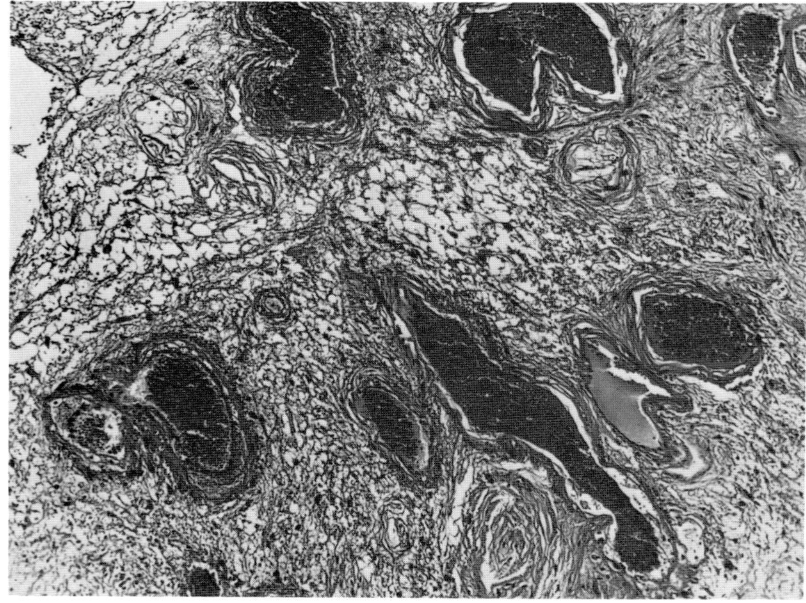

Figure 39. Usually tumor blood vessels are of medium size, as these are. (H & E × 90)

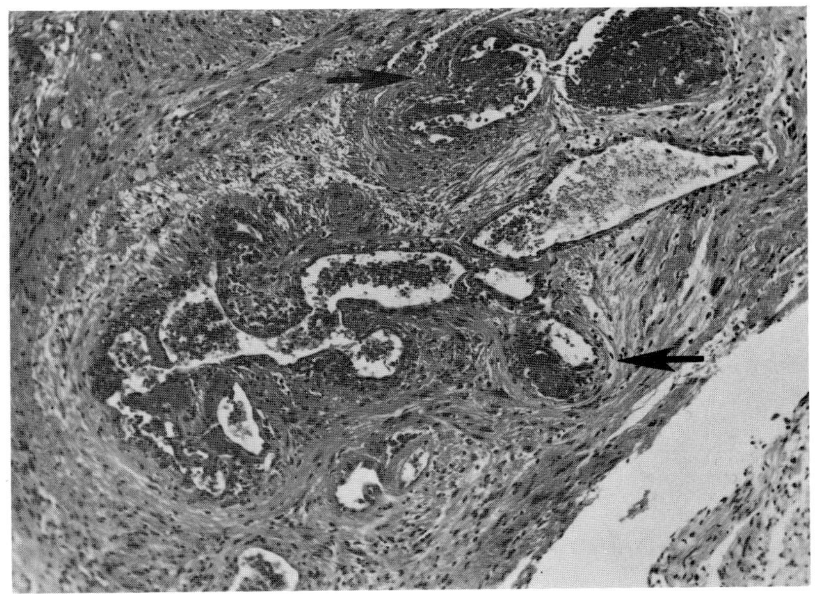

Figure 40. Thrombi (arrows) in various stages of organization. (H & E × 144)

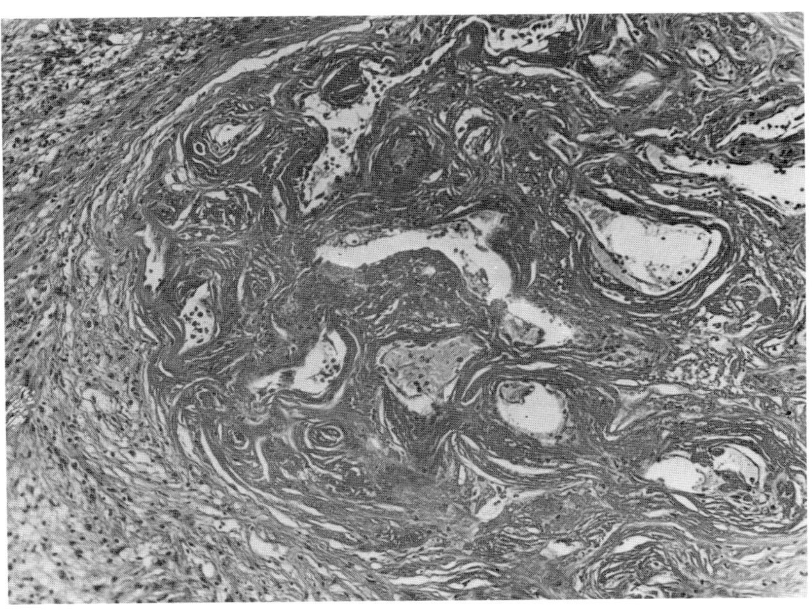

Figure 41. Hyalinized blood vessel walls (H & E × 144)

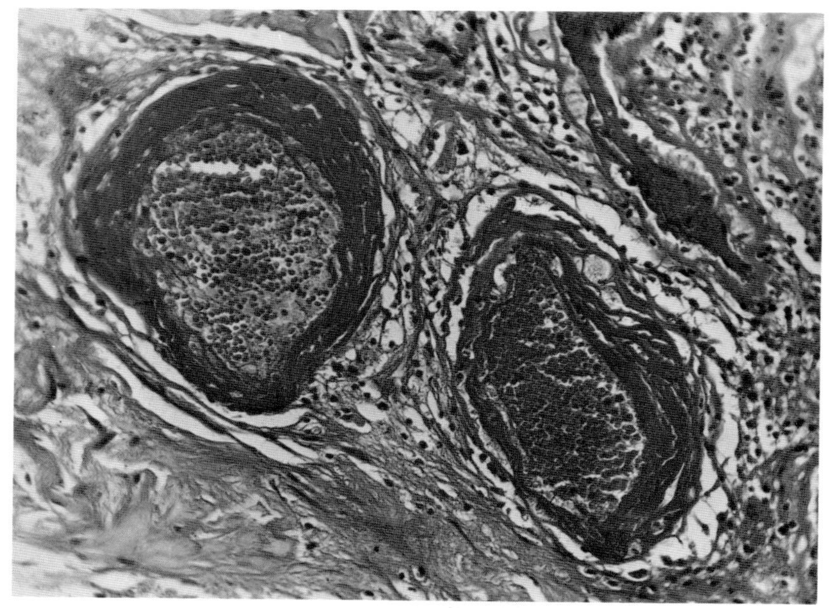

Figure 42. Bright eosinophilic appearance of vessel walls, apparently from fibrin, is typical of schwannomas. (H & E × 216)

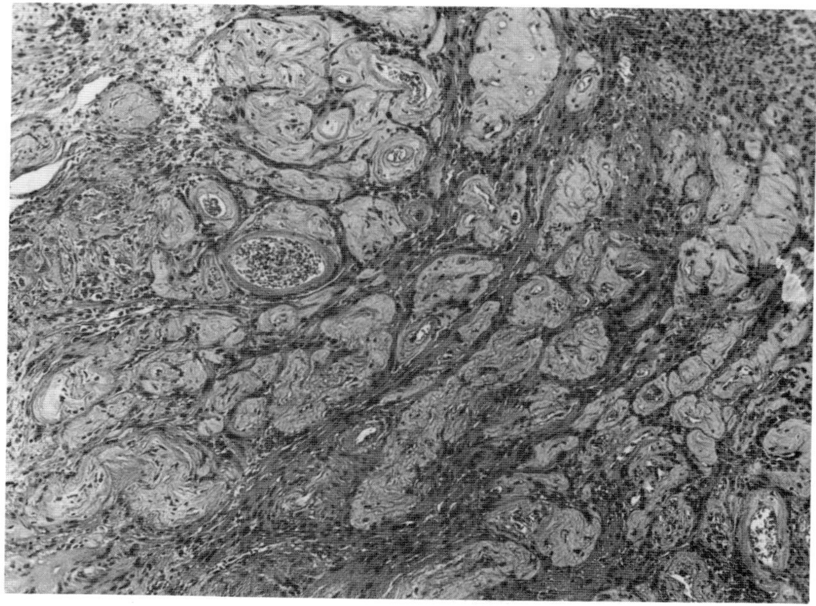

Figure 43. Hyalinized blood vessels barely recognizeable as vessels. (H & E × 144)

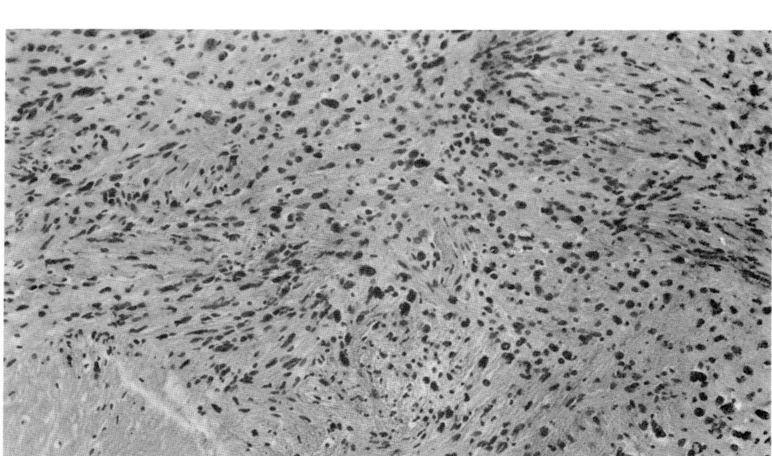

Figure 51. Moderate nuclear pleomorphism adjacent to necrosis (bottom left). (H & E × 162)

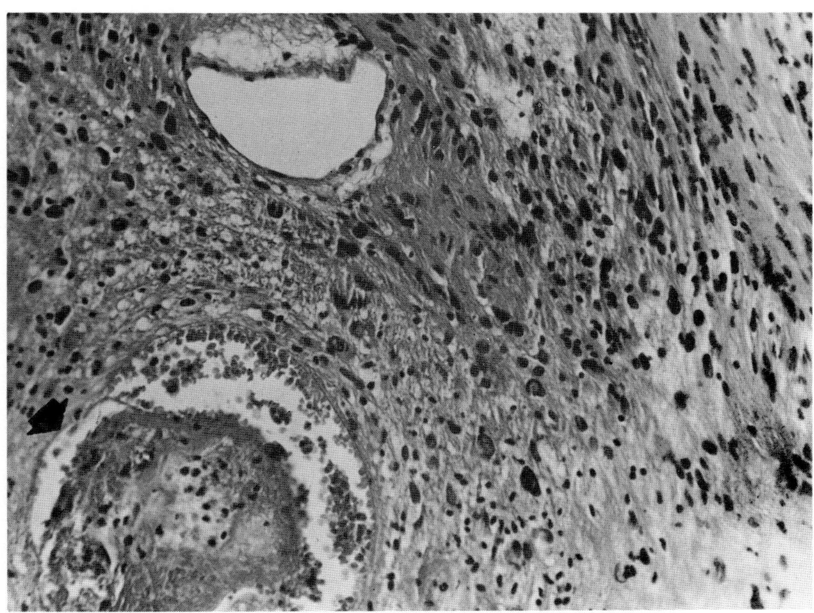

Figure 52. Moderate nuclear pleomorphism adjacent to thrombus (arrow). Same case as Figure 51. (H & E × 288)

tumor (Figure 61). Some of these are probably bone fragments from the auditory canal, but similar irregular calcifications may occur within the tumor, away from the edges. Other patterns are seen, such as those depicted in Figure 62, with broader and finely stippled calcifications. Even osseous metaplasia with central fatty bone marrow is possible (Figure 63).

We have not observed tumors with melanin deposits, but such have been described (35).

Focally, acoustic tumors may have an appearance resembling primary brain tumors, i.e., various gliomas as well as meningiomas. Figure 64 shows a halo around cells in the tumor resembling oligodendroglioma. The patterns in Figures 65 and 66 certainly resemble low-grade gliomas. An otherwise typical schwannoma may have areas of palisading around blood vessels (Figure 67), and such perivascular cuffing is reminiscent of glioblastoma, ependymoma, and oligodendroglioma. In other instances a schwannoma resembles the fibroblastic or transitional types of meningioma.

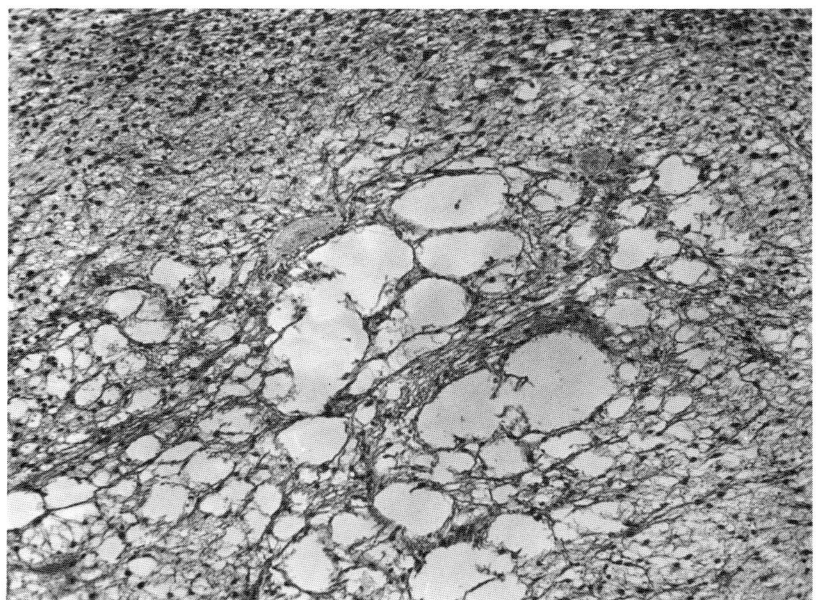

Figure 53. Microcystic change developing in Antoni B area of schwannoma. (H & E × 144)

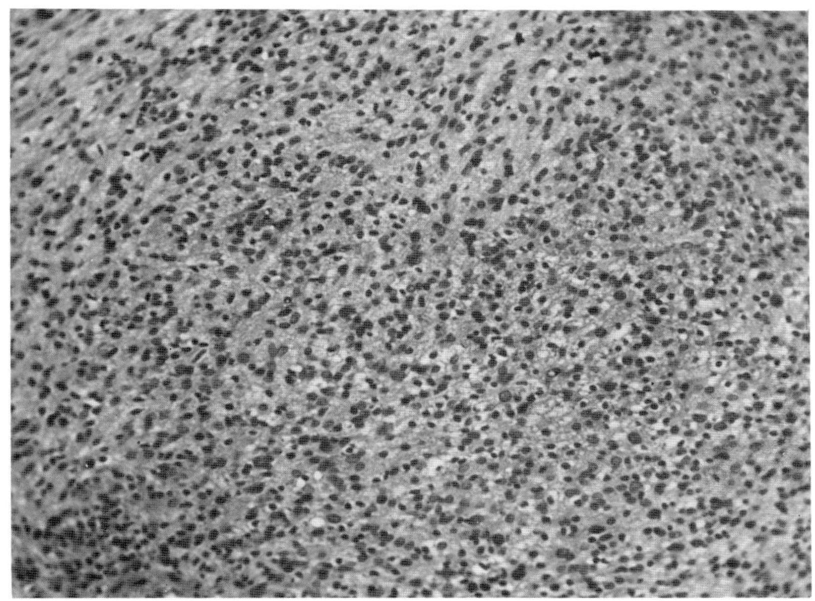

Figure 66. Same case as Figure 65, different area, also resembling low grade glioma. (H & E × 216)

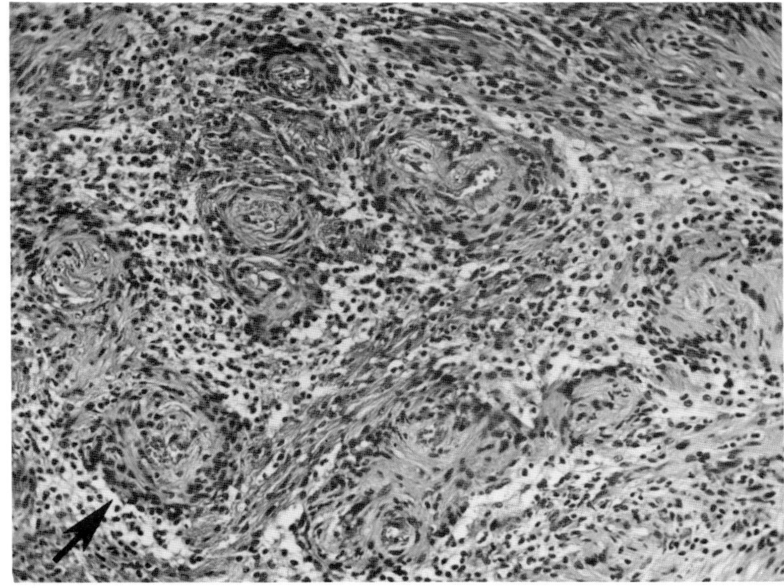

Figure 67. Perivascular cuffing (arrow) mimics glioblastoma multiforme, ependymoma and oligodendroglioma. (H & E × 225)

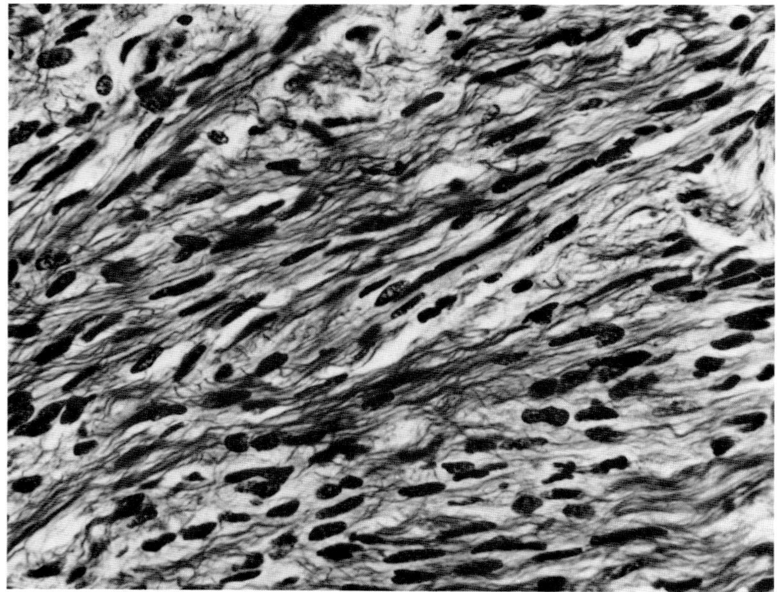

Figure 68. Silver reticulum stain of acoustic schwannoma. Numerous argyrophilic fibers parallel to the spindle cells of the tumor (×576)

Tumors in von Recklinghausen's disease may have special features and are discussed separately (see "von Recklinghausen's Disease and Multiplicity").

Schwannomas do not show a proliferation of nerve fibers as an actual part of the tumor. The acoustic (or other nerve) is often stretched over the tumor. Some twigs of the nerve may enter the tumor, as can be seen on Bodian stain. Fibers of the nerve of origin may be in the deeper aspect of the tumor, but they are not thought to be actually part of the neoplastic process and may have grown in from another location. Tumors in von Recklinghausen's disease may have a somewhat different distribution of neurites (see below).

Reticulum stain on an acoustic tumor often demonstrates numerous argyrophilic delicate fibers parallel to the long axis of the tumor cell (Figure 68). The nature of these argyrophilic fibers has been in question, and possibly basement membrane material plays a role in this staining (32). Not all areas of the tumor will show reticulum on silver stain.

ELECTRON MICROSCOPY

Electron microscopic studies of these tumors reveal some characteristic ultrastructural features, but there is still some disagreement about the principal cell of origin. Although participation by the perineurial cell cannot be entirely excluded, most feel the Schwann cell is the neoplastic element (31, 32).

The principal cell (Figures 69 and 71) in these tumors is an elongated cell with the morphologic features of a Schwann cell, forming extremely thin interdigitating cell processes. Basement membrane material covers the cell and its processes and coats the plasmalemma (cell membrane) (32). The cytoplasm contains fine filaments and glycogen particles among the other cell organelles. In schwannomas, basement

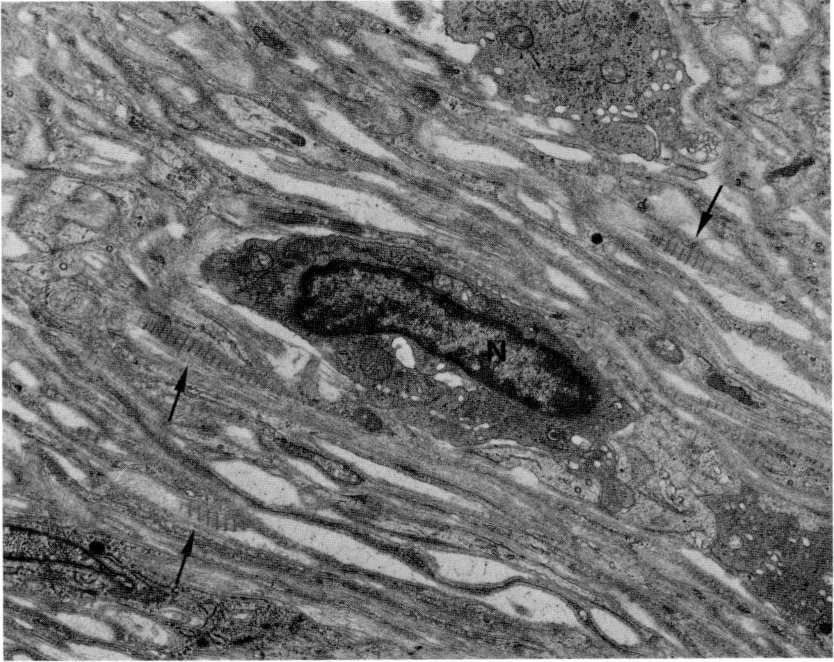

Figure 69. Antoni A area of acoustic schwannoma, electron micrograph. Numerous elongated cells and processes, with nucleus (N) of one cell in center. Many intercellular Luse bodies present, some of which are indicated (arrows). (×7,380) (Tissue in Figures 69–72 fixed in 2% buffered glutaraldehyde and stained with uranyl acetate and lead citrate).

membrane surrounds tumor cells and their processes. In gliomas, basement membrane has not been demonstrated. Meningiomas have basement membrane, but the membrane envelops the surface of groups of cells, rather than individual tumor cells, as in the schwannoma (6).

The Antoni B cell is a basement membrane coated cell, but it contains large numbers of organelles, mitochondria and dense bodies, and vacuoles. This is compatible with a high degree of metabolic activity (30) (Figure 70).

The intercellular areas of these tumors are another region of note. The extracellular space may contain some bundles of collagen fibrils. Normal collagen has cross-striation periodicity of 700 Å (range 640–710 Å) (28). There is also fine granular and filamentous material.

A characteristic finding in these tumors is the banded fusiform fibers identified in the intercellular spaces. Described by Luse (36) as pointed at each end with cross-banding between 1200–1500 Å, they are now referred

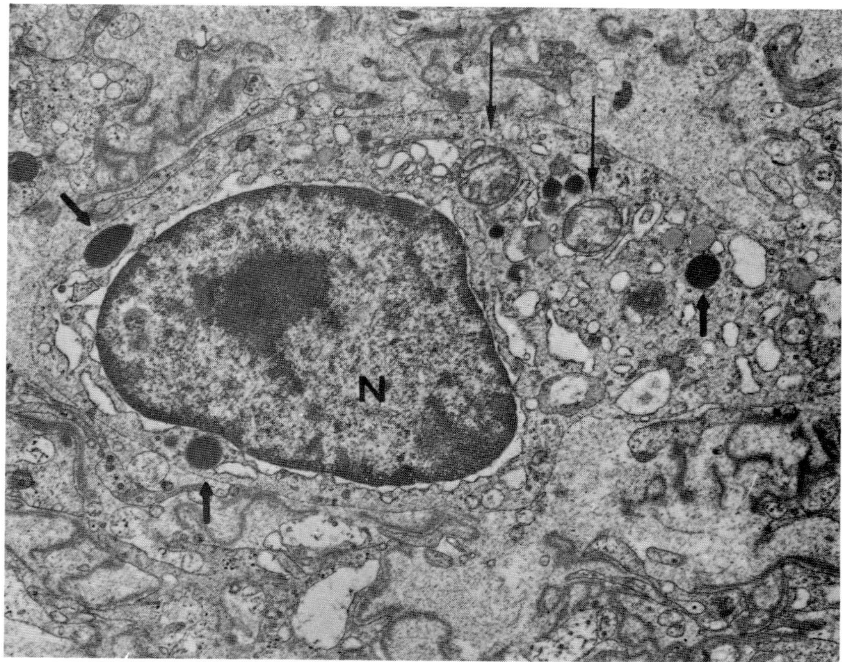

Figure 70. Electron micrograph showing cytoplasmic features of Antoni B cell. Nucleus (N), dense bodies (short arrows) and mitochondria (long arrows). (×7,560)

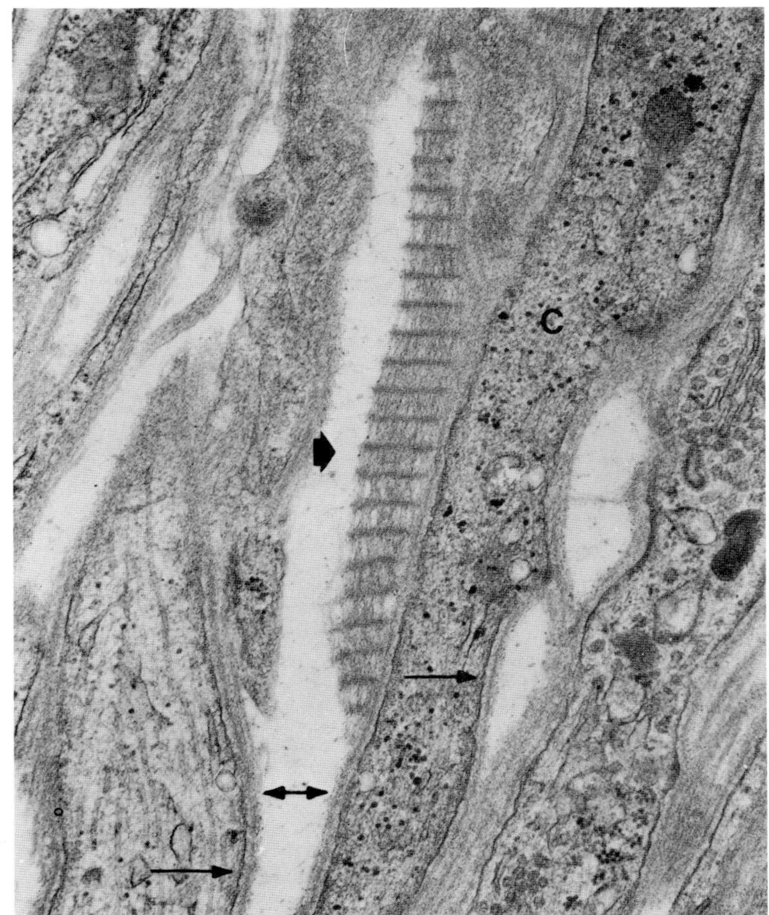

Figure 71. Electron micrograph, Antoni A area of acoustic schwannoma. Elongated cell (C), Luse body (short arrow) blending into basement membrane (double-headed arrow), and plasmalemma (long arrows). (×30,000)

to as Luse bodies (Figures 69, 71 and 72). These structures are also well described by Friedmann (27).

Cravioto's ultrastructural study (31) of 50 acoustic tumors showed these banded fusiform fibers, with 1200-Å repeating macroperiods in the extracellular space of the dense areas of every tumor studied. These fibers probably represent a form of long spacing collagen (31, 37). Cravioto and Lockwood (37) further described these as averaging 3 μm

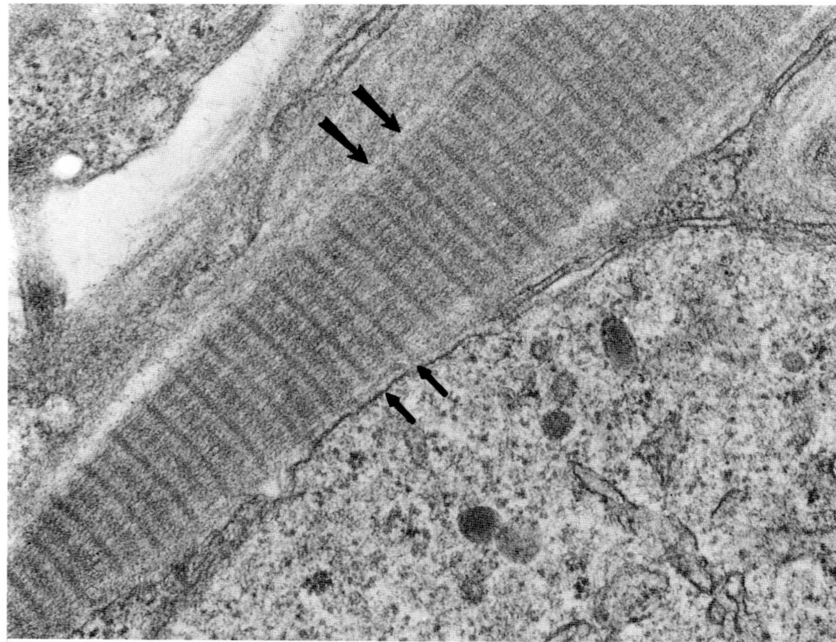

Figure 72. Portion of Luse body, electron micrograph. Narrow dense cross bands (small arrows) and wider less dense cross bands (large arrows). (×40,890)

in length and 0.5 μm in diameter, with two distinct cross-striated lines (narrower dense line, 300 Å, and a less dense line, 500 Å). The main periodicity (between dense bands) ranged from 550 Å to 1400 Å. Basement membrane material could be followed into the banded structures and was thought to be forming part of it.

It has been stated that "neurilemmoma" cells lack what is probably the only pathognomonic feature of normal Schwann cells: mesoaxons. In this respect they resemble the perineurial cell (29). We have seen a few probable mesoaxons in our electron micrographs of acoustic tumors.

An interesting feature in schwannomas is that the blood vessels have been found to be of the fenestrated type (38). Possibly this may explain the findings seen in radiologic studies (tumor blush on angiography or contrast enhancement of the tumor on computed tomography). Also, the role of fenestrae, as related to the elevated spinal fluid protein associated with these tumors, is worth considering (38).

TISSUE CULTURE

The classic study of Murray and Stout (33) showed that distinctive types of Schwann cell could be cultured from type A and type B areas of human schwannomas. The cells from type A and B areas each had different growth characteristics, but both were regarded as having the same cellular origin—Schwann cells. Those derived from type B tissue had a more pronounced liquefactive action on culture media than did those of type A. This may have some bearing on the disposition of type B tissue to undergo cystic degeneration. Previously, type B was thought to be a degenerative phase of type A, yet, when cultivated in vitro, the cells did not die but in fact were highly active metabolically (33). Murray and Stout also concluded that the "neurilemmoma" is of Schwann cell origin and no typical fibroblasts appeared in the outgrowths. The collagen and reticulum in these tumors, therefore, are presumably formed under Schwann cell influence. After Murray and Stout's original report in 1940, the similar in vitro behavior of two examples of cerebellopontine angle tumor was confirmed (39), including production of reticulum in the vicinity of Schwann cells, not fibroblasts.

Cravioto and Lockwood (40) studied 50 acoustic tumors in tissue culture with observance of four main cell types. No conclusion could be reached regarding the origin of the collagen and reticulum fibers. Their ultrastructural study of acoustic tumors (37) showed that in vivo and in vitro cell processes were frequently surrounded by basement membrane and that there was formation of fusiform banded fibers (Luse bodies).

Tissue cultures of 12 acoustic schwannomas (41) yielded two tumor cell types, frequently bridged by transitional forms. One cell type in culture corresponded to Antoni type B and the other to Antoni type A. Also emphasized in this study was the ability of the Schwann cell in vitro to become a macrophage with phagocytic properties.

Therefore, tissue culture, as well as electron microscopic findings of Antoni B type cells, tends to disprove the previous impression that Antoni B tissue is merely a degenerative form of type A.

MALIGNANT TUMORS

Malignant schwannomas of the eighth nerve must be extremely rare. In our review of the microscopic sections of approximately 1,000 acoustic tumors, we have not diagnosed any as malignant, nor in subsequent follow-up have any proven to be malignant.

Since the terminology of malignant tumors arising in nerve is somewhat confusing, a definition of malignant schwannoma and nerve sheath fibrosarcoma (neurofibrosarcoma) seems justified.

A malignant schwannoma (28) is a malignant neoplasm of nerve sheath origin, thought to be of Schwann cell origin, that locally infiltrates and also metastasizes. It may occur sporadically but it usually is found in patients with von Recklinghausen's disease. An erroneous diagnosis of malignant schwannoma can be made either by calling a benign schwannoma malignant or by mistaking fibrosarcoma and leiomyosarcoma for nerve sheath neoplasms. The term "malignant schwannoma" is acceptable if its use is restricted to those variants of malignant nerve sheath tumor that show distinctive features of Schwann cell differentiation. If the term is restricted in that sense, it seldom will be used. Microscopically malignant schwannomas are composed of plump spindle cells, mitoses are present and may be numerous, nuclei are hyperchromatic, there is increased cellularity, and areas of necrosis may occur.

A nerve sheath fibrosarcoma (28) is the most common type of malignant neoplasm found in association with neurofibromatosis. The tumor cells are thought to be fibroblasts; however, it is not known whether the lesion may be in part or totally of Schwann cell origin. Microscopically, the pattern is that of a cellular, poorly differentiated fibrosarcoma.

Although schwannomas arising from peripheral nerves have been reported to undergo malignant transformation in exceptional instances, it is difficult to find documented examples of malignant change in an intracranial or intraspinal schwannoma.

Nager (42) was unable to find any report of malignant degeneration of eighth nerve tumors, and, according to Zulch (3) malignant transformation occurs only in the peripheral "neurinomas" of von Recklinghausen's disease.

Ash (43) states that malignant deterioration of the acoustic nerve tumor occurs occasionally and also that malignant melanoma has been reported as arising from the melanoblasts that are occasionally included in the tumor.

Malignant transformation of a vestibular schwannoma in a 9-year-old girl has been described by Schuknecht (11). In that case, a schwannoma of the vestibular nerve was in continuity with a malignant tumor that had invaded the petrous bone and destroyed part of the internal auditory canal. The malignant schwannoma was described as being highly cellular, with hyperchromatic nuclei and numerous mitotic figures.

DIFFERENTIAL DIAGNOSIS

Acoustic tumors are the most frequent tumors of the cerebellopontine angle. Gonzalez Revilla (5) reviewed 205 tumors in the cerebellopontine recess and found that 78% were "neurinomas" (eighth nerve tumors except for a few), 6.3% meningiomas, 6.3% cholesteatomas, 5.9% gliomas, and the remaining 3.5% abscesses and miscellaneous tumors. There are, however, numerous tumors and pathological conditions that may occur in or near that region and pose a problem in differential diagnosis. Most of these are mentioned as space-occupying lesions, but they may be distinguished by clinical means, grossly or microscopically, and therefore do not present real diagnostic problems. Those that are of special interest are discussed subsequently (vide infra).

Space-occupying angle lesions would include cholesteatomas (primary cholesteatomas more often simulate acoustic tumors than do the secondary), dermoids, teratomas, chordoma, and choroid plexus tumor. Metastatic malignant neoplasm is always a possibility. On review of the previously published reports of secondary malignant tumors of the temporal bone, Schuknecht found the most common primary sites of origin, in order of frequency, to be breast, kidney, lung, stomach, larynx, prostate, and thyroid gland (44). Leukemias and lymphomas can involve this area, as can tumors from adjacent areas, e.g., lymphoepitheliomas. Neoplasm to neoplasm metastasis is possible, e.g., bronchogenic carcinoma metastasizing to an acoustic "neurinoma" (45).

Vascular lesions may affect the eighth nerve, including aneurysms, compression of nerve by a crossing artery, and AV malformation. We have encountered several cases of a peculiar tumor composed of numerous irregular vascular channels with thick walls (Figure 73). These lesions have been up to 1 cm in diameter and have been located in or near the internal auditory canal. The exact classification is as yet undetermined, but the possibilities considered are cavernous hemangioma and vascular hamartoma or malformation. They may be of dural sinus origin. Clinically they present as acoustic tumors (or as seventh nerve tumors with facial weakness). Grossly, they are red-pink and spongy, which is unlike a schwannoma. Other lesions may simulate cerebellopontine angle tumor: e.g., arachnoiditis, abscesses, arachnoid cyst, and granulomas, including tuberculosis, parasites, and hematomas. Histologically leiomyomas may resemble schwannomas, but a leiomyoma in this location would be extremely unusual. Rarely, a melanotic schwannoma can occur (35). Schwann cells are derived from neural crest and probably bring melanoblasts with them. Therefore, if one encounters a tumor with melanotic cells, a primary as well as metastatic tumor should be considered.

By far the most practical problem in differential diagnosis (in terms of frequency of occurrence and gross and microscopic appearance) is differentiating meningioma from acoustic schwannoma. Although small biopsies of acoustic tumors received from surgery are characteristic 90 to 95% of the time (Figure 7), meningiomas may have the same pale yellow semi-translucent appearance. Meningiomas may even be bright yellow (Figure 74), as one would more typically expect from a histiocytic area of acoustic tumor. Later, the larger gross specimen of acoustic tumor is usually typical, but it can be more tan-white and rubbery, like meningioma, and meningioma can resemble typical acoustic tumor. Microscopically, meningiomas may have numerous patterns. The menin-

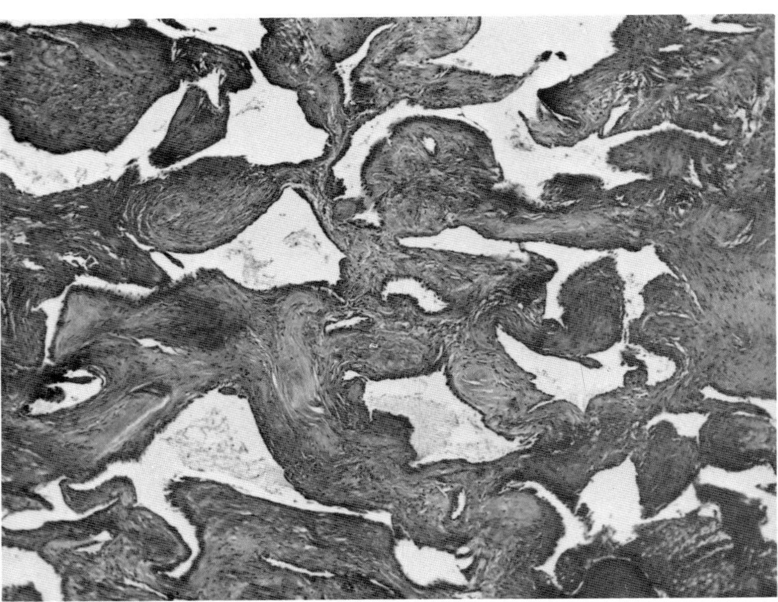

Figure 73. Cavernous hemangioma, or vascular hamartoma or malformation, composed of numerous irregular dilated channels with thick walls (see text). This is not a schwannoma. (H & E × 61.2)

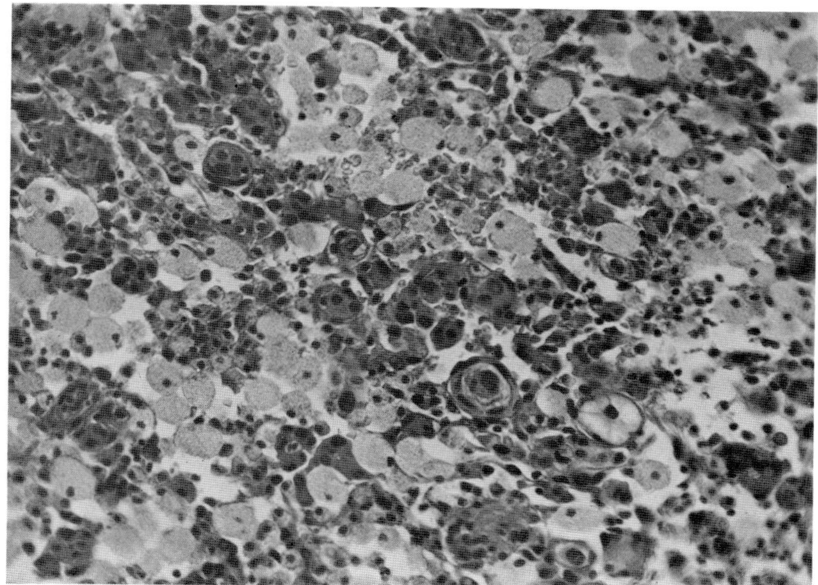

Figure 74. Meningioma containing histiocytes, specimen grossly yellow. (H & E × 288)

gothelial or psammomatous meningiomas are usually easy to recognize microscopically, but the fibrous and transitional types may be difficult to distinguish from schwannoma. This may be especially true on frozen section or particularly when only small fragments of tissue are received. Schwannomas can have whorls mimicking meningioma (Figures 26 and 27). When the entire tumor becomes available, the problem is usually resolved.

Various gliomas may occur in this region and may even extend from the brainstem along the eighth nerve and present as an eighth nerve tumor. Since a portion of an acoustic tumor may resemble a glioma (Figures 64–67), this again may be a problem, especially on frozen section or in a small biopsy. Areas of schwannomas may have vascular patterns resembling capillary hemangioma, glomus tumor, or cavernous hemangioma (Figures 36–38).

VON RECKLINGHAUSEN'S DISEASE AND MULTIPLICITY

Von Recklinghausen's disease presents three forms that appear relatively distinct: a central form, with multiple intracranial and intraspinal tumors; a peripheral form, which is associated with cafe au lait patches; and a visceral form. There may, of course, be some overlap (32).

In von Recklinghausen's disease, vestibular schwannomas occur in about 5% of reported cases and are nearly always bilateral (11). It is generally considered that most bilateral acoustic schwannomas are part of von Recklinghausen's disease. Bilateral acoustic tumors are so classic a feature of this disease that, in rare cases where they are the sole finding, the manifestation may be interpreted as a forme fruste of the disease.

The earliest recorded examples of bilateral recess tumors in association with central neurofibromatosis appear to have been those of Wishart (46) in 1822 and those of Knoblauch (47).

Gardner and Turner (48) studied a family in which von Recklinghausen's disease in the form of bilateral acoustic tumors had been transmitted through generations. It was assumed that all family members

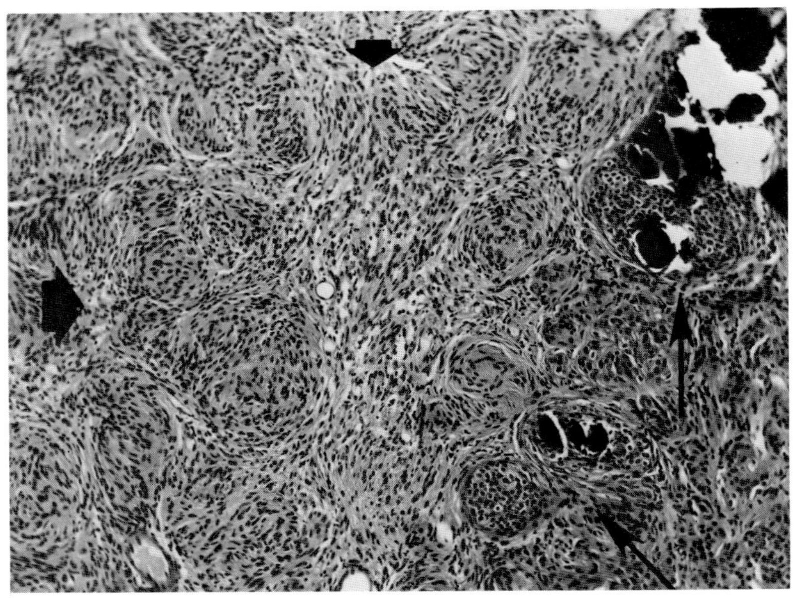

Figure 75. *Acoustic tumors and meningiomas in von Recklinghausen's disease* (*Figures 75–82*). One of multiple pieces of tissue received during acoustic tumor surgery. Nests of meningothelial cells with psammoma bodies (long arrows), mixed with whorled areas (large broad arrow), probably meningioma, and other areas (small broad arrow) in the center which are difficult to distinguish from schwannoma. (H & E $\times$ 135)

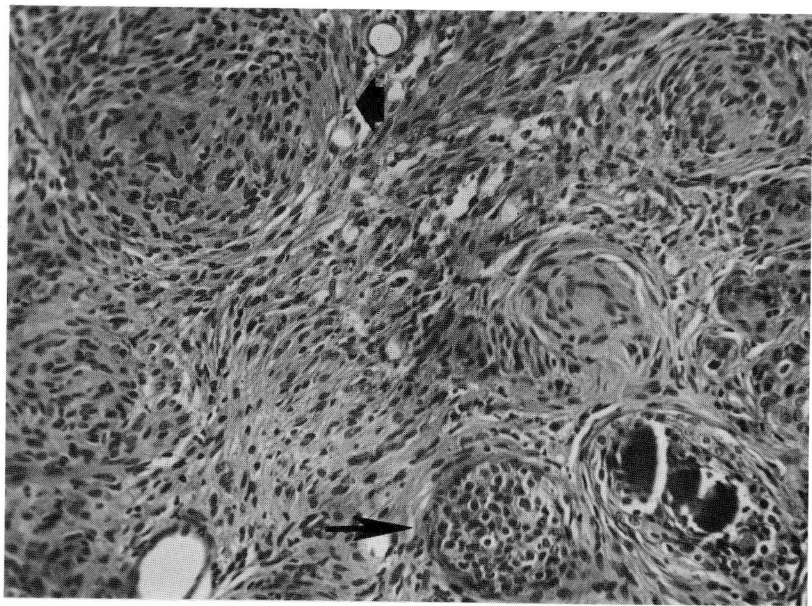

Figure 76. Higher power of Figure 75. Meningothelial nests (long arrow) with psammoma bodies, whorled cells (short broad arrow), probably meningioma, and areas in the center similar to schwannoma. (H & E × 252)

who were deaf, or deaf and blind, had bilateral acoustic tumors. In the six members on whom operation or necropsy was performed, this assumption was proved correct.

Figures 8 and 9 show the specimen from a 53-year-old man with bilateral acoustic tumors (right previously operated). After complete autopsy, the only other indication of von Recklinghausen's disease was a small schwannoma in a nerve near the temporal bone, and multiple small schwannomas in the cauda equina and in a few of the cervical spinal roots, so that the main manifestation of the disease was bilateral acoustic schwannomas.

We have not been able to appreciate any gross difference in appearance between the unilateral and bilateral tumor as they are received from surgery.

One of the interesting phenomena, however, in von Recklinghausen's disease is that there may be one or multiple schwannomas involving an individual nerve or any of numerous nerves, as well as one or multiple meningiomas. Schwannomas and meningiomas may be present in the same surgical specimen as collision tumors or as separate individual lesions. One may or may not be able to distinguish the two grossly.

Microscopically, in most cases of von Recklinghausen's disease the acoustic schwannoma is identical on routine H & E stain to any of the usual unilateral tumors. Occasionally, however, tumors in von Recklinghausen's disease may show areas that appear to be intermediate in pattern between meningioma and schwannoma (Figures 75–78). Actually, this is not surprising, since the cells in both schwannomas and meningiomas originate from the neural crest. Occasionally, in some cases of otherwise typical unilateral schwannoma, there are areas that have cross-features between meningioma and schwannoma. Whether in these cases this is part of von Recklinghausen's disease or just variance in microscopic pattern is only a matter of speculation. It is, however, always possible that there is a small, as yet undetected, contralateral schwannoma.

The other common feature in von Recklinghausen's disease is the multiplicity of meningiomas. Often these are tiny or microscopic and

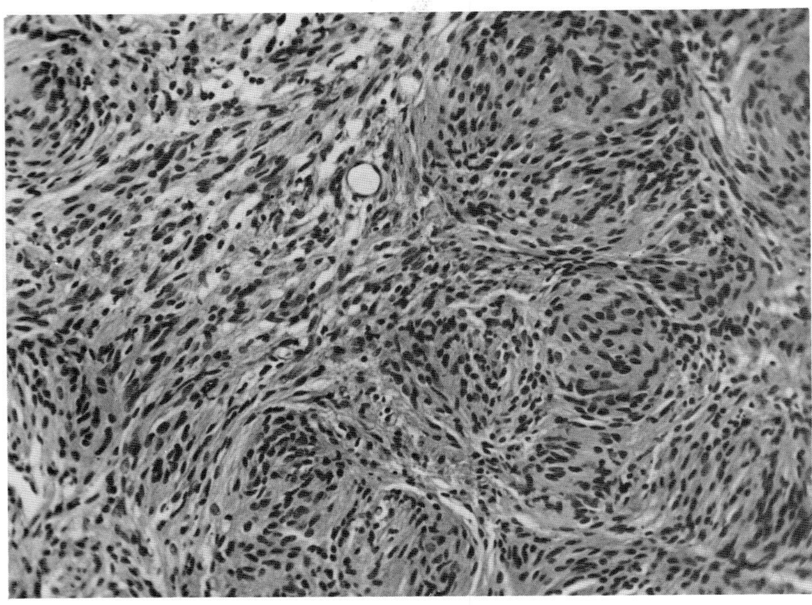

Figure 77. Same case as Figure 75. Whorled areas (right) more resemble meningioma, and elongated cells (left) are intermediate in pattern between meningioma and schwannoma (H & E × 252)

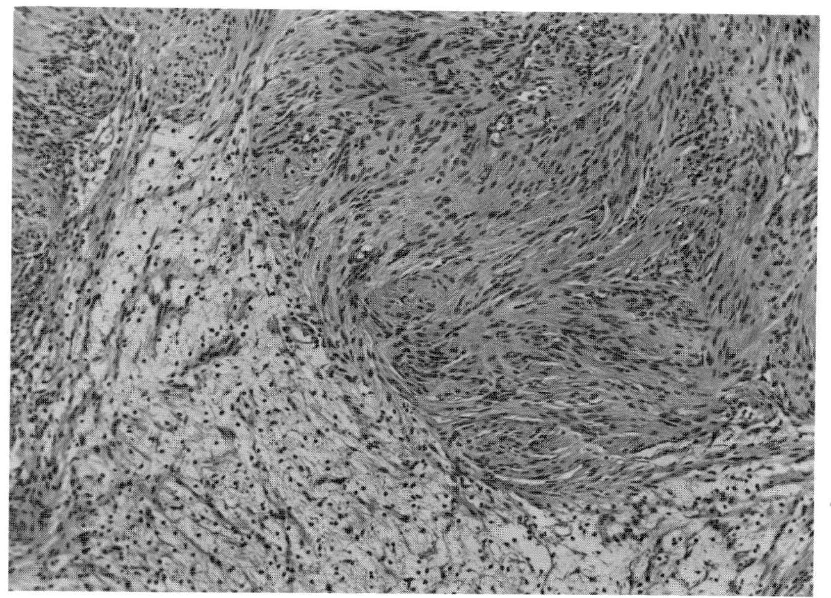

Figure 78. Same case as Figure 75, showing typical schwannoma at the edge of the tissue (Antoni A, top right, Antoni B, bottom left). (H & E × 144)

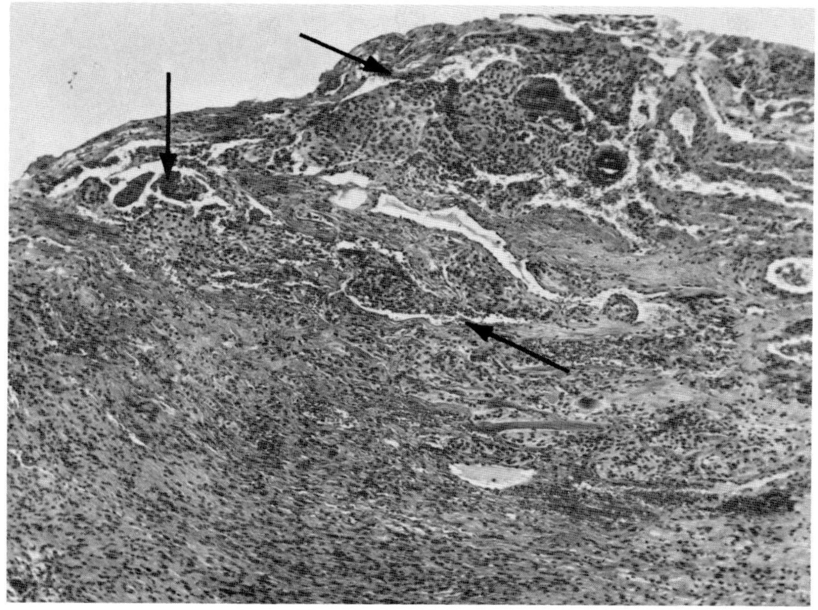

Figure 79. Multiple micromeningiomas (or meningeal proliferations) (arrows) at the edge of a schwannoma (bottom). (H & E × 99)

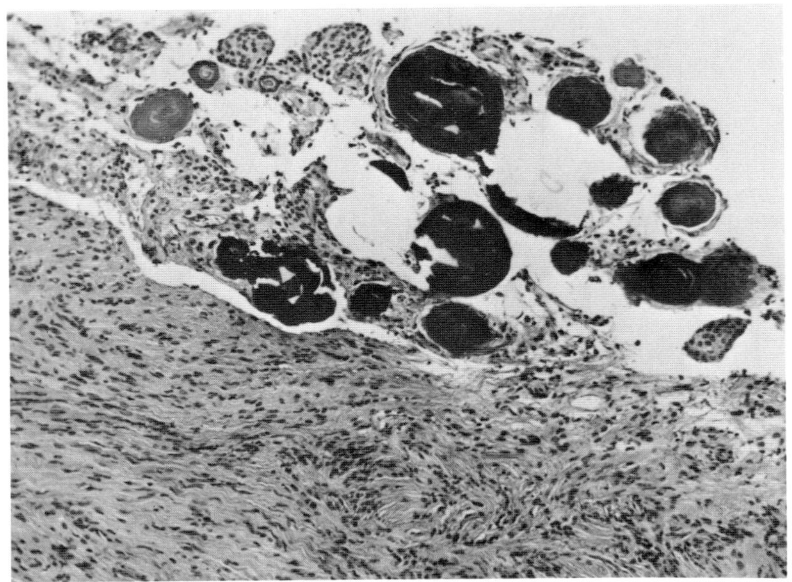

Figure 80. Same case as Figure 79, different area. "Micromeningioma" with psammoma bodies (top) at edge of a schwannoma (bottom). (H & E × 144)

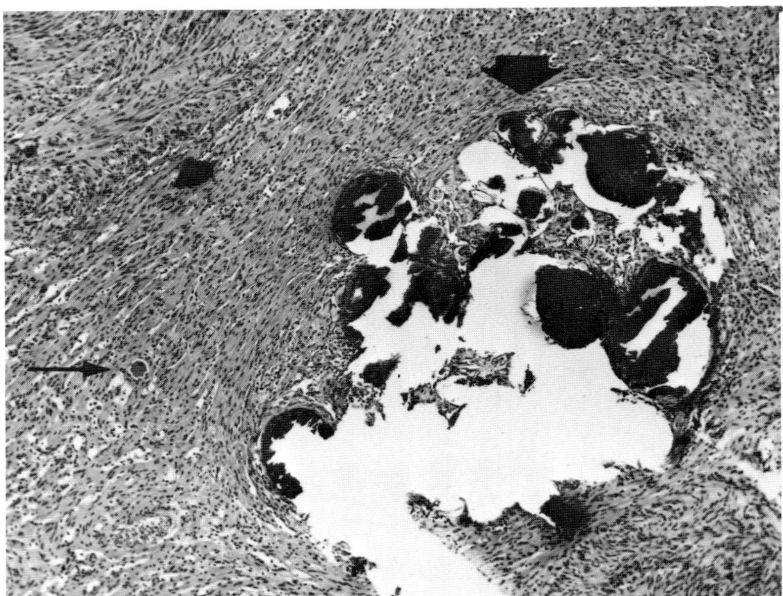

Figure 81. Same case as Figures 75–78, different sample of tissue. Meningioma (broad arrow) with psammoma bodies is surrounded by schwannoma. (Artefactual fracturing due to calcification) Ganglion cell (long arrow) entrapped by schwannoma. (H & E × 72)

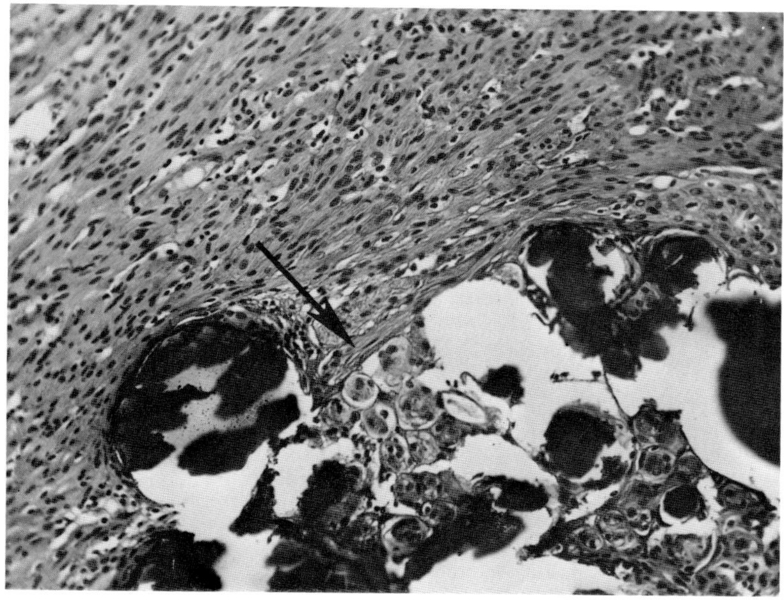

Figure 82. Higher power of Figure 81. Meningothelial meningioma (arrow) with psammoma bodies. Schwannoma at top. (H & E × 180)

may be considered focal meningeal proliferations or "micromeningiomas." They often occur at the edge of an otherwise typical example of schwannoma (Figures 79 and 80). Meningiomas may be microscopically intermixed with schwannoma (Figures 81 and 82). The meningiomas can, of course, be large.

In von Recklinghausen's disease, on routine H & E stain the acoustic tumor appears similar to that in the unilateral case. As described by Linthicum (49, 50), Bodian stain for neurites shows that, in the unilateral case, usually the axons of the nerve are spread out over the surface of the tumor, and the nerve is compressed or stretched with a pressure effect so that there is apparent loss of function. In the bilateral or von Recklinghausen's case, as indicated by Bodian stain, the nerve fibers are more intact and not compressed to one side, but rather are separated by the growing tumor. Although these fibers are distorted and separated by the tumor, they can apparently function. This may explain why the patient in a bilateral case may have relatively good hearing in spite of the presence of a large tumor, while in the ordinary unilateral tumor there will be earlier hearing loss, and when the tumor is smaller.

ACKNOWLEDGMENT

The authors wish to thank Drs. Raymond B. Wuerker and John O. Erickson of the Veterans' Administration Hospital, Long Beach, California, for providing the electron micrographs.

REFERENCES

1. Cushing, H. 1932. Intracranial Tumors. Charles C Thomas, Springfield, Ill.
2. Walshe, F. 1931. Intracranial tumours: A critical review. Quart. J. Med. 24:587.
3. Zulch, K. 1957. Brain Tumors: Their Biology and Pathology. Springer Publishing Co., New York.
4. Hoessly, G. F., and Olivecrona, H. 1955. Report of 280 Cases of Verified Parasagittal Meningioma. J. Neurosurg. 12:614.
5. Revilla, A. G. 1948. Differential diagnosis of tumors at the cerebellopontile recess. Bull. Johns Hopkins Hosp. 83:187.
6. Pool, L. J., Pava, A. A., and Greenfield, E. C. 1970. Acoustic Nerve Tumors—Early Diagnosis and Treatment, 2nd Edition. Charles C Thomas, Springfield, Ill.
7. Sandifort, E. 1777. Observationes anatomico-pathologicae. Lugduni Batavorum, Chapter IX, pp. 116–120. (Cited in Refs. 9 and 12.)
8. Leveque-Lasource, A. 1810. Observation sur un amaurosis et un cophosis. . . . J. gen de med., chir. et pharm., XXXVII, pp. 368–378. (Cited in Ref. 9.)
9. Cushing, H. 1963. Tumors of the Nervus Acusticus and the Syndrome of the Cerebellopontile Angle. Hafner Publishing Co., New York and London. (Reprint: originally published 1917.)
10. Bell, C. 1830. The Nervous System of the Human Body. London, Appendix of Cases, CXII–CXIV. (Cited in Ref. 9.)
11. Schuknecht, H. F. 1974. Pathology of the Ear. Harvard University Press, Cambridge, Mass.
12. Information Center for Hearing, Speech and Disorders of Human Communication. 1971. Acoustic Neurinoma: Present Status and Research Trends. The Johns Hopkins Medical Institutions, Baltimore, Maryland. (Dec.) (Distributed by National Technical Information Service, U.S. Department of Commerce, 5285 Port Royal Road, Springfield, Virginia.)
13. Skinner, H. A. 1929. The origin of acoustic nerve tumors. Brit. J. Surg. 16:440–463.
14. Henschen, F. 1915. Zur Histologie und Pathogenese der Kleinhirnbruckenwinkeltumoren. Arch. Psychiat. lvi. (Cited in Ref. 13.)
15. Hardy, M., and Crowe, S. J. 1936. Early asymptomatic acoustic tumor. Report of six cases. Arch. Surg. 32(2):292–301.
16. Leonard, J., and Talbot, M. 1970. Asymptomatic acoustic neurilemmoma. Arch. Otolaryngol. 91:117.
17. Stewart, T. J., Liland, J., and Schuknecht, H. F. 1975. Occult schwannomas of the vestibular nerve. Arch. Otolaryngol. 101(2):91–95. (Feb.)

18. Gussen, R. 1971. Intramodiolar acoustic neurinoma. Laryngoscope 81:1979–1984.
19. Wanamaker, H. H. 1972. Acoustic neuroma: Primary arising in the vestibule. Laryngoscope 82(6):1040–1044. (June)
20. Naunton, R., and Petasnick, J. 1970. Acoustic neurinomas with normal internal auditory meatus. Arch. Otolaryngol. 91:437–443.
21. Stout, A. P. 1949. Tumors of the Peripheral Nervous System. Armed Forces Institute of Pathology Fascicle No. 6, First Series.
22. Verocay, J. 1908. Multiple geschwulste als Systemerkrankung am nervosen Apparate. Festch. Chiari (Wien und Leipzig.) Braunmuller, 278. (Cited in Ref. 6.)
23. Mallory, F. B. 1919. The type cell of the so-called dural endothelioma. J. Med. Res. 41:349.
24. Antoni, N. R. E. 1920. Uber Ruckenmarkstumoren und Neurofibrome, pp. 234–311. Bergmann, Munich. (Cited in Ref. 6).
25. Masson, P. 1923. Les Tumeurs, p. 568. Maloine, Paris. (Cited in Ref. 6.)
26. Stout, A. P. 1935. The peripheral manifestations of the specific nerve sheath tumor (neurilemmoma). Am. J. Cancer 24:751.
27. Friedmann, I. 1974. Pathology of the Ear, pp. 213–223. Blackwell Scientific Publications, Oxford.
28. Harkin, J. C., and Reed, R. J. 1969. Tumors of the Peripheral Nervous System. Armed Forces Institute of Pathology Fascicle No. 3, Second Series.
29. Ackerman, L. 1974. Surgical Pathology, 5th Edition. C. V. Mosby Co., St. Louis.
30. Russell, D. S., and Rubinstein, L. J. 1977. Pathology of Tumors of the Nervous System, 4th Edition. The Williams & Wilkins Co., Baltimore.
31. Cravioto, H. 1969. The ultrastructure of acoustic nerve tumors. Acta Neuropathol. (Berl.) 12:116–140.
32. Rubinstein, L. J. 1972. Tumors of the Central Nervous System. Armed Forces Institute of Pathology Fascicle, No. 6, Second Series.
33. Murray, M., and Stout, A. P. 1940. Schwann cell vs. fibroblast as the origin of the specific nerve sheath tumor. Am. J. Pathol. 16:41.
34. Pineda, A., and Feder, B. H. 1967. Acoustic neuroma: A misnomer. Am. Surg. 33(1):40–43. (Jan.)
35. Dastur, D. K., Sinh, G., and Pandya, S. K. 1967. Melanotic tumor of the acoustic nerve. Case report. J. Neurosurg. 27:166.
36. Luse, S. A. 1960. Electron microscopic studies of brain tumors. Neurol. 10:881–905.
37. Cravioto, H., and Lockwood, R. 1968. Long spacing fibrous collagen in human acoustic nerve tumors. J. Ultrastruc. Res. 24:70–85.
38. Hirano, A., Dembitzer, H. M., and Zimmerman, H. M. 1972. Fenestrated blood vessels in neurilemmoma. Lab. Invest. 27(3):305.
39. Murray, M. R. 1942. Comparative data on tissue culture of acoustic neurilemmomas and meningiomas. J. Neuropathol. Exp. Neurol. 1:123.
40. Cravioto, H., and Lockwood, R. 1969. The behavior of acoustic neuroma in tissue culture. Acta Neuropathol. (Berl.) 12:141.
41. Lumsden, C. E. 1971. The study by tissue culture of tumors of the nervous system. In: D. S. Russell and L. J. Rubinstein (eds.), Pathology of

Tumors of the Nervous System, 3rd Edition. The Williams & Wilkins Co., Baltimore.
42. Nager, G. T. 1969. Acoustic neurinomas, pathology and differential diagnosis. Arch. Otolaryngol. 89:68–95. (Feb.)
43. Ash, J. E. 1960. Pathology of the ear. In: G. M. Coates and H. P. Schenck (eds.), Otolaryngology, Volume 1, Chapter 4. W. F. Prior Co., Inc., Hagerstown, Maryland.
44. Schuknecht, H. F., Allam, A. F., and Murakami, Y. 1968. Pathology of secondary malignant tumors of the temporal bone. Ann. Otol. Rhinol. Laryngol. 77:5.
45. Le Blanc, R. A. 1974. Metastasis of bronchogenic carcinoma to acoustic neurinoma. Case report. J. neurosurg. 41:614–617. (Nov.)
46. Wishart, J. 1822. Cases of tumors in the skull, dura mater and brain. Edinb. M. & S. J., XVII, 393–397. (Cited in Ref. 9.)
47. Knoblauch. 1843. De neuromate et gangliis accessoriis. Inaug. Dissert. Frankfort. (Cited by Adrian, C., 1903, listed in Ref. 9.)
48. Gardner, W. J., and Turner, O. 1940. Bilateral acoustic neurofibromas. Arch. Neurol. Psychiat. 44(1):76–99. (July)
49. Linthicum, F. H. 1972. Unusual audiometric and histologic findings in bilateral acoustic neurinomas. Ann. Otol. Rhinol. Laryngol. 81(3):433. (June)
50. Linthicum, F. H. 1978. Personal communication.

Acoustic Tumors
Volume I, *Diagnosis*
Edited by W. F. House and C. M. Luetje

Section III

EVALUATION OF THE ACOUSTIC TUMOR PATIENT

Chapter 7

Acoustic Tumors: Selected Histories and Patient Reviews

Malcolm D. Graham, M.D.*
Professor of Otorhinolaryngology, University of Michigan, Ann Arbor

---

Acoustic tumors are benign, encapsulated tumors arising from the eighth cranial nerve, usually the vestibular division, within the internal auditory canal (1). Murray and Stout (2), in 1942, reported that Schwannian tumor cells cultivated in vitro could be shown to form reticulin fibers. Since then, acoustic tumors have been considered to arise as a result of neoplastic proliferation of the neurolemmal or Schwannian nerve sheath cells of the eighth cranial nerve.

While the acoustic tumor usually arises from the superior vestibular nerve, it may arise from the inferior vestibular nerve (3) or cochlear nerve (4), either deep within the internal auditory meatus or in the posterior fossa (5). These variations must be borne in mind when considering the signs and symptoms elicited during history-taking from an acoustic tumor suspect.

As the tumor grows, it characteristically extends medially out of the internal auditory canal into the posterior cranial fossa and eventually

* Mailing address: Department of Otorhinolaryngology, 1405 E. Ann St., Ann Arbor, Michigan 48109

impacts into the cerebellopontine angle (Figures 1–3). The rate of growth varies considerably, but generally there is inexorable progression of symptoms and signs as the tumor enlarges (6). As pointed out by Sheehy (7), the eighth nerve symptoms, with rare exceptions, are the first indications of a developing acoustic neuroma. However, there is no typical pattern. Unilateral sensorineural hearing loss, tinnitus, dizziness, and fullness in the ear are suggestive of an acoustic tumor, and the patient should be completely evaluated for this lesion. The symptoms may be insidious or abrupt in onset and may fluctuate from time to time, and the patient may indeed become asymptomatic for an interval, only to have a recrudescence of symptoms at a later date. An acoustic tumor may develop in a patient already suffering from otosclerosis, chronic ear disease, or Meniere's disorder, thereby making diagnosis even more challenging. Only by maintaining a high index of suspicion, by thoroughly assessing all acoustic tumor suspects, and by being aware of the infinite variety of ways in which this capricious tumor may present will the ultimate diagnosis of an acoustic tumor be made. Since the publication of the first and second acoustic tumor monographs (8,9) summarizing our experience with the diagnosis and treatment of the first sixty-two and later of two hundred patients with acoustic tumors, there

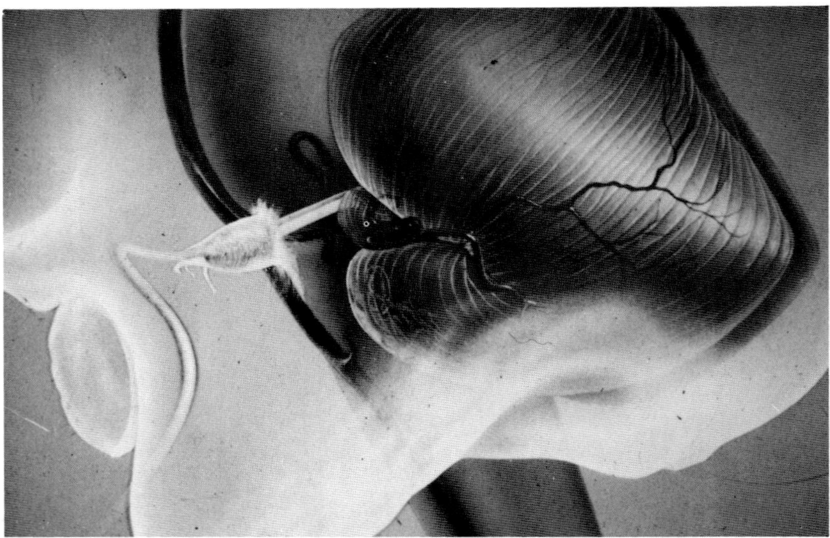

Figure 1. Intracanalicular tumor.

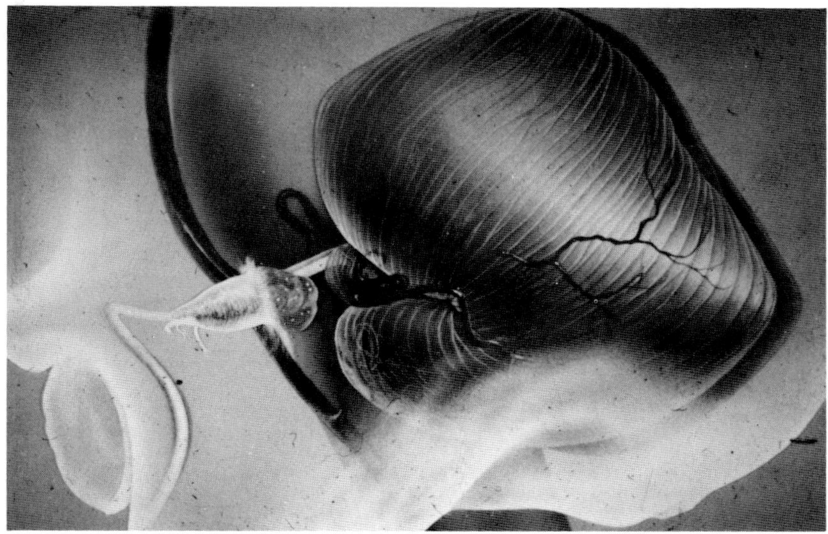

Figure 2. Acoustic tumor protruding into posterior fossa.

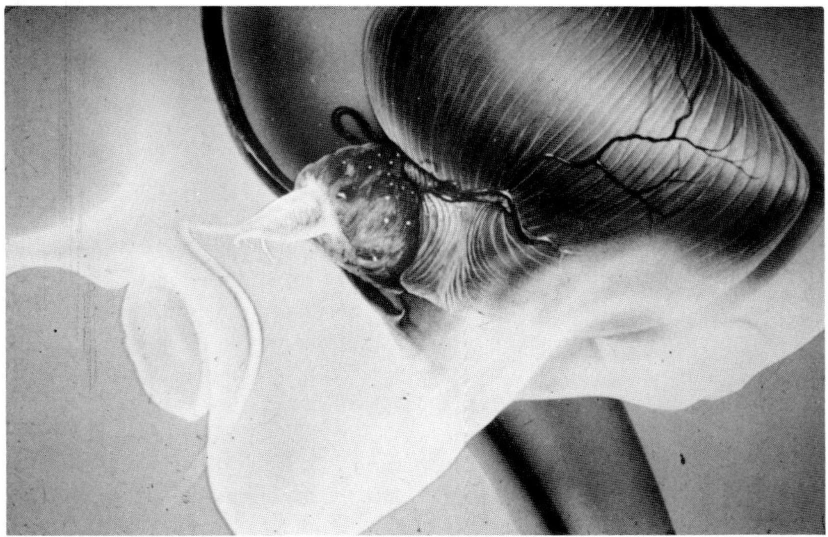

Figure 3. Tumor impacted into brainstem.

has been a general appreciation of the diagnostic features of the "typical" acoustic tumor. However, as stated earlier, their presentation may be infinitely varied.

The intent of this chapter is threefold: to review briefly the evolution of the diagnostic techniques that have been practiced since 1960, to review the evolution of surgical techniques over this same period of time, and to present selected case histories to illustrate the great variability of presenting signs and symptoms in patients harboring an acoustic tumor. Detailed descriptions of diagnostic techniques and surgical approaches are covered in other chapters of this book.

DIAGNOSTIC TECHNIQUES—A REVIEW

While audiometric, vestibular, neurologic, and radiologic studies have formed the basis for the diagnosis of an acoustic neuroma since 1961, there have been significant changes in techniques and emphasis (9). Air and bone conduction, speech, and Bekesy and SISI audiometry have been routinely used since 1960. However, since 1975 Bekesy and SISI testing have been superseded by stapedial reflex testing (10) and brainstem auditory response testing (11) because of their much higher reliability. Initially, vestibular response was assessed by the minimal ice-water cold caloric test, but since 1965 electronystagmography has been routinely used (12). While well-taken petrous pyramid x-rays in multiple views still form the basis for initial radiographic assessment, since 1963 definitive diagnosis of a tumor has been made with a positive contrast medium Pantopaque (iophendylate) posterior fossa myelography (13). This study was uniquely valuable and consistently used for definitive diagnosis until 1975. By this time, computerized cranial tomography (EMI or CAT scan) was available and rapidly superseded Pantopaque myelography as the initial definitive test for acoustic neuroma. This preference arose for several reasons: tomography is a non-invasive technique; it frequently allows differentiation between acoustic neuroma, meningioma, and congenital cholesteatoma of the posterior fossa; and it also allows assessment of brainstem shift and ventricular system obstruction by tumor. However, the CAT scan is deficient in not delineating small tumors and on occasion not detecting large ones. Therefore, if suspicion remains after a negative scan, the Pantopaque posterior fossa myelography is performed. Because myelography has become less frequently performed, the opportunity to obtain cerebrospinal fluid has been infrequent and therefore less reliance is placed on this index.

SURGICAL APPROACHES—A REVIEW

Surgical approaches too have evolved over the past 15 years. Initially, William House operated on the patient in the upright position and all tumors were approached via the middle cranial fossa. Soon, the translabyrinthine approach evolved and the patient was placed in the supine position on the operating table. The translabyrinthine approach was preferred over the middle fossa approach for several reasons: a more direct access to the tumor bed in the posterior fossa was possible, greater control of bleeding in the posterior fossa was obtainable, and there was better identification of and less encroachment on the operating field by the facial nerve. By 1962, only small intracanalicular acoustic tumors were removed by the middle fossa approach. All other tumors were removed via the translabyrinthine approach.

In 1965, in an attempt to gain more exposure for large tumor removals, the transsigmoid approach was evolved. Here the sigmoid sinus was ligated and reflected, giving more exposure of the posterior fossa and more exposure of the tumor and the cerebellopontine angle. However, the direct retraction of the cerebellum was followed by edema and often by postoperative ataxia. By 1968, it was realized that these complications could be avoided by greater bone removal posterior to the sigmoid sinus, thus allowing extradural retraction of the cerebellum without the necessity for ligating the sigmoid sinus. Formerly, large tumors with cranial nerve involvement and/or increased intracranial pressure were removed in two stages. Initially, a suboccipital decompression was performed and 10 to 14 days later the translabyrinthine removal was completed. Because of the morbidity and occasional mortality from the suboccipital decompression itself, this procedure was generally abandoned by 1975. Since then, the translabyrinthine approach has been used for any tumor in the posterior fossa, while the middle fossa is reserved for small intracanalicular tumors in patients with serviceable hearing.

CASE HISTORIES

The following case reports are provided to emphasize unusual or atypical features in the signs, symptoms, and test results in patients with acoustic tumors. The discussions accompanying the case reports identify the unusual aspects of the case histories and illustrate how the routine tests usually lead to early suspicion of an acoustic tumor.

CASE 1

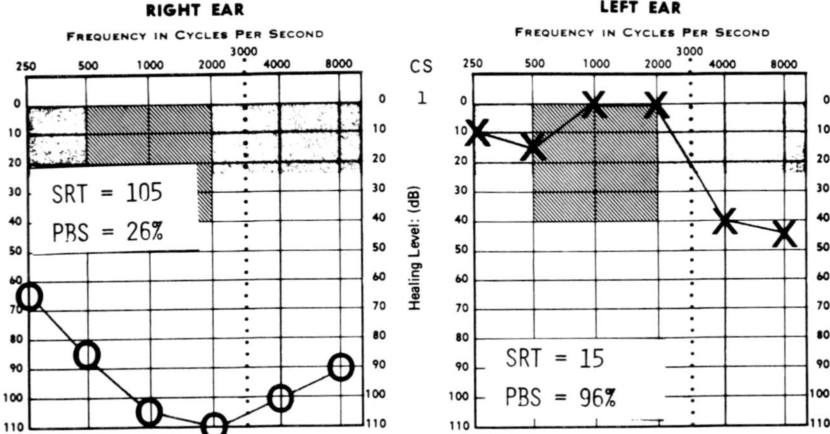

Summary—Hearing loss on the right noted for 24 years. A two-stage removal was performed using a transsigmoid approach.

History—This 56-year-old man noted a progressive hearing loss over 24 years in the right ear. He also complained of recent sharp twinges of pain in the right ear.

Examination—Normal exam except for eighth nerve findings.

Eighth nerve findings—Pure tone 105 dB high tone loss, right. Discrimination 26%, Bekesy type IV, SISI 0% at 500, tone decay complete at 250–20, 500–25.

Vestibular—30% reduced vestibular response, right.

Cerebrospinal fluid protein—124 mg/100 ml.

Petrous pyramid x-ray—Enlarged internal auditory canal right.

Pantopaque—3-cm mass in right cerebellopontine angle.

Surgery—On March 19, 1968, a transsigmoid removal of an acoustic neuroma was attempted. Surgery was stopped after 4 hr because of an increased respiration and elevation of the temperature. Several small pledgets of Surgicel were placed in the wound and it was closed. Three days later, the patient was returned to surgery. The previously placed Surgicel was then removed and a 2-cm tumor was exposed in the angle. The tumor was only slightly adherent to the brain and was totally removed without event and with preservation of the facial nerve.

Comment—In spite of a 24-year history of hearing loss, the ENG revealed only a 30% reduced vestibular response. However, the unilateral sensorineural hearing loss and abnormal petrous pyramid x-rays prompted the myelogram, which confirmed the diagnosis. The transsigmoid approach is no longer utilized.

CASE 14

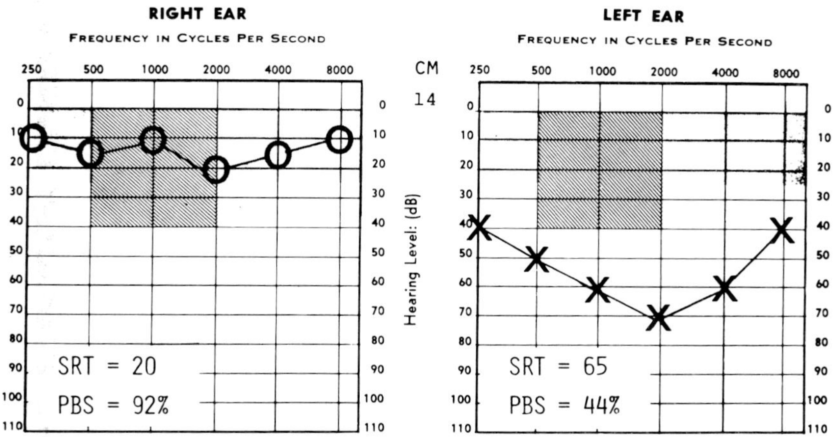

Summary—Hearing loss on the left of 2 years' duration. Small acoustic neuroma, left, was removed by the middle fossa approach with preservation of hearing.

History—This 30-year-old woman had noticed a hearing loss on the left side of 2 years' duration, with some dizziness 7 months earlier but none at the time of initial examination. Tinnitus was intermittently present on the left.

Examination—Normal except for eighth nerve findings.

Eighth nerve findings—Flat 65 dB sensorineural hearing loss on the left with 44% discrimination.

Vestibular—Normal electronystagmographic recording.

Petrous pyramid x-rays—Enlarged internal auditory canal on the left.

Pantopaque—Intracanalicular lesion, left internal auditory canal.

Surgery—On September 9, 1968, a middle fossa total removal of an acoustic neuroma was performed uneventfully. The neuroma was approximately 3 × 7 mm in size and originated from the inferior vestibular nerve.

Postoperative course—Uneventful. She had a mild facial paralysis on the involved side postoperatively that cleared completely by 6 months. Postoperative pure tone audiogram remained at the same level. However, her discrimination score improved from 44% to 92%.

Comment—In spite of this tumor being small, the unilateral sensorineural hearing loss and abnormal x-rays were highly suggestive of an acoustic neuroma. The Pantopaque study was confirmatory. This small tumor originated from the inferior vestibular nerve, thereby not producing a reduced vestibular response. The middle cranial fossa approach was utilized to remove this tumor. Hearing was preserved and discrimination score improved.

CASE 20

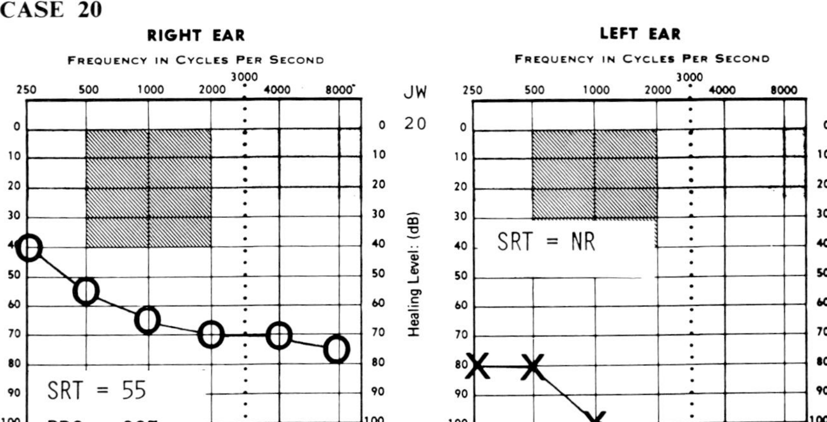

Summary—Progressive hearing loss on the left of 8 years' duration with a lifetime bilateral hearing loss. Transsigmoid total removal of an acoustic tumor.

History—This 32-year-old pharmacist was initially seen in 1962 with a progressive hearing loss and tinnitus noted in both ears. His right ear was the better ear at that time, with a 50 dB loss, and his left ear had a 90 dB loss. He stated that he had a lifelong hearing loss on the left but it has progressively worsened over the last 8 years. It was initially diagnosed as a congenital sensorineural hearing loss and a hearing aid was prescribed. He returned in 1968 complaining of frequent unsteadiness and episodic vertigo.

Examination—Normal except for eighth nerve findings and fifth cranial nerve findings. Cerebellar signs were also present.

Eighth nerve findings—Hearing tests revealed a predominantly high-tone loss of 95 dB on the left with 0% discrimination. SISI 80% at 1 Hz, 60% at 500 Hz.

Fifth nerve findings—Corneal reflex and nasal tickle sensation decreased.

Cerebellar—Slight dysmetria was noted on the left hand movements.

Cerebrospinal fluid proteins—11 mg/100 ml.

Vestibular—Normal ENG.

Petrous pyramid x-rays—Showed a widening of the internal auditory meatus on the left.

Pantopaque—Showed a 2-cm filling defect in the posterior fossa.

Surgery—A transsigmoid removal of the acoustic tumor was carried out. The tumor measured approximately 2 cm in the cerebellopontine angle and was very fibrous and extremely vascular. Removal was total, with preservation of the facial nerve. There were no vital sign changes and estimated blood loss was 1,200 cc with 1,000 cc blood replacement. The patient tolerated the procedure well.

Comment—This young adult had a lifelong bilateral sensorineural hearing loss with an 8-year history of worsening hearing on the left. In spite of unsteadiness, the ENG was normal. However, neurologic examination, audiometry, and x-ray studies were abnormal. The diagnosis was confirmed by a Pantopaque study.

CASE 40

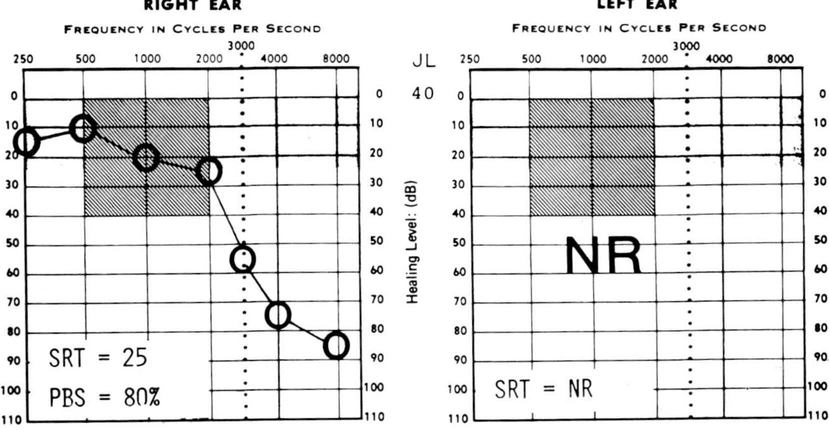

Summary—A progressive hearing loss on the left was noted 4 years prior to surgery. Increased intracranial pressure was also noted before surgery. A two-stage removal was performed using the translabyrinthine approach.

History—Four years prior to surgery, this 63-year-old man noted progressive hearing loss. He had noted severe progressive unsteadiness for three months and numbness of the left cheek four 4 to 5 months. He had complaints of frequent headaches for the last 2 months, experienced early in the morning, with occasional sharp twinges of pain in the left side on the neck.

Examination—Normal except for fifth and eighth nerve findings and bilateral papilledema.

Eighth nerve findings—No hearing in the left ear.

Fifth nerve findings—Decreased corneal reflex and diminished sensation over the left cheek.

Vestibular—There is 100% reduced vestibular response on the left.

Petrous pyramid x-rays—Left internal auditory canal enlarged.

Pantopaque—Revealed a large left cerebellopontine angle filling defect.

Surgery—Stage one: Suboccipital craniectomy and laminectomy, cervical I and II. On April 25, 1969, a suboccipital decompression was performed. During this procedure, the patient experienced a precipitous drop in blood pressure to 80 mm Hg. The blood pressure returned to normal levels as the procedure continued. Throughout the remainder of the operation, the blood pressure fluctuated. The patient tolerated the procedure well and left the operating room in good condition. Stage two: On May 5, 1969, via the translabyrinthine approach, the acoustic tumor was totally removed. The patient tolerated the procedure very well. There were no vital sign changes during the surgery. Blood loss was approximately 500 cc.

Comment—This individual had only a 4-year history of hearing loss, yet a large tumor with fifth cranial nerve involvement and papilledema was present. The usual tests were abnormal. In spite of the two-stage procedure, significant vital sign changes occurred during the initial decompression.

CASE 60

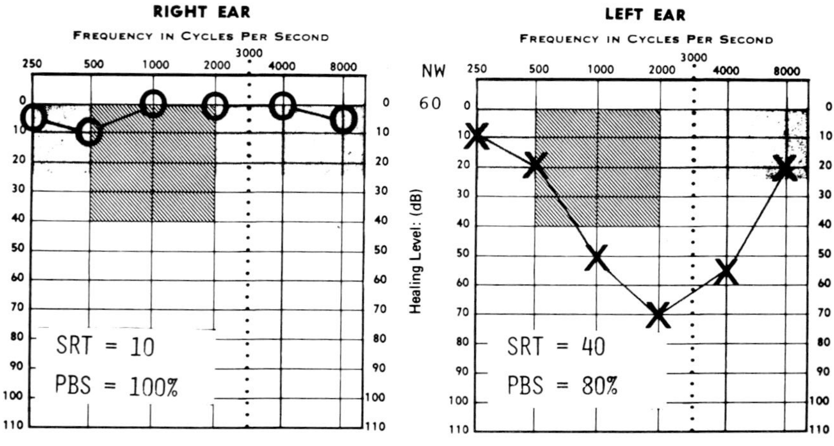

Summary—A hearing loss on the left and tinnitus were noted 18 months prior to surgery. Translabyrinthine approach total removal was performed.

History—This 36-year-old woman noted a ringing in the left ear and hearing loss 18 months prior to surgery. Other complaints were slight pressure in the left ear and occasional unsteadiness. She stated that she had had headaches over the left frontal parietal area for many years, but they had been more severe and associated with nausea in the past few months.

Examination—Normal except for eighth and seventh nerve findings.

Eighth nerve findings—Pure tone 40 dB left predominantly high tone loss. Discrimination 80%, Bekesy type II, SISI 4000–100%, 1000–100%, tone decay 2 Hz = 35 dB, 4 Hz = 40 dB.

Seventh nerve findings—Ear canal sensations (Hitselberger sign) decreased.

Vestibular—41% reduced vestibular response on the left.

Petrous pyramid x-rays—Enlarged left internal auditory canal.

Pantopaque—2-cm filling defect, left cerebellopontine angle.

Surgery—A translabyrinthine approach total removal of an acoustic neuroma was accomplished. The tumor filled the internal auditory canal and extended into the cerebellopontine angle about 1.5 cm. The facial nerve was somewhat stretched but was intact at the end of the procedure.

Comment—This young woman had a very short history of hearing loss and tinnitus. However, audiometric, vestibular, and radiographic tests were all suggestive of a cerebellopontine angle lesion. A fairly large tumor was confirmed by Pantopaque study.

CASE 66

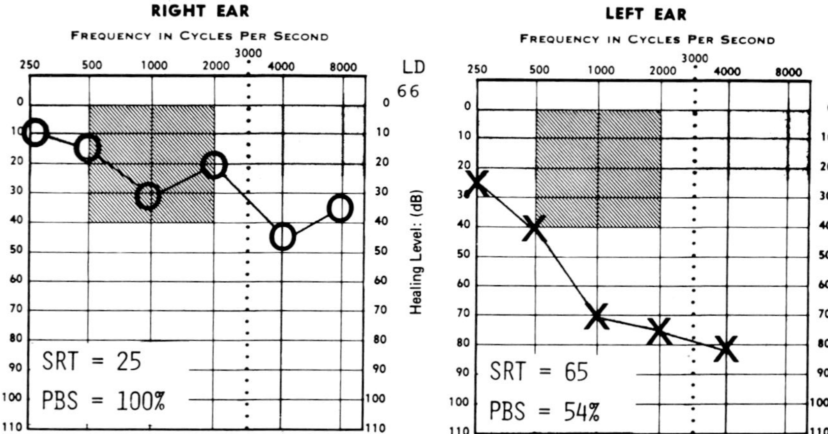

Summary—Hearing loss of 10 years' duration. Translabyrinthine removal of acoustic neuroma, left.

History—This 63-year-old man noticed a progressive hearing loss on the left of 10 years' duration. This was associated with constant tinnitus and some unsteadiness.

Examination—Normal save for eighth nerve signs, decreased corneal reflex, left, and failure to perform the tandem Romberg.

Eighth nerve findings—High-tone 65 dB sensorineural hearing loss, left, with 54% discrimination, type IV Bekesy, and 0% SISI score at 2,000 Hz.

Vestibular—16% reduced vestibular response, left, with 5° spontaneous nystagmus to left.

Petrous pyramid x-rays—Enlarged internal auditory canal, left.

Pantopaque—2-cm cerebellopontine angle mass, left.

Surgery—On September 29, 1969, left translabyrinthine total removal of an acoustic neuroma was performed uneventfully. Estimated blood loss was 350 cc. Facial nerve continuity was preserved. There were no vital sign changes.

Postoperative course—Uneventful save for immediate postoperative complete facial paralysis that has persisted for a period of 3 years. Hypoglossal facial anastomosis was recommended. However, the patient has declined further surgical intervention.

Comment—While this patient's pure tone speech audiograms, electronystagmography and plain x-ray findings were rather typical for acoustic neuroma, the 10-year history with a 2-cm tumor illustrates the very variable growth rate of these lesions. In spite of the moderate tumor size and preservation of continuity of the facial nerve at surgery, the immediate postoperative facial paralysis and its persistence for 3 years illustrate the unpredictability of the course of facial nerve recovery in acoustic tumor surgery.

CASE 71

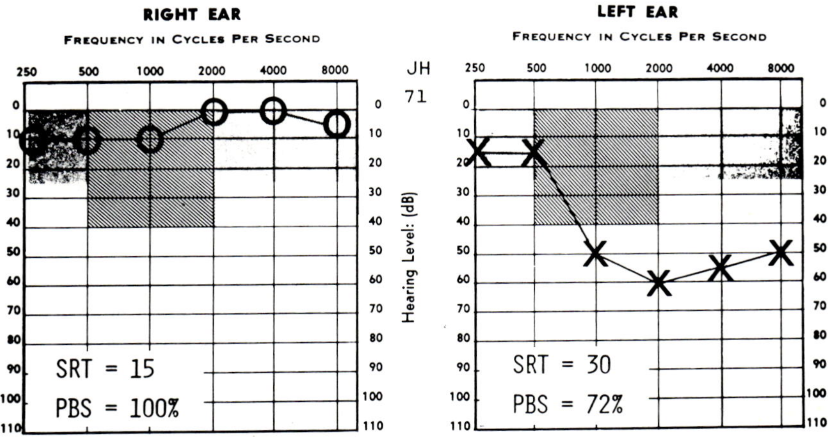

Summary—Four-month history of hearing loss in the left ear. Translabyrinthine removal of acoustic neuroma on the left was accomplished uneventfully.

History—This 23-year-old woman noticed a 4-month history of hearing loss, sudden in onset, with constant tinnitus but without unsteadiness, fluctuation of hearing, or pressure in the ear.

Examination—Normal save for eighth nerve findings.

Eighth nerve findings—High tone sensorineural hearing loss, 30 dB, with 72% discrimination, left.

Electronystagmography—53% reduced vestibular response on the left.

Petrous pyramid x-rays—Enlarged internal auditory canal, left.

Pantopaque—2-cm filling defect, left cerebellopontine angle.

Cerebrospinal fluid protein—50 mg/100 ml.

Surgery—On November 14, 1969, a total removal of a 2-cm acoustic neuroma was accomplished by the translabyrinthine approach. Estimated blood loss was 350 cc. No blood replacement and no vital sign changes occurred during surgery.

Postoperative course—Uneventful. No facial nerve weakness postoperatively.

Comment—This patient demonstrates a short symptomatic history in a young adult, with significant reduction in vestibular response on electronystagmography in spite of the absence of imbalance. Here, utilizing the audiometric, vestibular, and x-ray studies, presumptive diagnosis of an acoustic neuroma was made. The presence of this lesion was confirmed by Pantopaque studies of the posterior fossa.

CASE 86

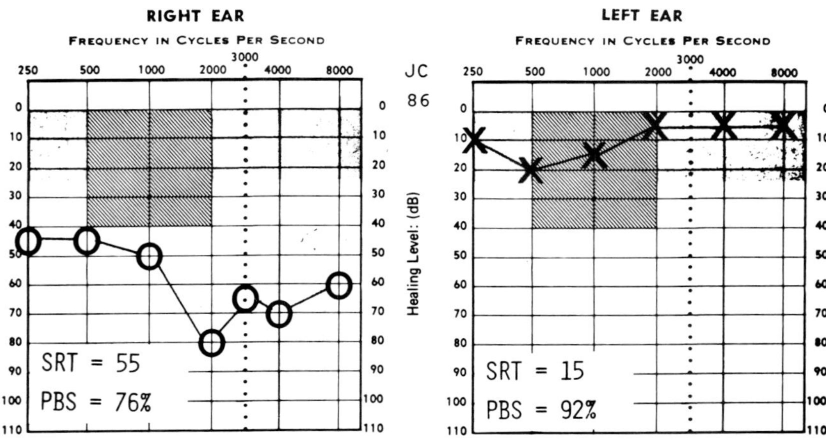

Summary—Hearing loss on the right of 1 year's duration. Two-stage total removal of a 4-cm acoustic neuroma was performed.

History—This 18-year-old woman noticed a hearing loss on the right side of 1 year's duration with constant tinnitus and some slight unsteadiness.

Examination—Normal save for eighth nerve findings and decreased corneal reflex on the right.

Eighth nerve findings—Flat 55 dB sensorineural hearing loss, right, with 76% discrimination, Bekesy type II, and a SISI score of 30% at 1 kHz.

Vestibular—100% reduced vestibular response on the right with 7° spontaneous right beating nystagmus.

Petrous pyramid x-rays—Enlarged internal auditory canal, right.

Pantopaque—Pantopaque myelogram revealed a 4-cm cerebellopontine angle lesion on the right.

Surgery—Right suboccipital decompression was performed on February 2, 1970, and on February 6, 1970, total removal of a 4-cm acoustic neuroma via the translabyrinthine approach was accomplished. Estimated blood loss was 2,500 cc and blood replacement was 2,500 cc. Patient's pulse slowed on two occasions transiently, considerable swelling of the brainstem was obvious at the time of surgery, and the patient was apneic on one occasion for 1 min.

Postoperative course—Her postoperative course was uneventful save for a complete facial paralysis that gradually recovered completely save for slightly decreased function of right forehead motion.

Comment—In spite of this woman's young age and short history, she had a large tumor in the right cerebellopontine angle. All three diagnostic tests—audiometric, vestibular, and radiographic—were abnormal and pointed to an acoustic neuroma. Her surgical course, vital sign changes, and heavy blood loss are typical of larger tumor removals.

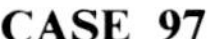

CASE 97

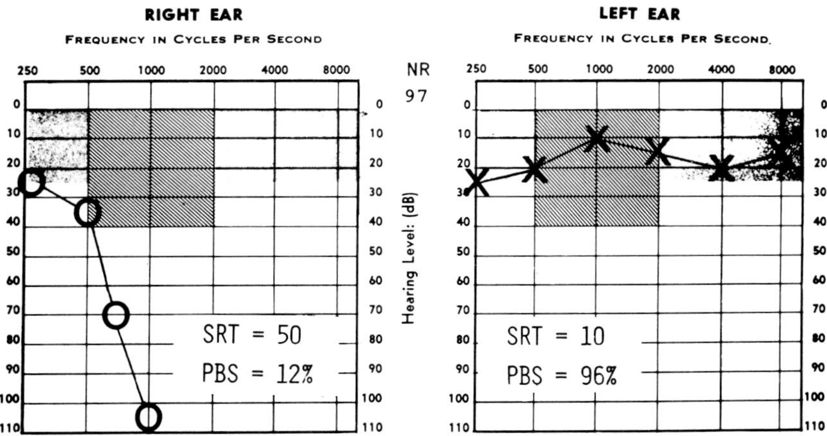

Summary—Decreased hearing on the right of 8 years' duration. A small acoustic neuroma was totally removed by the translabyrinthine approach.

History—This 57-year-old woman noticed a hearing loss and tinnitus 8 years earlier with some unsteadiness at the onset of her hearing loss but no dizziness since its onset.

Examination—Normal save for eighth nerve findings.

Eighth nerve findings—Right high frequency sensorineural hearing loss of 50 dB with 12% discrimination.

Vestibular—Normal electronystagmographic recording.

Petrous pyramid x-rays—Normal and symmetric internal auditory canals bilaterally.

Pantopaque—Revealed a small filling defect in the lateral aspect of the right internal auditory canal.

Surgery—On March 16, 1970, this patient underwent total removal of a small acoustic neuroma via the translabyrinthine approach. It appeared to arise from the inferior vestibular nerve and measured approximately 0.7 cm in diameter. Her operative and postoperative courses were uneventful, with normal facial nerve function.

Comment—In spite of the small tumor in this instance, this patient's symptoms were relatively long-term. The lesion was apparently small enough not to result in an enlargement of the internal auditory canal on the involved side, and its origin from the inferior vestibular nerve accounted for her normal electronystagmography. However, the possibility of an acoustic neuroma prompted the posterior fossa myelographic study, which, in this instance, substantiated the diagnosis of an intracanalicular neoplasm.

CASE 100

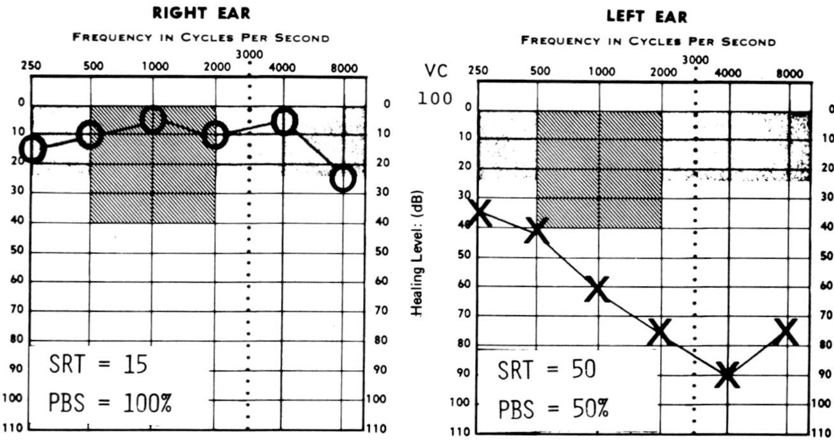

Summary—Hearing loss of 10 years' duration. Two-stage removal via the translabyrinthine approach.

History—This 47-year-old woman was seen with complaints of hearing loss on the left for 10 years, and pain around the left ear. In November, 1969, a left stapedectomy was performed with no subsequent improvement in hearing. Tinnitus began after surgery. Other complaints were numbness of the face and visual disturbances.

Examination—Normal except for findings related to fifth and eighth nerves.

Eighth nerve findings—Pure tone 50 dB high tone loss, left. Discrimination 50%, Bekesy type II, SISI 95% at 2 kHz, 100% at 4 kHz (with 67–70 NBN).

Fifth nerve findings—Corneal reflex decreased, decreased sensation first and second divisions.

Cerebrospinal fluid protein—35 mg/100 ml.

Vestibular—Reduced vestibular response 100% on the left.

Petrous pyramid x-ray—Left internal auditory canal enlarged.

Pantopaque—2-cm filling defect, left cerebellopontine angle.

Surgery—Stage one: On April 9, 1970, a suboccipital craniectomy was carried out. Stage two: On April 25, 1970, via the translabyrinthine approach, total tumor removal of a 2.5-cm tumor was accomplished with preservation of the facial nerve. No vital sign changes occurred during surgery.

Comment—This patient had a previous stapedectomy in the ear harboring an acoustic tumor. In spite of having had no vertigo she had 100% reduced vestibular response on the left. Of interest is the finding that, in spite of a large tumor being present, the cerebrospinal fluid protein was normal. Audiologic, vestibular, and radiographic studies were abnormal and pointed to the presence of a cerebellopontine angle lesion.

CASE 111

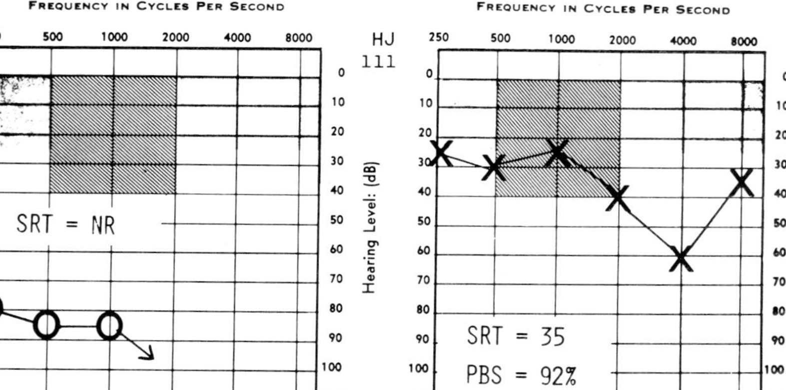

Summary—Right-side hearing loss of 4 years' duration. A planned subtotal removal of right acoustic neuroma was performed.

History—This 73-year-old woman had progressive hearing loss on the right with progressively worsening imbalance of 4 years' duration. She had fallen on several occasions and was becoming progressively incapacitated and unable to care for herself. Tinnitus was constant on the right.

Examination—Normal save for eighth nerve findings and poor cerebellar coordination testing results on the right.

Eighth nerve findings—No recordable hearing, right.

Vestibular—100% reduced vestibular response, right, with 3° of spontaneous nystagmus to the left.

Petrous pyramid x-rays—Enlarged internal auditory canal, right, with some petrous apex erosion.

Pantopaque—3.5-cm filling defect in the right cerebellopontine angle.

Surgery—On June 9, 1970, planned subtotal right translabyrinthine acoustic tumor removal was performed. Tumor removal was intracapsular. Approximately 80% of the tumor volume was recovered. Her operative course was uneventful.

Postoperative course—Uneventful. Facial nerve function was normal. Within 12 months her balance was considered normal and she was able to function independently.

Comment—While this patient's findings are typical of an acoustic tumor, the management of such a lesion in the aged presents a great problem if incapacitating unsteadiness and imbalance are present.

Here a planned subtotal removal of a large acoustic tumor was performed, which involved a labyrinthectomy, partial removal of the tumor mass, and resultant decompression of the posterior fossa. As illustrated in this patient, there is frequently great improvement in the balance, allowing these previously incapacitated individuals to be self-sufficient for the remainder of their lives.

CASE 121

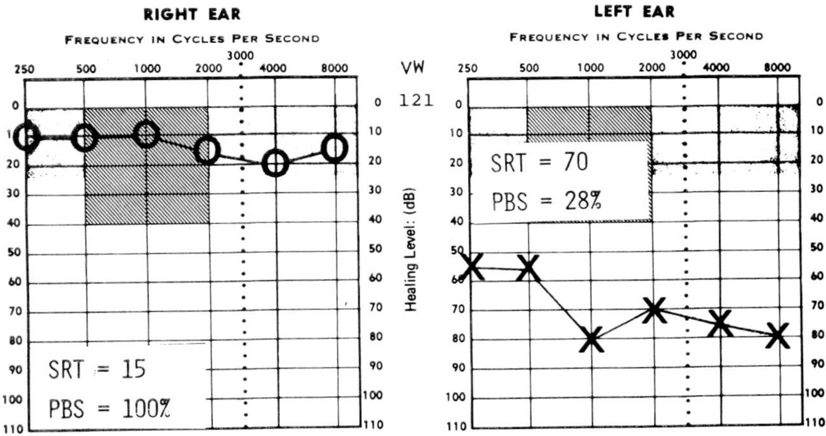

Summary—A progressive hearing loss was noted on the left for 5 months. A translabyrinthine approach was used for total removal of an acoustic tumor.

History—This 30-year-old man was seen with the complaint of progressive hearing loss of 5 months' duration. He also complained of a constant ringing in the left ear.

Examination—Normal except for findings related to the eighth nerve.

Eighth nerve findings—Pure tone 70 dB, flat loss, left. Discrimination 28%, Bekesy type II, SISI 65% at 1 k Hz, 70% at 2 kHz.

Vestibular—Reduced vestibular response, left, 85%.

Petrous pyramid x-ray—Left internal auditory canal enlarged.

Pantopaque—2-cm filling defect noted in the left cerebellopontine angle.

Surgery—A 2-cm tumor was removed from the cerebellopontine angle via the translabyrinthine approach. There was some bleeding from the brainstem, however. No vital sign changes occurred during this procedure and the patient tolerated the surgery well.

Comment—This young man had a fairly large tumor. ENG was markedly abnormal in spite of the absence of a subjective imbalance. All the routine tests were abnormal, pointing to a cerebellopontine angle lesion.

CASE 141

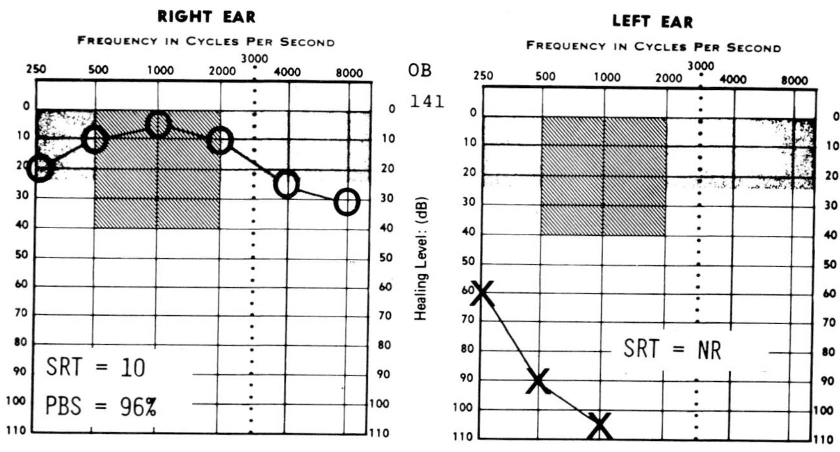

Summary—Hearing loss on the left side with dizziness intermittently, of 15 years' duration. Left acoustic neuroma removed by the trans-labyrinthine approach.

History—This 60-year-old woman has had a 15-year history of progressive hearing loss on the left with continuous tinnitus and intermittent dizzy spells.

Examination—Normal except for eighth nerve findings.

Eighth nerve findings—Complete hearing loss, left.

Vestibular—Normal electronystagmography recording.

Petrous pyramid x-rays—Enlarged internal auditory canal on the left.

Cerebrospinal fluid protein—29 mg/100 ml.

Pantopaque—Filling defect, left cerebellopontine angle, approximately 1.5 cm.

Surgery—On January 20, 1971, translabyrinthine acoustic tumor removal was performed on the left, with total removal of a 1.5-cm neuroma.

Postoperative course—Uneventful. Normal facial nerve function post-operatively.

Comment—In spite of 15 years' history of progressive hearing loss and dizziness, the acoustic tumor was only 1.5 cm in size and electronystagmography was entirely normal. However, the combination of unilateral sensorineural hearing loss and a large internal auditory canal prompted Pantopaque study, with confirmation of a cerebellopontine angle lesion.

CASE 142

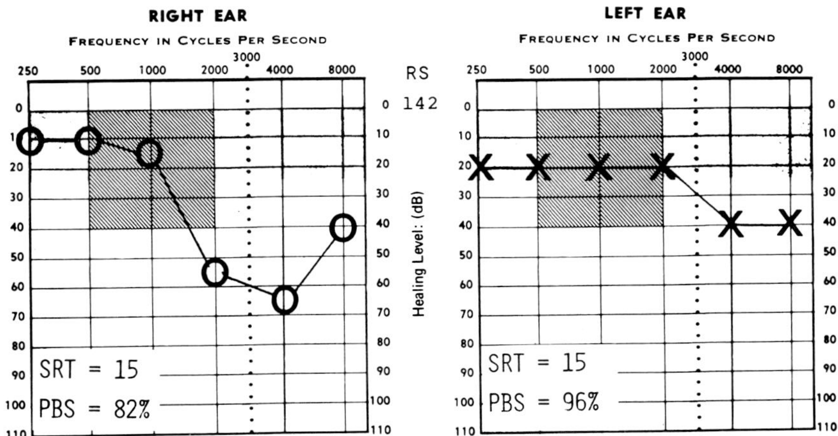

Summary—Progressive hearing loss and tinnitus of 18 months' duration. Translabyrinthine approach with a total removal of an acoustic tumor.

History—This 40-year-old man first noticed a ringing in the left ear 5 years ago. No hearing loss had been noted.

Examination—Exam was normal except for findings related to eighth nerve.

Eighth nerve findings—Pure tone 15 dB, high tone loss. Discrimination 96%, Bekesy type II, SISI 0% at 4 kHz, 0% at 1 kHz, tone decay 500–0, 10 dB at 2 kHz, 10 dB at 2 kHz, 10 dB at 3 kHz, 10 dB at 4 kHz.

Cerebrospinal fluid protein—39 mg/100 ml.

Vestibular—Reduced vestibular response on the left, 64%.

Petrous pyramid x-ray—Left internal auditory canal slightly enlarged.

Pantopaque—2.5-cm tumor mass noted in left cerebellopontine angle.

Surgery—On January 6, 1971, a translabyrinthine removal was carried out. The tumor was mobilized off the surrounding structures and the brainstem with only minimal bleeding. The total removal of a 2.5-cm acoustic neuroma with preservation of the facial nerve was accomplished.

Comment—Here only a mild hearing loss was present. In spite of the absence of subjective unsteadiness, ENG showed a significant 64% reduced vestibular response. While the tumor was medium in size, the cerebrospinal fluid protein was normal.

CASE 152

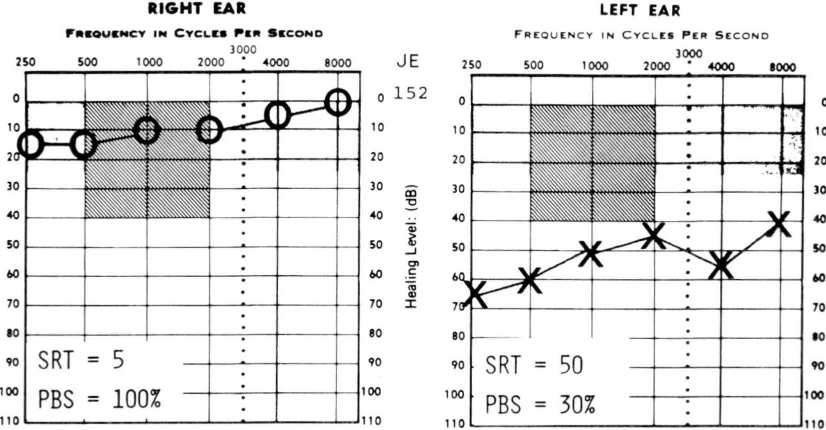

Summary—One-year history of fullness and decreased hearing on the left side. Acoustic neuroma removed uneventfully via translabyrinthine approach.

History—This 22-year-old woman had a 1-year history of fullness and decreased hearing in the left ear. There was no dizziness, but she had Bell's palsy for one and a half months during one of her pregnancies two and a half years previously.

Examination—Normal save for eighth nerve findings.

Eighth nerve findings—50 dB flat, pure tone sensorineural hearing loss, left, with 30% discrimination. Type III Bekesy, SISI 0% at 1,000 kHz.

Vestibular—35% reduced vestibular response on the left.

Petrous pyramid x-rays—Enlarged internal auditory canal, left.

Pantopaque—1.5-cm cerebellopontine angle tumor on the left.

Surgery—On March 2, 1971, a left translabyrinthine removal of acoustic neuroma was performed. Total removal was accomplished of a

medium-sized tumor. Estimated blood loss was 500 cc. The facial nerve was preserved. No vital sign changes during surgery.

Postoperative course—Uneventful postoperative course with normal facial nerve function.

Comment—This patient is young. Unilateral sensorineural hearing loss with poor discrimination would lead one to suspect the possibility of acoustic neuroma. The abnormal x-rays and the slightly reduced vestibular response on the left are suggestive evidence of an acoustic neuroma. The presence of this lesion was confirmed by Pantopaque studies.

CASE 159

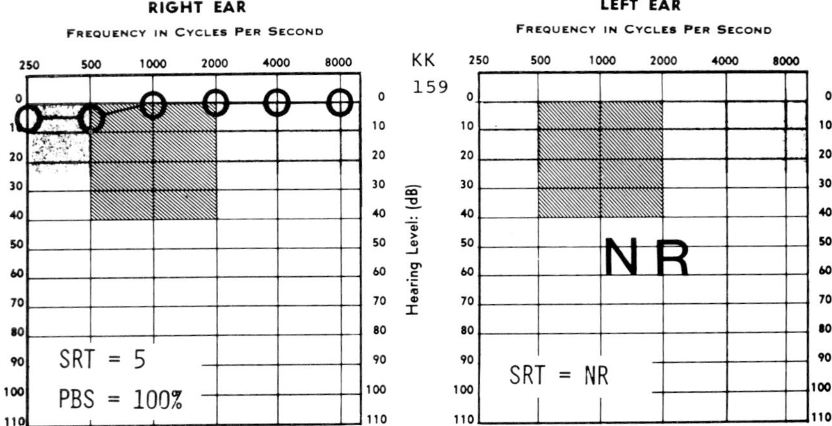

Summary—Hearing loss on the left of 5 months' duration. An acoustic neuroma was removed by a left translabyrinthine approach.

History—This 12-year-old girl noticed a progressive hearing loss on the left side of 5 months' duration. Four months before being seen she had had a high temperature with dizziness and subsequent tinnitus. Slight unsteadiness was a problem with position change.

Examination—Normal save for eighth nerve findings.

Eighth nerve findings—No recordable hearing, left.

Vestibular—100% reduced vestibular response on the left.

Petrous pyramid x-rays—Enlarged internal auditory canal, left.

Pantopaque—3-cm posterior fossa filling defect on the left.

Cerebrospinal fluid protein—32 mg/100 ml.

Surgery—On April 5, 1971, a left translabyrinthine approach removal of

a 3-cm acoustic tumor was performed. Facial nerve integrity was preserved. Estimated blood loss was 1,300 cc; blood replacement was 1,000 cc. Her operative course was smooth.

Postoperative course—Smooth. She had almost total facial paralysis immediately postoperatively; by two years postoperatively she had recovered except for some right forehead weakness.

Comment—This 12-year-old girl represents one of the youngest patients we have managed with acoustic neuroma. She had a large tumor in spite of her short history, and while the unilateral sensorineural hearing loss, abnormal electronystagmography, and enlarged internal auditory canal on plain films were pathognomonic of acoustic neuroma, it is interesting to note her normal cerebrospinal fluid protein level.

CASE 162

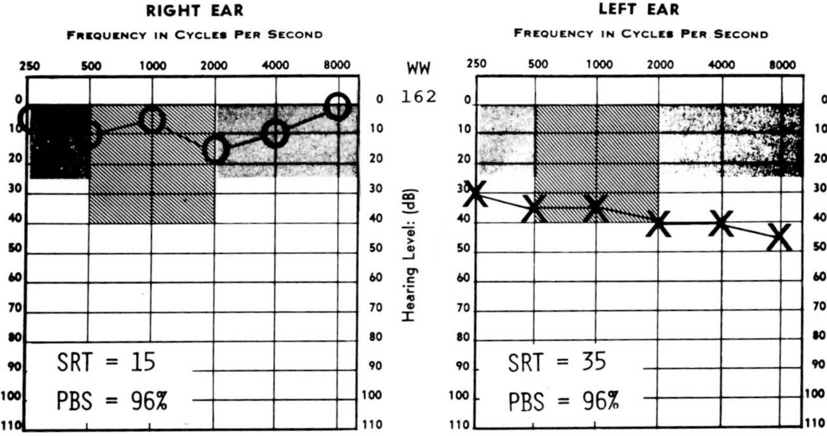

Summary—Sudden hearing loss occurred 9 months prior to being seen. Total removal of a large acoustic neuroma was accomplished by the translabyrinthine approach.

History—This 32-year-old man experienced a sudden hearing loss on the left 9 months earlier. There was occasional tinnitus on the left but no episodes of unsteadiness.

Examination—Unremarkable save for eighth nerve findings on the left.

Eighth nerve findings—Flat 35 dB sensorineural hearing loss, left, with 96% discrimination. Bekesy type I.

Vestibular—Electronystagmography revealed a 30% reduced vestibular response on the left.

Petrous pyramid x-rays—Showed a large internal auditory canal on the left.

Pantopaque—5-cm filling defect, left cerebellopontine angle.

Surgery—On April 9, 1971, this patient underwent total removal of a 4- to 5-cm acoustic neuroma via the translabyrinthine approach. Its origin appeared to be from the inferior vestibular nerve. There were no vital sign changes. Estimated blood loss was 2,500 cc; blood replacement was 2,500 cc. Facial nerve integrity was preserved.

Postoperative course—Uneventful except for mild facial paresis on the operated side. This recovered and facial nerve function was normal at the end of 1 year.

Comment—This patient illustrates the growth of a large tumor in a young adult, with only minimal symptoms of short duration and a history suggesting that the tumor arose in the cerebellopontine angle initially rather than deep in the internal auditory canal. The tumor origin from the inferior vestibular nerve is consistent with a relatively normally functioning vestibular system on testing. However, complete evaluation of this unilateral sensorineural hearing loss resulted in finding a large internal auditory canal on petrous pyramid x-rays, which was highly suggestive of an acoustic neuroma.

CASE 175

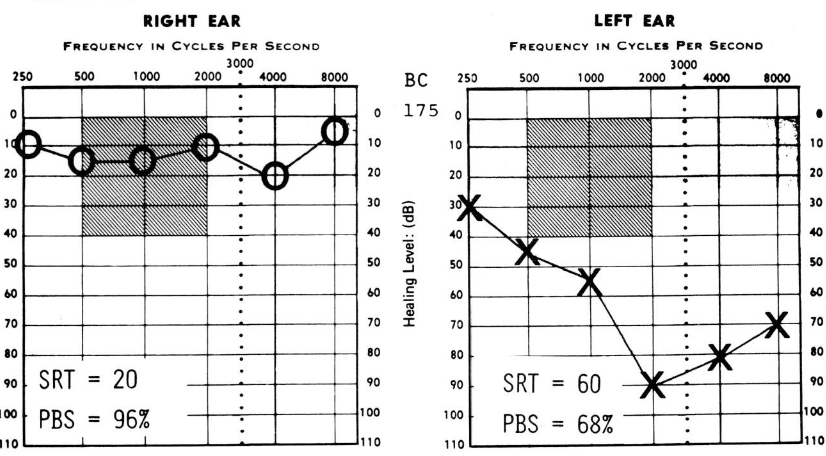

Summary—Hearing loss on the left side of 2 years' duration. Total removal of acoustic neuroma accomplished by left translabyrinthine approach.

History—This 51-year-old woman had noted a hearing loss of 2 years' duration on the left. Seven years earlier, a gunshot explosion near the left ear gave her some temporary hearing loss. Tinnitus was constant on the left and there was some fullness and fluctuation on the left side.

Examination—Normal save for eighth nerve findings.

Eighth nerve findings—High-tone 60 dB sensorineural hearing loss, left, with 68% discrimination.

Vestibular—Normal electronstagmograhic findings.

Cerebrospinal fluid protein—46 mg/100 ml.

Pantopaque—1.5-cm filling defect, left cerebellopontine angle.

Surgery—On June 21, 1971, a translabyrinthine total removal of acoustic neuroma was performed on the left. Estimated blood loss was 500 cc. There was no blood replacement. Facial nerve continuity was preserved.

Postoperative course—Her postoperative course was uneventful, with normal facial nerve function.

Comment—In spite of a gunshot explosion near the left ear earlier and in spite of normal electronystagmography findings, the internal auditory canal x-rays were pathognomonic for an acoustic neuroma on the left, which was proved subsequently by posterior fossa Pantopaque study.

CASE 192

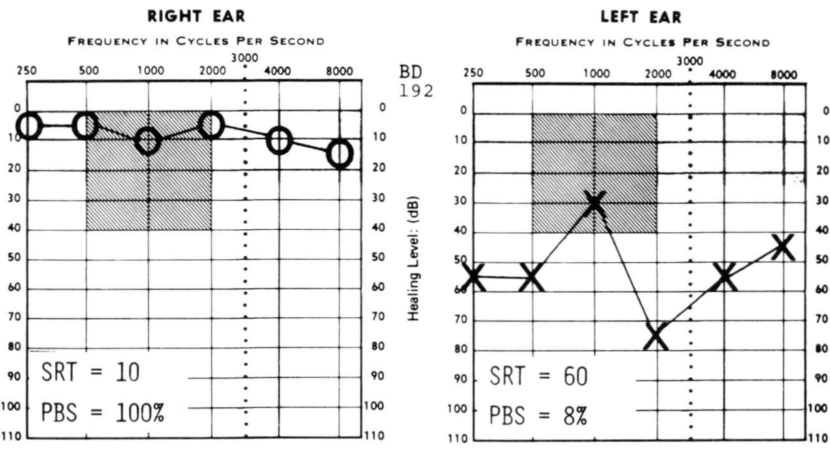

Summary—Left hearing loss of two years' duration. Left translabyrinthine acoustic tumor removal was performed.

History—This 42-year-old man noted a progressive hearing loss on the left of 2 years' duration with intermittent tinnitus. Six years earlier, he had an episode of severe vertigo lasting several months but accommodating to the point where he was asymptomatic.

Examination—Normal save for eighth nerve findings.

Eighth nerve findings—Flat 60 dB sensorineural hearing loss, left, with 8% discrimination, Bekesy type II, and SISI 100% at 2 kHz.

Vestibular—100% reduced vestibular response on the left with 5° of spontaneous nystagmus to the left.

Petrous pyramid x-rays—Normal and symmetric internal auditory canals bilaterally.

Pantopaque—1.5-cm filling defect, left cerebellopontine angle.

Surgery—On August 24, 1971, left translabyrinthine total removal of an acoustic neuroma was performed. His surgical course was uneventful, with an estimated blood loss of 400 cc without blood replacement.

Postoperative course—Uneventful. There was no facial weakness.

Comment—While this patient presented with a unilateral sensorineural hearing loss with poor speech discrimination rather typical of an acoustic neuroma, his history of vertigo several years earlier was a little unusual and might have been interpreted as being a vestibular neuronitis. In spite of his freedom from dizziness at the time of his initial visit, electronystagmography revealed markedly abnormal findings. In spite of his normal plain x-ray films, the combination of the unilateral sensorineural hearing loss and abnormal vestibular function on electronystagmography required Pantopaque study of the posterior fossa. This in turn was diagnostic of a cerebellopontine angle lesion on the left.

CASE 198

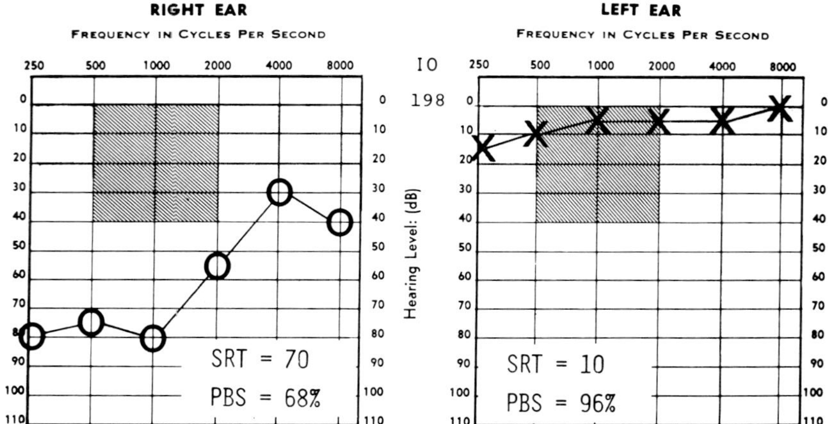

Summary—Hearing loss on the right of 6 months' duration. An acoustic neuroma on the right was removed by the translabyrinthine approach.

History—This 24-year-old woman noticed a progressive hearing loss on the right of 6 months' duration. No fullness or fluctuation had been noticed and only mild occasional unsteadiness on arising. Constant high-pitched tinnitus on the right side.

Examination—Normal save for eighth nerve findings.

Eighth nerve findings—Low frequency 70 dB sensorineural hearing loss with 68% discrimination, right.

Vestibular—71% reduced vestibular response on the right.

Petrous pyramid x-rays—Large internal auditory canal on the right.

Cerebrospinal fluid protein—21 mg/100 ml.

Pantopaque—Filling defect, intracanalicular, right.

Surgery—On September 9, 1971, total removal of an acoustic neuroma on the right was performed by the translabyrinthine approach. The intraoperative period was uneventful. Facial nerve integrity was preserved. On September 20, 1971, she underwent closure of a persistent cerebrospinal fluid leak. However, the cerebrospinal leak persisted and repeat closure was performed on September 30, 1971. This resulted in cessation of her leak. Otherwise, postoperatively she has done well, with normal facial nerve function.

Comment—This young patient with a short history had a small tumor and yet had great hearing and vestibular function losses. Her cerebrospinal fluid leak, which required two attempts at closure, demonstrates not only that cerebrospinal fluid leak is a complication following translabyrinthine acoustic tumor removal but occasionally may be difficult to stop.

CASE 240

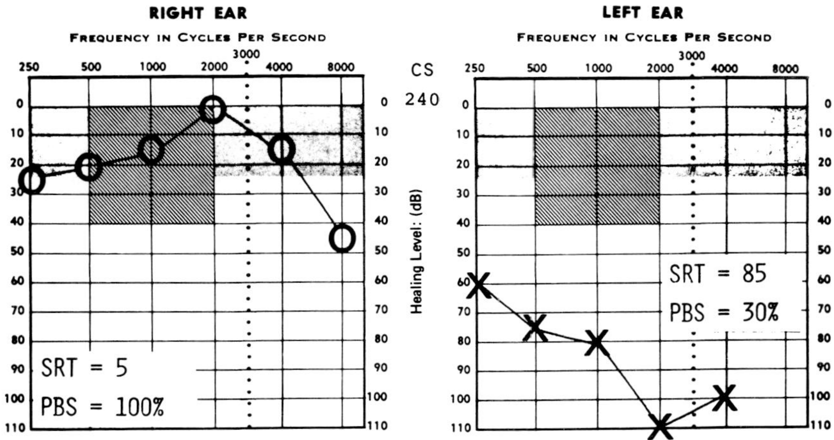

Summary—Seven-year history of gradual hearing loss, constant tinnitus, precipitated by a 3-month attack of dizziness. Translabyrinthine approach with total removal was performed.

History—This 49-year-old woman first developed a hearing problem in 1965. The problem was ushered in with a severe bout of dizziness, lasting 3 or 4 months, during which she was completely incapacitated. She had dizzy spells since that time, all of lesser intensity.

Examination—Findings normal except for eighth nerve.

Eighth nerve findings—Pure tone 85 dB, discrimination 30% left, Bekesy type IV, SISI 0% at 1 kHz, 0% at 1500 Hz, tone decay 500-15, 1 kHz, 1500-20 (complete decay).

Cerebrospinal fluid protein—25 mg/100 ml.

Vestibular—Reduced response, 100%.

Petrous pyramid x-ray—Left internal auditory canal enlarged.

Pantopaque—Filling defect on the left measuring approximately 1 cm.

Surgery—On February 22, 1972, through a translabyrinthine approach, the tumor was completely removed. The patient had no vital sign changes during the procedure. Facial nerve was preserved.

Comment—The acute onset of symptoms associated with 3 months of severe dizziness is unusual and might lead one to suspect a lesion of vascular or viral etiology. However, a full routine test battery was highly suggestive of a cerebellopontine angle lesion.

CASE 242

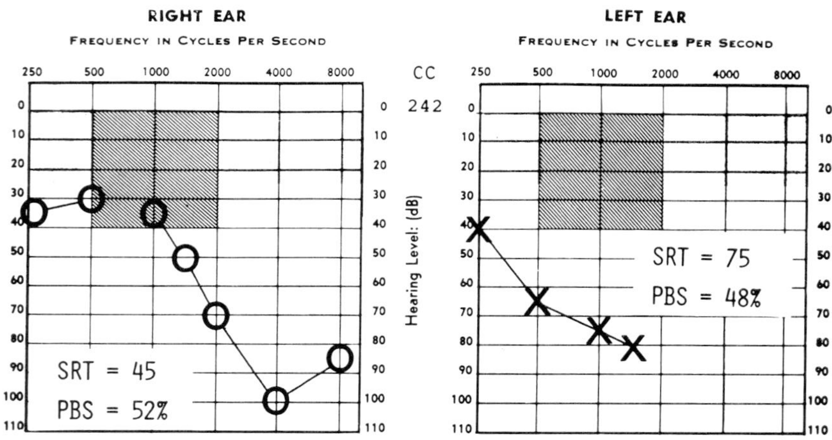

Summary—Hearing loss on the left of 8 years' duration. A medium-sized tumor was removed on the left via the translabyrinthine approach.

History—This 50-year-old man began to lose hearing on the left side 8 years ago and on the right 4 years ago. Tinnitus had been constant on both sides. He had suffered from left Bell's palsy 6 years earlier with good recovery in a few weeks' time. He had been exposed to noise over a prolonged period from both helicopter engines and firearms. He had not suffered imbalance.

Examination—Unremarkable except for eighth nerve findings.

Eighth nerve findings—High frequency sensorineural hearing loss bilaterally, 75 dB on the left with 48% discrimination, 45 dB on the right with 52% discrimination.

Vestibular—100% directional preponderence to the right.

Petrous pyramid x-rays—Slight internal auditory canal enlargement on the left.

Pantopaque—1-cm cerebellopontine angle filling defect, left.

Cerebrospinal fluid protein—79 mg/100 ml.

Surgery—On March 14, 1972, a left translabyrinthine acoustic neuroma removal was performed. Total removal was accomplished with preservation of the facial nerve. There were no vital sign changes. Estimated blood loss was 250 cc with no blood replacement.

Postoperative course—Uneventful. Normal facial nerve function preserved.

Comment—This man had bilateral hearing loss that was suggestive of the effects of chronic noise exposure, which he had experienced for many years. The examiner must be most suspicious in cases where concomitant hearing losses, such as those of chronic noise exposure, chronic ear disease, and otosclerosis, or of temporal bone trauma, are present. Plain x-rays of the internal auditory canals revealed asymmetry, which led to the performance of a Pantopaque study and definitive diagnosis of a cerebellopontine angle lesion on the left.

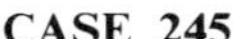

CASE 245

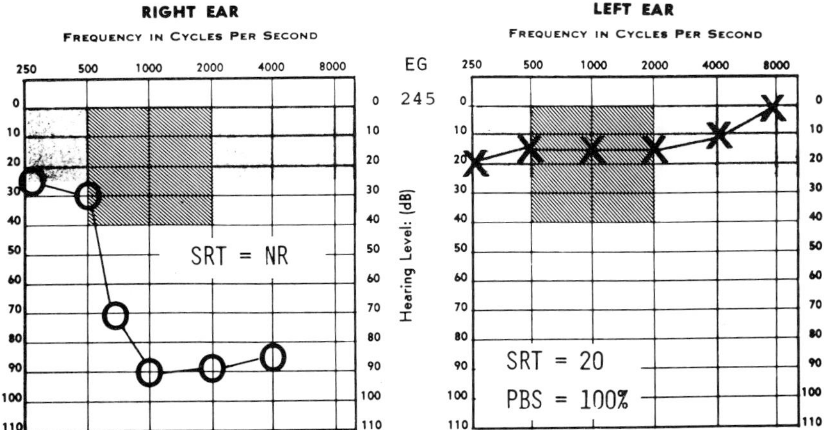

Summary—Hearing loss was noted on the right side for one and a half months prior to a translabyrinthine removal of an acoustic neuroma on the right side.

History—This 52-year-old woman noticed a hearing loss on the right side associated with constant tinnitus for one and a half months. She had had some unsteadiness for approximately 3 months but was free of it at the time of examination.

Examination—Normal except for eighth nerve findings, right.

Eighth nerve findings—Mid- and high-frequency sensorineural hearing loss of 67 dB with 0% discrimination.

Vestibular—Normal electronystagmographic recording.

Petrous pyramid x-rays—Enlarged right internal auditory canal.

Pantopaque—2- to 3-cm filling defect, right cerebellopontine angle.

Surgery—On March 27, 1972, a total removal of a 2.5-cm acoustic tumor on the right was accomplished by the translabyrinthine approach. Facial nerve integrity was preserved and estimated blood loss was 500 cc. No blood replacement.

Postoperative course—Uneventful, with normal facial nerve function.

Comment—This patient's course demonstrates the relatively short duration of symptoms in a middle-aged adult, significant with a medium-sized tumor.

CASE 246

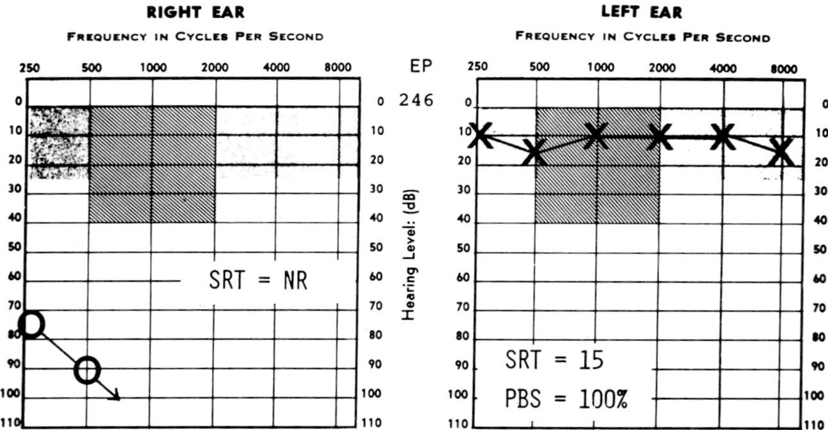

Summary—Hearing loss on the right side of 5 years' duration. Acoustic tumor removed by two-stage translabyrinthine approach.

History—This 57-year-old man noticed a progressive hearing loss on the right of 5 years' duration associated with a constant tinnitus. He had not noticed any imbalance.

Examination—Normal save for eighth nerve findings, right.

Eighth nerve findings—No recordable hearing, right.

Vestibular—100% reduced vestibular response, right.

Petrous pyramid x-rays—Enlarged internal auditory canal, right.

Pantopaque—4-cm filling defect, right cerebellopontine angle.

Surgery—On March 17, 1972, a suboccipital decompression was performed on the right, followed on March 27, 1972, by removal of an acoustic neuroma via the translabyrinthine approach. Estimated blood loss was 1,000 cc. There was a transient increase in blood pressure, which returned to normal within several minutes. Facial nerve integrity was preserved.

Postoperative course—Uneventful. About 75% facial paralysis on the right in the immediate postoperative period; by 1 year he had 10% facial weakness in all rami on the right. There was some mass action. The eye was able to close satisfactorily.

Comment—This 57-year-old man demonstrates the fairly rapid progressive growth of an acoustic neuroma, the interval being only five years from onset of symptoms to the presence of a 4-cm acoustic neuroma.

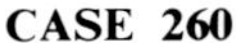

CASE 260

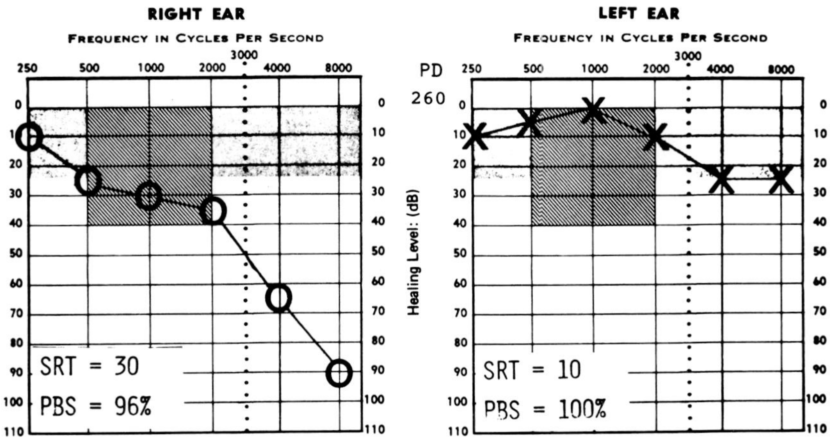

Summary—Fullness in the right ear for 1 year, tinnitus for 4 months, hearing loss for 1 month. A translabyrinthine total removal of an acoustic neuroma was accomplished.

History—This 38-year-old executive developed a hearing loss that was discovered 1 month ago while listening on the telephone. He noticed fullness in his ear and wanted his "ear cleaned out." He had tinnitus in his right ear and slight imbalance.

Examination—Normal except for eighth nerve findings.

Eighth nerve findings—Pure tone 30 dB high tone loss, right. Discrimination 96%, Bekesy type II, SISI 1000–100% at +65, 2000–100% at +65, tone decay 1 kHz-0, 2 kHz-0, 4 kHz-0.

Cerebrospinal fluid protein—73 mg/100 ml.

Vestibular—Reduced vestibular response on the right, 49%.
Petrous pyramid x-ray—Right internal auditory canal enlarged.
Pantopaque—Filling defect on the right measuring approximately 2 cm.
Surgery—On May 15, 1972, a total translabyrinthine removal of an acoustic neuroma was performed. During the removal, approximately 2,200 ml of blood were lost during a short period of time when the petrosal vein was entered. Bleeding was controlled with clips and Surgicel. There were no vital sign changes. Blood replacement was 1,000 cc. Facial nerve was preserved.
Comment—In spite of a short symptomatic history, audiometric, vestibular, and radiologic studies were abnormal. The complaint of "not being able to hear on the telephone," in spite of fairly good pure tone and speech audiometric test results, is suggestive of a retrocochlear lesion probably due to auditory fatigue.

CASE 280

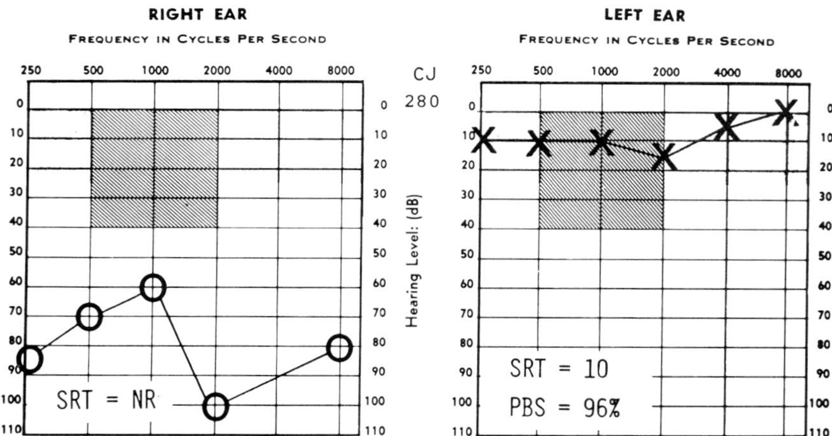

Summary—Hearing loss on the right of 3 months' duration. A 3-cm acoustic neuroma was removed from the right side via a translabyrinthine approach.
History—This 54-year-old woman had noticed a progressive hearing loss on the right of 3 months' duration. She had some slight unsteadiness and intermittent tinnitus on the right side. Within a month of the onset of her hearing loss, she had noticed some decreased sensation on the right side of her face.

Examination—Normal except for eighth nerve findings on the right, decreased corneal reflex, right, and decreased sensation, all rami, right fifth cranial nerve.

Eighth nerve findings—No recordable hearing, right.

Vestibular—100% reduced vestibular response, right.

Petrous pyramid x-rays—Enlarged internal auditory canal, right.

Pantopaque—2.5-cm filling defect, right cerebellopontine angle.

Cerebrospinal fluid protein—140.0 mg/100 ml.

Surgery—On August 15, 1972, a right translabyrinthine approach was utilized to totally remove a 2.5-cm acoustic neuroma. Her operative course was uneventful. Estimated blood loss 1,000 cc, with blood replacement of 1,000 cc. Facial nerve integrity was preserved.

Postoperative course—Her course was smooth. Total facial paralysis was present in the immediate postoperative period. Four years postoperatively, she had approximately three-quarters of facial nerve return of function on the operated side and is able to close her eye.

Comment—In spite of only a 3-month history of hearing loss, this patient had a large tumor that was extending to involve the fifth cranial nerve. Unilateral sensorineural hearing loss, abnormal x-rays, and electronystagmography all pointed to the possibility of a cerebellopontine angle lesion. This was confirmed by Pantopaque study.

CASE 300

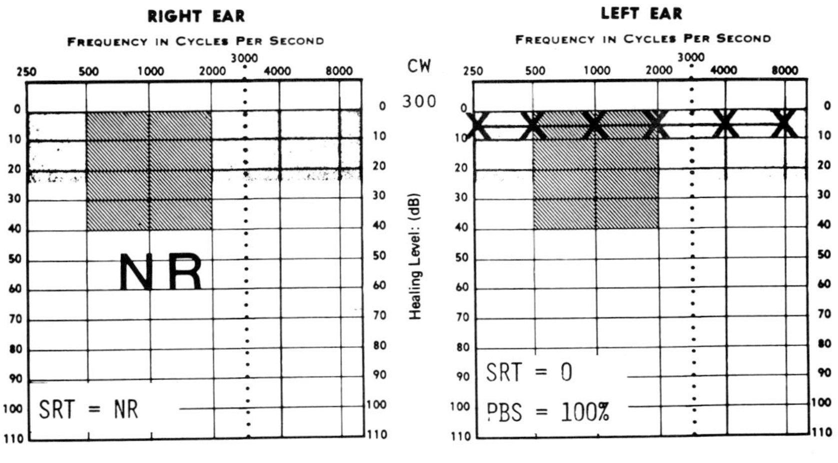

Summary—Hearing loss on the right side for one and a half years, associated with tinnitus. Translabyrinthine approach was accomplished for total removal of the tumor.

History—This 19-year-old student experienced a gradual hearing loss on the right side associated with a high-pitched tinnitus. Her balance was quite good except during sudden changes in position or during bouts of fatique, when she noticed some unsteadiness.

Examination—Normal except for eighth nerve findings.

Eighth nerve findings—No response in the right ear.

Cerebrospinal fluid protein—44 mg/100 ml.

Vestibular—Reduced vestibular response on the right, 53%.

Petrous pyramid x-rays—Right internal auditory canal enlarged.

Pantopaque—Filling defect on the right measuring 1.5 cm.

Surgery—A 1.5-cm acoustic tumor was totally removed via the translabyrinthine approach. It appeared that the tumor arose from the inferior vestibular nerve. No vital sign changes during surgery. Blood loss was approximately 250 cc. Facial nerve was preserved.

Comment—This young adult had a short history of symptoms; however, the hearing loss progressed rapidly. All tests were abnormal, presumptive evidence of a cerebellopontine angle lesion.

CASE 307

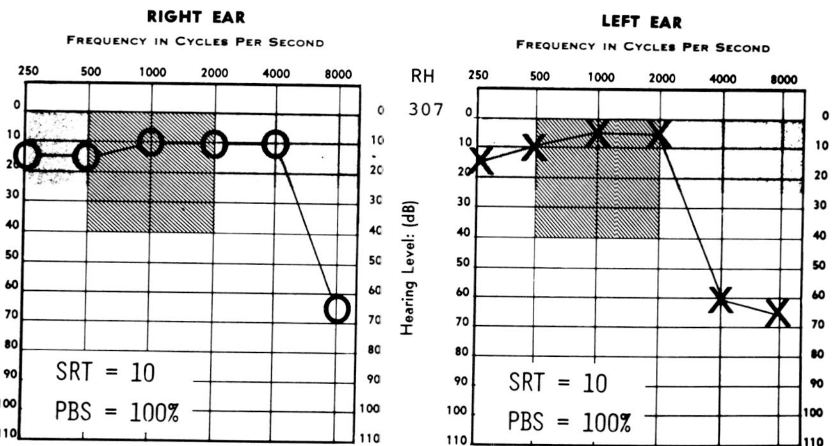

Summary—Progressive hearing loss on the left. Translabyrinthine removal of acoustic neuroma, left.

History—This 54-year-old woman was first seen September 4, 1970, with fullness and tinnitus in the left ear. There was some slight unsteadiness for about 9 months. There had been no hearing loss. Initially, her hearing was normal. Electronystagmography showed normally functioning vestibular systems bilaterally, and there were no abnormalities detected on petrous pyramid x-rays. She was treated with vasodilator medications and seen 1 year later, at which time she was still slightly unsteady. There were no objective changes. On October 20, 1972, she was seen for progressive hearing loss on the left and at that time had a 52 dB flat sensorineural hearing loss with 28% discrimination. Petrous pyramid x-rays were again normal. However, electronystagmography at this time revealed 100% reduced vestibular response on the left. Pantopaque study was performed, confirming a filling defect on the left.

Examination—Normal save for eighth nerve findings.

Eighth nerve findings—Initially, normal hearing on the left, progressing over 2 years to a flat 52 dB sensorineural hearing loss with 28% discrimination.

Vestibular—Initially, normally functioning vestibular system; within 2 years, 100% reduced vestibular response, left.

Petrous pyramid x-rays—Normal.

Pantopaque—1.5-cm filling defect, left cerebellopontine angle.

Cerebrospinal fluid protein—50 mg/100 ml.

Surgery—On January 2, 1973, a left translabyrinthine total removal of a 1.1-cm acoustic neuroma was performed uneventfully. Estimated blood loss was approximately 700 cc. There was no blood replacement. Facial nerve integrity was maintained. Postoperatively, there was 75% facial paresis on the left that recovered in 1 year with only a trace of mass action.

Comment—This patient demonstrates insidious onset of an acoustic neuroma. When she was initially seen, with symptoms of fullness in the left ear and unsteadiness, all tests were normal. Over a period of 2 years, hearing loss was demonstrable on the left and great reduction in vestibular response on the left was detected on repeat electronystagmography. This patient demonstrates well the need for follow-up examination and repeat testing if indicated.

CASE 312

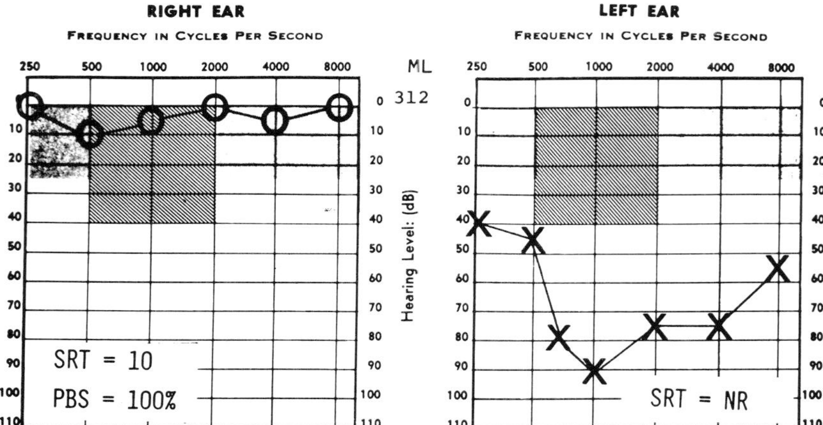

Summary—Three and a half year history of hearing loss on the left. Large acoustic neuroma was removed from the left cerebellopontine angle in a two-stage translabyrinthine removal.

History—This 42-year-old man had noticed a hearing loss on the left side of three and a half years' duration with occasional tinnitus. He had had no unsteadiness.

Examination—Normal except for eighth nerve findings.

Eighth nerve findings—Trough-shaped 70 dB sensorineural hearing loss with 0% discrimination, type III Bekesy, and 0% SISI, left.

Vestibular—100% reduced vestibular response on the left and 7° of spontaneous nystagmus to the right.

Petrous pyramid x-rays—Enlarged internal auditory canal on the left.

Pantopaque—2- to 3-cm filling defect, left cerebellopontine angle.

Surgery—On January 15, 1973, this patient underwent a left translabyrinthine acoustic tumor removal. After removal of approximately 60% of the tumor mass and elevation of the posterior inferior lobe of the tumor, his blood pressure increased to 180 mm Hg systolic. All cottonoids were removed and his systolic blood pressure decreased to 150 mm Hg. On further manipulation, the identical blood pressure changes occurred. Therefore, surgery was terminated at this point, and plans were made for a second stage later for total removal. He had approximately 50% facial paresis on the left following this initial surgery. On June 28, 1973, he underwent second-stage translabyrinthine removal of acoustic neuroma. Total removal of the tumor was accomplished, with 1,400 cc of blood lost, and 1,500 cc of blood replaced. Only two brief episodes of blood pressure elevation to 140 mm Hg were encountered.

Postoperative course—He did well. Facial nerve function, which had returned to normal prior to the second stage, remained normal postoperatively.

Comment—This patient had a rather typical history for an acoustic neuroma. Unpredictably, he demonstrated significant vital sign changes during his first operation. At this point, surgery was terminated, with a second stage planned in 4 to 6 months. Usually, at the second operation manipulations identical to those that provided significant vital sign changes in the first surgery can be performed without significant recurrence of the problem and total removal may be accomplished.

CASE 320

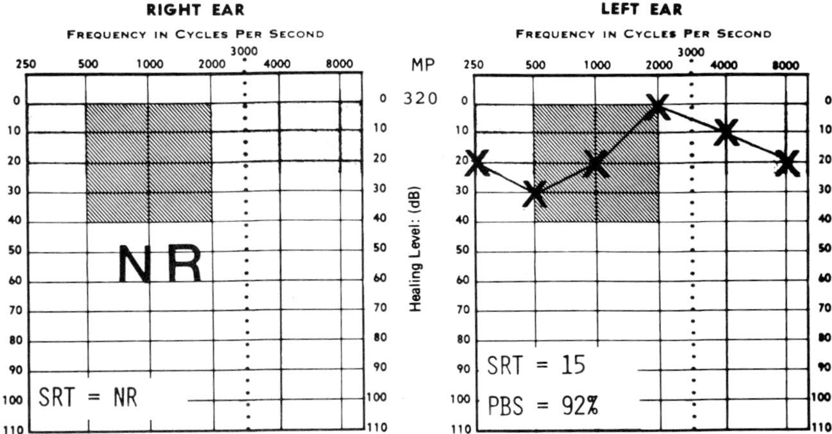

Summary—Gradual hearing loss, right, associated with tinnitus for 5 years. Translabyrinthine approach with total removal.

History—This 43-year-old woman noted that she had not been able to use the telephone on the right side for about 5 years. The hearing loss was associated with severe tinnitus on the same side. She had not suffered from unsteadiness.

Examination—Normal except for signs related to the fifth and eighth nerves.

Eighth nerve findings—No response in the right ear.

Fifth nerve findings—Hypesthesia over the right cheek and a decreased corneal reflex on the right.

Cerebrospinal fluid protein—70 mg/100 ml.

Vestibular—Reduced vestibular response on the right, 55%.

Petrous pyramid x-rays—Normal.

Pantopaque—There was a filling defect on the right measuring approximately 2 cm.

Surgery—A total tumor removal was accomplished via the translabyrinthine approach. The facial nerve was preserved.

Comment—While a significant hearing loss was present, the x-rays were normal. However, a significant reduced vestibular response in the absence of dizziness suggested a cerebellopontine angle lesion. This was confirmed by Pantopaque study.

CASE 340

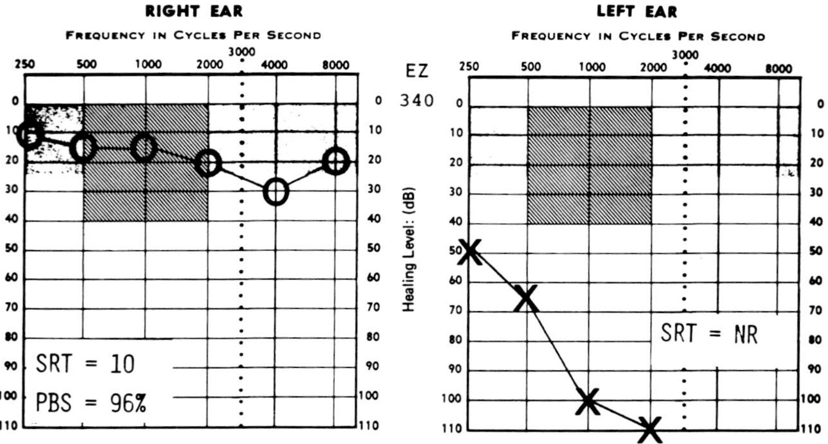

Summary—Hearing loss in the left ear for 5 years. Translabyrinthine approach on two occasions: a partial, then a total, removal of an acoustic tumor.

History—This 43-year-old man developed an insidious onset of hearing loss on the right side that was first interpreted as Meniere's disease. He was given several histamine treatments that were of little help. The hearing loss fluctuated but the general course was progressive. He experienced some imbalance.

Examination—Normal except for signs related to eighth nerve findings.

Eighth nerve findings—Pure tone 92 dB, no discrimination, Bekesy type III, SISI 500-0%, tone decay 500-45.

Cerebrospinal fluid protein—340 mg/100 ml

Petrous pyramid x-rays—Both internal auditory canals appeared larger than normal, the left showing questionable inferior lip erosion.

Pantopaque—Filling defect on the left, measuring approximately 3 cm.

Surgery—Stage one: On June 13, 1973, a translabyrinthine approach was carried out. The tumor was very extensively gutted so that the capsule collapsed quite well. During an attempt to remove the tumor from the posterior superior pole, the blood pressure went up rather precipitously from 110 to 160. On removal of the packs, the pressure gradually came back down. There were no respiratory changes. Because of the vascularity of the tumor and because of its adherence to surrounding structures, it was decided to do a partial removal at that time. It was necessary to place one pack of Surgicel along the inferior pole, where a rather large vein was located. The tumor in the internal auditory canal was not removed. Fat was taken from the abdomen and packed over the opening in the dura. Stage two: On November 7, 1973, the previous postauricular incision was opened and the fat was removed from the cavity. It was possible to obtain total tumor removal without vital sign changes. There was considerable bleeding during the procedure, about 2,500 cc in toto, which was replaced during the operation.

Comment—This patient initially presented with symptoms suggestive of endolymphatic hydrops (Meniere's disorder). However, examination with audiometric, vestibular, and radiographic testing pointed to a cerebellopontine angle lesion etiology. The surgical course illustrates the difficulties that may be encountered in the large tumor removals.

CASE 367

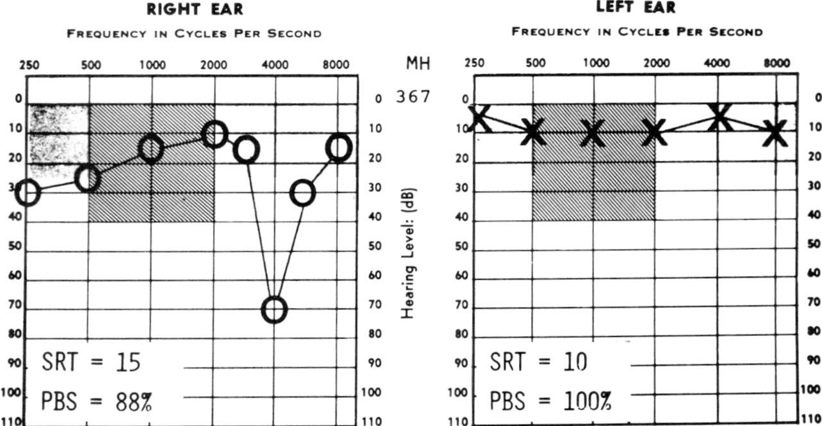

Summary—Hearing loss on the right for 1 year with dizziness for 3 months. Total removal of a right acoustic neuroma was accomplished by the translabyrinthine approach.

History—This 40-year-old woman had noted some constant unsteadiness with positional aggravation for 3 months. She had noticed her hearing on the right had been less acute over the telephone for the past year. Tinnitus was present constantly on the right.

Examination—Normal save for eighth nerve findings.

Eighth nerve findings—15 dB speech reception threshold on the right with 88% discrimination. Marked 4,000 cycle dip to 70 dB.

Vestibular—100% reduced vestibular response on the right with 3.5° of spontaneous nystagmus to the left.

Petrous pyramid x-rays—Enlarged internal auditory canal on the right.

Pantopaque—1.5-cm filling defect, right cerebellopontine angle.

Surgery—On July 26, 1973, a right translabyrinthine removal of an acoustic neuroma was performed. Total removal of a 1.5-cm tumor, with preservation of the facial nerve, was effected. Estimated blood loss was 500 cc. There was no blood replacement. There were no vital sign changes during surgery.

Postoperative course—Uneventful save for immediate onset of complete paralysis of the right facial nerve, which necessitated spring insertion for eyelid closure. After 2 years, she had minimal voluntary function of the right face.

Comment—In spite of minimal sensorineural hearing loss on the right, electronystagmography and petrous pyramid x-rays substantiated the likelihood of a cerebellopontine angle lesion on the right side. This was confirmed by Pantopaque studies.

CASE 395

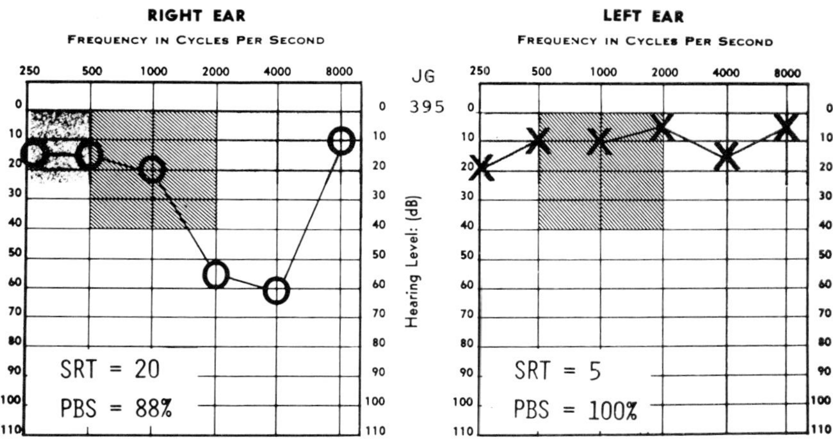

Summary—Hearing loss on the right of 6 months' duration. Intracanalicular tumor removed via the middle fossa approach with preservation of hearing.

History—This 28-year-old man noticed a hearing loss on the right side of 6 months' duration with intermittent tinnitus. He had previous noise exposure with heavy machinery. He did not notice any imbalance.

Examination—Normal save for eighth nerve findings.

Eighth nerve findings—20 dB SRT with 88% discrimination, right, but with marked 4,000 cycle dip to 60 dB.

Vestibular—28% reduced vestibular response on the right (within normal range).

Petrous pyramid x-rays—Enlarged internal auditory canal, right.

Pantopaque—Intracanalicular filling defect, right internal auditory canal.

Surgery—On December 13, 1973, a middle fossa removal of a 1-cm acoustic neruoma was performed on the right. The tumor appeared to originate from the inferior vestibular nerve. Facial nerve integrity was preserved. Estimated blood loss was 450 cc. There were no vital sign changes.

Postoperative course—Uneventful, with normal facial nerve function and preservation of hearing.

Comment—Short duration of symptoms in a young man with an audiogram highly reminiscent of noise trauma to the ear. In spite of the small lesion in this instance, petrous pyramid x-rays revealed an enlarged internal auditory canal on the involved side. The normal vestibular test results are typical of lesions originating from the inferior vestibular nerve. This patient illustrates the ideal to which we aim: early diagnosis of a small lesion that can be removed via the middle cranial fossa with preservation of serviceable hearing.

CASE 428

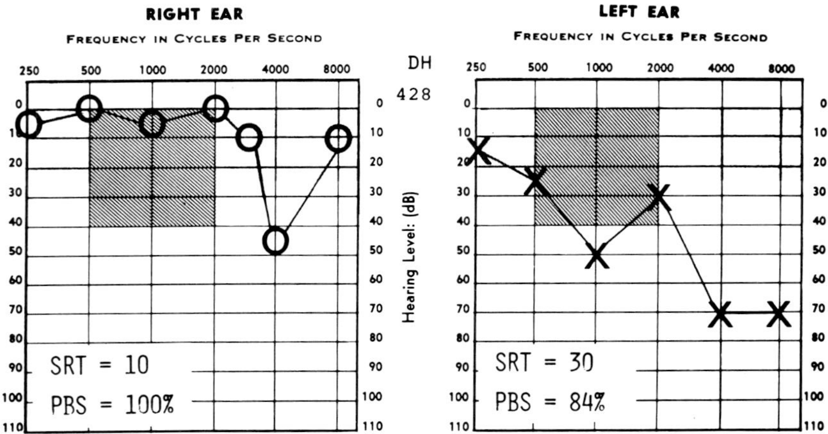

Summary—Hearing loss on the left side for 1 year. Middle fossa removal of an acoustic neuroma was performed with preservation of hearing.

History—This 35-year-old man noticed a mild hearing loss on the left side 1 year prior to his initial visit. He had noticed constant tinnitus but no unsteadiness.

Examination—Normal save for eighth nerve findings on the left.

Eighth nerve findings—Sloping 30 dB sensorineural hearing loss with 84% discrimination, left.

Vestibular—63% reduced vestibular response on the left with 3.5° of spontaneous nystagmus to the left.

Petrous pyramid x-rays—Enlarged internal auditory canal on the left.

Pantopaque—Intracanalicular lesion on the left.

Surgery—On April 18, 1974, a left middle fossa total removal of an 8-mm acoustic neuroma was performed. It appeared to originate from the superior vestibular nerve. There were no vital sign changes during surgery. Approximately 600 cc of blood loss with no blood replacement.

Postoperative course—Uneventful, with preservation of hearing at the preoperative level and normal facial nerve function.

Comment—In spite of this lesion being small, all routine tests were suggestive of an acoustic tumor. The removal of the tumor with preservation of serviceable hearing represents an ideal situation.

CASE 436

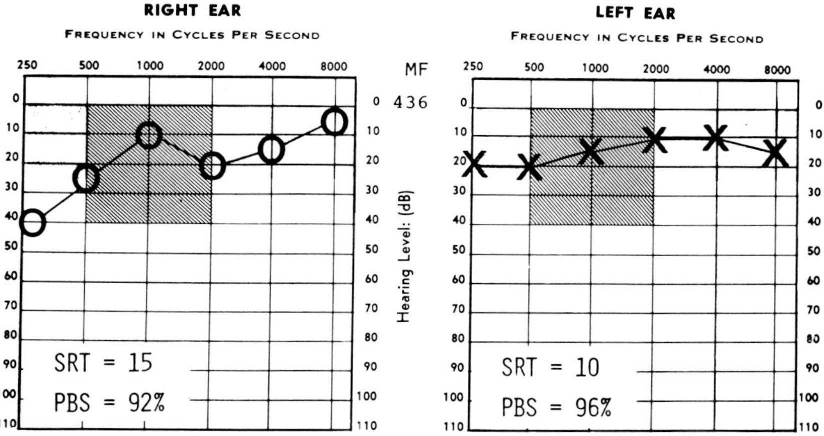

Summary—Hearing loss on the right of 9 months' duration, only noticed on the telephone. Total removal of a large acoustic neuroma by the translabyrinthine approach was accomplished.

History—This 20-year-old woman had noticed a hearing loss of 9 months' duration only in telephone conversations. She noticed some numbness in the right gums and cheek of about a year's duration and occasional positional dizziness.

Examination—Revealed bilateral early papilledema.

Eighth nerve findings—15 dB SRT, right, with 92% discrimination with only minimal low frequency sensorineural hearing loss.

Vestibular—81% reduced vestibular response on the right.

Petrous pyramid x-rays—Enlarged right internal auditory canal.

Pantopaque—Revealed a well-circumscribed 4.0-cm filling defect in the right cerebellopontine angle.

Surgery—On May 3, 1974, a 4.5-cm acoustic neuroma was totally removed via the right translabyrinthine approach. The tumor was very adherent to the cerebellum and brainstem. There was approximately 1,500 cc of blood loss and 1,000 cc of blood replacement. Facial nerve was preserved intact.

Postoperative course—Uneventful. Postoperatively she had an immediate complete facial paralysis on the operated side, with some recovery at 18 months, including the ability to close the eye, but voluntary facial function was absent.

Comment—This patient illustrates the presence of a large tumor in a young adult with a very short symptomatic history. The inability to hear on the telephone despite good hearing on the involved side has been encountered on several occasions in patients with acoustic tumors. In spite of essentially normal hearing, electronystagmography and petrous pyramid x-rays were abnormal, thereby substantiating the likely diagnosis of a cerebellopontine angle lesion. In this patient, angiography was performed in lieu of posterior fossa Pantopaque study because of bilateral papilledema indicative of increased intracranial pressure.

ACKNOWLEDGMENTS

I am most grateful to Ms. Nanette Teausant for her help in acquiring the data for this chapter. To Mr. Lawrence Irwin, Ms. Annette Florance, and Ms. Cynthia Smith for their help in manuscript preparation, and to Mrs. Diane Churchill, who prepared the audiometric illustrations for publication, my sincere thanks.

REFERENCES

1. Dykstra, P. C. 1964. The pathology of acoustic neuromas. Arch. Otolaryngol. 80:605–616.
2. Murray, M. R., and Stout, A. P. 1942. Demonstration of formation of reticulin by Schwannian tumor cells *in vitro*. Amer. J. Pathol. 18:585–589.
3. Linthicum, F. H. Personal communication.
4. Nager, G. 1964. Association of bilateral VIIIth nerve tumors with meningiomas in von Recklinghausen's disease. Laryngoscope 74:1220.
5. House, W. F. Personal communication.
6. House, W. F. 1968. Case summaries. Arch. Otolaryngol. 88:586–591.
7. Sheehy, J. L. 1968. The neuro-otologic evaluation. Arch. Otolaryngol. 88:592–597.
8. House, W. F. (Ed.) 1964. Transtemporal bone microsurgical removal of acoustic neuromas. Arch. Otolaryngol. 80:597–796.

9. House, W. F. (Ed.) 1968. Monograph II: Acoustic Neuroma. Arch. Otolaryngol. 88:575–718.
10. Sheehy, J. L., and Inser, B. E. 1977. Acoustic reflex test in neuro-otologic diagnosis. Arch. Otolaryngol. 103:152–158.
11. Selters, W. A., and Brackmann, D. E. 1977. Acoustic tumor detection with brain stem electrical response audiometry. Arch. Otolaryngol. 103:181–187.
12. Linthicum, F. H., and Churchill, D. 1968. Vestibular test results in acoustic tumor cases. Arch. Otolaryngol. 88:604–607.
13. Scanlan, R. L. 1964. Positive contrast medium (iophendylate) in diagnosis of acoustic neuroma. Arch. Otolaryngol. 80:698–706.

Acoustic Tumors
Volume I, *Diagnosis*
Edited by W. F. House and C. M. Luetje

Chapter 8

Neuro-Otologic Evaluation

James L. Sheehy, M.D.*

Clinical Professor of Otorhinolaryngology, University of Southern California School of Medicine, Los Angeles; also, Affiliated with the Ear Research Institute and the Otologic Medical Group, Inc., Los Angeles

---

Eighth nerve symptoms, with rare exceptions, are the first indication of a developing acoustic tumor. A high index of suspicion combined with a thorough neuro-otologic evaluation should make diagnosis of this tumor possible when it is relatively small; ideally, when it is still localized to the internal auditory canal.

This chapter describes neuro-otologic evaluation, details of which appear in subsequent chapters. This chapter also discusses the symptoms produced by this histologically benign but clinically malignant tumor.

SYMPTOMATOLOGY

An acoustic tumor produces symptoms and findings by pressure on both blood vessels and nerve tissue and, when it is quite large, by blocking the cerebrospinal fluid (CSF) absorption mechanism. When they result from

* Mailing address: 256 South Lake Street, Los Angeles, California 90057

interference with blood supply, these symptoms and findings may be of dramatically sudden onset, simulating a cochlear or inner ear problem or basilar vertebral insufficiency. Accordingly, they may fluctuate or they may seem to respond to medical treatment.

The symptoms resulting from pressure on neural tissue may be insidious and difficult to detect in the early phases if the physician does not maintain a high index of suspicion. An example of this type of symptom is severe impairment of discrimination, which may develop before evidence of pure tone threshold shift, or the finding of an almost functionless vestibular labyrinth in an individual with normal hearing and little or no history of unsteadiness.

An acoustic tumor may grow to a moderate size without producing striking symptoms in one patient, yet it may produce a multitude of symptoms (and findings), despite its small size, in another patient. There is no typical clinical pattern (1).

Every patient who has "inner ear" symptoms should be suspected of having an acoustic tumor. These symptoms may be minimal (unilateral tinnitus), may be typical of an end-organ disturbance (Meniere's disease, cochlear hydrops), or may be of sudden onset (so-called vascular accident of the inner ear). Each demands a complete evaluation: auditory, vestibular, neurological, and roentgenographic. Only in this way can an acoustic tumor be diagnosed early, while it is still confined to the internal auditory canal.

AUDITORY FINDINGS

Auditory symptoms and findings are the first to develop in most acoustic tumor cases.

Symptoms

We suspect that tinnitus is often the earliest symptom of an acoustic tumor, even though only 11% of our patients reported it as such. Over 80% had tinnitus when the tumor was diagnosed.

Unilateral hearing impairment may develop gradually or suddenly, and the hearing may fluctuate. Often there is a more marked discrimination impairment than one would anticipate from the pure tone threshold. We have also seen acoustic tumor cases with normal hearing for pure tones but no discrimination.

Evaluation

Auditory evaluation of inner ear problems involves, besides pure tone audiometry, a determination of speech discrimination and tests for auditory fatigue and loudness function. Characteristically in cases of acoustic tumor one would expect a unilateral sensorineural hearing impairment with poorer speech discrimination than would be anticipated from the pure tone findings, abnormal auditory fatigue or adaptation (tone decay), and normal loudness function (absence of recruitment) (2).

During the early 1960s, as otologists were becoming more alert to the diagnosis of acoustic tumors, the Bekesy and small increment sensitivity index (SISI) tests were used regularly in this evaluation. One anticipated a type III or IV Bekesy audiogram with a low SISI score. Unfortunately, only 47% of the first 500 acoustic tumor cases operated at the Otologic Medical Group, Inc., showed the anticipated auditory responses to all tests. In large tumors, 63% had classic auditory findings (2).

When impedance audiometry came into use as a routine clinical test, it became apparent that the acoustic reflex text was a rapid, inexpensive, easily performed objective test for both auditory fatigue and loudness function. Furthermore, this test yielded a higher percentage of positive results than other auditory tests (1).

As a result of these findings, in 1975 we discontinued the routine use of Bekesy and SISI tests in the neuro-otologic evaluation of cases with suspected tumors. Impedance audiometry was used whenever the hearing level was 75 dB or less or 500 and 1,000 Hz. Eighty-eight percent of confirmed tumor cases tested since 1975 showed absence or decay of the acoustic reflex.

A recent addition to the battery of auditory tests is brainstem electric response audiometry (BERA). Responses have been positive (wave V delayed or absent) in over 95% of the acoustic tumor cases tested to date. BERA is currently being performed on all confirmed tumors prior to surgery (for test evaluation purposes) and on all cases in which the routine neuro-otologic evaluation leaves us with considerable doubt about the presence of a tumor (3).

Summary

When a patient develops unilateral tinnitus or unilateral sensorineural hearing impairment, he is immediately suspected of having an acoustic tumor unless the onset is quite clearly associated with acoustic trauma, head injury, mumps, or some acute infectious disease. Even then one should not rule out this possibility. Unusually severe discrimination impairment or acoustic reflex decay should make the clinician even more suspicious of a retrocochlear etiology. It is necessary to look at the overall pattern of the auditory test battery.

VESTIBULAR FINDINGS

Vestibular symptoms are present in 69% of our acoustic tumor cases and are recorded as the initial symptom in 11%. Vestibular dysfunction, however, is not always present in these cases.

Symptoms

The vestibular system is capable of a limited number of responses (i.e., vertigo, unsteadiness) to a wide variety of stimuli. Furthermore, a clinical picture may be confused by the rather rapid suppression of symptoms. An example of this is the long-standing minimal unsteadiness that may follow a sudden episode of vertigo in an individual with progressive vestibular paralysis from a tumor.

The presence of any symptoms from the vestibular apparatus and its central connections warrants an evaluation. At one time we were content to make the diagnosis of Meniere's disease without complete evaluation in cases of episodic vertigo associated with fluctuating low-tone sensorineural hearing impairment and tinnitus. We have since learned that an acoustic tumor may produce just these symptoms. Similarly, in the past we frequently did not thoroughly evaluate the patient with episodic vertigo and normal hearing, or the older individual with presbycusis and persistent postural vertigo or unsteadiness. Acoustic tumors may also produce these symptoms.

There are no typical symptoms from the vestibular apparatus or pathways that clearly differentiate, by themselves, between a peripheral and central origin of the symptoms. Although episodic vertigo and the syndrome of benign paroxysmal nystagmus are usually of peripheral origin, each case requires a complete evaluation if we are to pinpoint the cause of the dizziness and diagnose the early acoustic tumor.

The most common vestibular symptom in our confirmed tumor cases is unsteadiness, present in 65%. A "Dizziness Questionnaire" (4) is helpful in bringing symptoms to light. It may also help the patient to recall any auditory or neurological symptoms that may have been overshadowed by more recent developments in his symptomatology.

Evaluation

Evaluation of the vestibular apparatus, as it relates to a cerebellopontine angle lesion, is performed primarily to determine the presence or absence of function. We use electronystagmography.

A reduced or absent vestibular response on one side is found in the majority of acoustic tumor cases. Unfortunately, there are other conditions that may produce similar results: vestibular neuronitis syndrome, "vascular accident" of the inner ear, and Meniere's disease. Therefore, this finding is not diagnostic of an acoustic tumor but merely an anticipated finding, fitting into the overall clinical picture.

Normal vestibular findings suggest that the problem at hand is not an acoustic tumor, but they do not rule out the possibility of this or some other cerebellopontine angle lesion. Over 50% of our small tumors have vestibular responses within the range of normal.

Summary

Every patient with unilateral sensorineural hearing impairment or symptoms from the vestibular pathways should have his vestibular apparatus tested in an appropriate manner. A reduced response is found in 82% of acoustic tumor cases.

NEUROLOGICAL FINDINGS

An acoustic tumor will produce easily recognizable neurological symptoms and findings as it enlarges to involve other cranial nerves, the brainstem, and the cerebellum. Our objective is to make the diagnosis before the tumor reaches such proportions, and thereby greatly decrease the mortality and morbidity associated with the surgery.

The reader should note that in this text about 50% of our cases do not have any objective neurological findings aside from those of the eighth nerve. When there are such findings, they may be limited to the trigeminal nerve. This absence of neurologic signs is an indication of a high index of suspicion and of relatively early diagnosis. However, a careful neurological examination is important with regard to subsequent decisions in connection with the technique of radiographic examination and surgical approach to the tumor.

Symptoms

Many years ago it was unusual to diagnose an acoustic tumor before it had produced gross neurological signs and increased intracranial pressure. In fact, it was stated that the diagnosis could not be made prior to this time. As recently as 30 years ago it was thought that the diagnosis should not be made until there was total deafness, loss of all labyrinthine function, and cerebellar signs. Twenty years ago it was frequently difficult to find a neurosurgeon who would operate on an acoustic tumor (or make a definite diagnosis) before the tumor had involved the trigeminal nerve and produced an elevated CSF protein. This hesitancy to make the diagnosis or to operate was related to both the lack of diagnostic tools and the rather significant morbidity and mortality associated with surgery.

We still see patients with gross neurological symptoms due to acoustic tumors, but these findings are not common in the otologist's practice. It is nonetheless important to query the patient regarding facial numbness, clumsiness, difficulty with speech or swallowing, and headache. These questions have been incorporated into the Dizziness Questionnaire (4). These symptoms, confirmed by examination, more clearly establish the diagnosis in questionable cases and help to indicate the size of the tumor.

Examination

The otologist must develop the habit of performing a neurological examination of the cranial nerves and cerebellum as part of his routine evaluation of any patient presenting with "inner ear" symptoms, insignificant as they may seem. The otologist is in the fortunate position of being able to do much of this routinely in connection with his examination of the tongue, palate, throat, and larynx (ninth, tenth, and twelfth nerves).

The otologist must take time to test corneal sensitivity in all such patients. The trigeminal nerve is the first nerve outside the internal auditory canal to become involved as the tumor enlarges.

The otologist must become proficient with the ophthalmoscope. Patients complaining of dizziness or headache should have the eyegrounds observed for papilledema and nystagmus. When nystagmus is observed, the vestibular testing will require electronystagmography for accuracy. If papilledema is noted, neurological consultation is indicated.

The cerebellar tests usually performed are the finger-to-nose and the Romberg. Positive findings may suggest a large tumor or a brainstem or cerebellar problem.

A determination of the CSF protein is normally deferred until the time of posterior fossa myelography. This used to be considered a good preliminary screening test, but we have learned that the protein is within the normal range in 48% of our acoustic tumor cases (80% of small tumors). Even when CSF protein is elevated, there are usually many other findings that more clearly indicate the presence of a cerebellopontine angle tumor.

Finally, the facial nerve should be mentioned. For some reason not completely clear, facial weakness of a magnitude to be observed clinically is a late finding, despite the fact that the nerve is involved early by the tumor in the internal auditory canal. This early involvement may be

Chapter 9

Results of Auditory Tests in Acoustic Tumor Patients

E. W. Johnson, Ph.D.*

Director of Audiology, Otologic Medical Group, Inc., Los Angeles; also, Affiliated with the Ear Research Institute, Los Angeles

---

Audiology has made significant contributions to the differential diagnosis of acoustic tumors. The first written report on the auditory aspects of acoustic tumors is credited to Gradenigo (1) in 1893. He wrote that a vibrating tuning fork could be heard for only a few seconds in patients with acoustic tumors.

Subsequent to this report of tone decay, Carhart (2), Hallpike and Hood (3), Pestalozza and Cioce (4), and Palva (5) established that excessive adaptation to a pure tone stimulus is frequently associated with retrocochlear lesions. The investigators described this phenomenon in

* Mailing address: 2122 West Third Street, Los Angeles, California 90057

various terms: e.g., abnormal adaptation, threshold shift, perstimulatory fatigue, or tone decay.

Review of the literature revealed that the early reports on auditory findings in acoustic tumors primarily noted unilateral sensorineural hearing impairment. Some investigators associated a particular type of frequency loss pattern with the presence of a tumor. Eggston and Wolff (6), Cambon and Guilford (7), and Schuknecht (8) equated low frequency loss and near normal high frequency patterns with the occurrence of acoustic tumors. The study of 500 cases of acoustic tumors upon which this text is based does not confirm this assumption.

The basic battery of audiologic tests in the differential diagnosis of acoustic tumors has changed through the years. Currently, the procedure that yields the highest degree of positive results in acoustic tumors is electric response audiometry (ERA). Ninety-eight percent of those patients who have been given electrocochleographic tests have had positive results. This type of testing is discussed in Chapter 10 of this book. The second highest positive finding at the present time is in the use of impedance audiometry. ERA and impedance audiometry were not available for a large part of this series of 500 cases. Tests that were of great importance in the early development of diagnostic testing for acoustic tumors were Bekesy audiometry, SISI tests, and alternate binaural loudness balance tests. These three tests are rarely, if ever, used at the present time in the differential diagnosis of this type of patient.

The first report of auditory results in a large series of cases in surgically confirmed acoustic tumors was in 1964 (9). The basic audiologic test battery at that time included pure tone air and bone conduction tests, speech tests, adaptation tests, including modified tone decay (MTDT) and Bekesy audiometry, and the short increment sensitivity index (SISI) test. Subsequent auditory findings for the same battery of tests were reported in additional studies with larger patient populations (10–12).

This chapter follows the same format in reporting on the basic audiologic test battery applied to this group of 500 surgically verified acoustic tumors. In addition, this study includes the results of impedance audiometry.

PROCEDURE

All patients in this series were given pure tone air and bone conduction tests and speech tests at the time of their original examination. In most instances, a MTDT test was also carried out. Whenever test results were equivocal, additional testing was carried out at the same visit. Most of the patients received plain x-ray studies, neuro-otologic examination, electronystagmography, and iophendylate posterior fossa myelography to complete their work-up. When all of the studies were completed, the diagnosis was confirmed, and the patient was scheduled for surgery, additional preoperative auditory tests were completed. These consisted of pure tone (air and bone) and speech tests in all cases. The MTDT tests were performed in many, but not all, cases. Bekesy and SISI tests were given in most cases with sufficient residual hearing to permit satisfactory test results. In a number of cases, repeat tests were spaced over a period of many months. In some patients test results changed from negative to positive during this time. Impedance audiometry was available only for the last 117 cases.

RESULTS

All patients in this series of 500 cases had unilateral sensorineural hearing impairments. Auditory tests were carried out in 499 of these 500 cases of unilateral acoustic tumors. One patient had been evaluated and diagnosed in another area of the country and reported directly to the hospital. Because surgery was carried out immediately, we have no auditory data on this patient.

Sixteen percent (78) of the 499 patients had a complete loss of hearing in the involved ear, and no auditory tests could be carried out. Other patients had great hearing losses that permitted only pure tone thresholds or pure tone and speech thresholds to be obtained. In some instances, patients could not repeat any spondee words but were able to respond to a number series. In those cases, an approximate threshold for speech was estimated.

PURE TONE PATTERNS

It was possible to obtain pure tone air conduction thresholds in 421 cases. The pure tone loss configuration was studied for each case to determine whether an important pattern would emerge. The audiograms were classified according to four different configuration groupings. A high tone loss was defined as a pattern that sloped from the low frequencies, with a loss of at least 25 dB, through the speech range and/or a total loss of hearing beyond 3,000 Hz. A pure tone pattern differing by not more than 10 dB through the speech range was classified as a flat type of loss. Configurations of good hearing in the high and low tones with elevated thresholds throughout the speech range were defined as

Table 1. Pure tone loss patterns (421 cases)

	N	Percent
High tone loss	275	65
Flat loss	92	22
Low tone loss	32	8
Trough-shaped loss	22	5

trough-shaped. Low tone loss patterns consisted of audiograms with reduced thresholds in the low frequencies and a rising curve into the speech range and the higher frequencies. All 421 cases could be classified into one of these four categories. An analysis of the pure tone loss pattern is shown in Table 1.

Sixty-five percent of the patients had a high frequency hearing loss. The second largest category was the flat type loss, accounting for approximately 22%. Low tone losses totaled 8% and trough losses were just 5%. In all of the previous studies, starting with the initial report of 53 cases (9), approximately two-thirds of all patients have fallen into the category of high frequency loss pattern.

Analysis of the pure tone loss patterns is interesting. Threshold pure tone ranged from 5 to 130 dB (no response). The mean pure tone threshold for the entire group was 66.52 dB. Table 2 relates the mean pure tone threshold to the pure tone pattern. No hearing was defined as no response to pure tones up to the limits of the audiometer at 130 dB. There were a few responses at 130 dB at some frequencies; these were considered to be in the no hearing category.

Table 3 relates pure tone pattern to the size of the tumor. The largest percentage of cases, whether the tumors were small, medium, or large, produced high frequency loss patterns. The data presented in Table

Table 2. Mean pure tone threshold related to pure tone pattern

Type of pattern	Mean pure tone threshold[a]
No hearing	129.59 dB
High	55.96 dB
Trough	54.18 dB
Low	56.72 dB
Flat	52.32 dB

[a] No hearing = no response to pure tones up to 130 dB.

Table 3. Pure tone pattern related to tumor size

Type of Pattern	Small N	Small Percent of total	Percent Small tumors	Medium N	Medium Percent of total	Percent Medium tumors	Large N	Large Percent of total	Percent Large tumors
No hearing	2	.4	7.7	25	5.1	8.4	47	9.6	27.6
High	11	2.2	42.3	196	39.8	66.2	66	13.4	38.8
Trough	2	.4	7.7	12	2.4	4.1	8	1.6	4.7
Low	1	.2	3.8	18	3.7	6.1	13	2.6	7.6
Flat	10	2.0	38.5	45	9.1	15.2	36	7.3	21.2

3 indicate a statistically significant relationship between the size of the tumor and the type of hearing loss pattern, with a probability level of .001, using a chi-square analysis.

Table 4 relates the mean pure tone threshold to the size of the tumor. The larger the tumor, the greater the mean pure tone threshold, as expected. There is a statistically significant relation between the size of the tumor and the pure tone loss threshold ($F = 15.13$, $P \leq .001$), using analysis of variance. This relation is probably due to the difference between the mean pure tone threshold for the large tumors and the smaller sizes.

SPEECH TEST RESULTS

Speech testing was carried out with spondee words taken from the W-1 word lists and monosyllabic words taken from the W-2 phonetically balanced (PB) word lists. Speech tests were accomplished in most instances by a tape recording (Los Angeles Foundation of Otology Tape Recording) (13). In a few cases the patient was unable to understand spondee words, and a number series was given by live voice to estimate the speech awareness level.

Table 4. Mean pure tone threshold related to size of tumor

Size of tumor	Mean pure tone threshold (dB)[a]
Small	59.35
Medium	60.31
Large	77.68

[a] NR = 130 dB.

In some instances of slight to moderate pure tone hearing loss, the patient was unable to establish a speech recognition threshold (SRT) and produced 0% discrimination for the PB word lists. One patient established a pure tone threshold of 25 dB with an SRT of 35 dB and a PB score of 0%. Another high frequency loss case had a pure tone average of 18 dB throughout the speech range. An SRT was established at approximately 30 dB, but the patient did not understand PB words at any level of the audiometer. In a third instance, a pure tone threshold that averaged 13 dB resulted in an SRT of 27 dB and a PB score of only 4%.

Table 5 is a summary of the speech discrimination test results in 418 cases. PB scores were divided into four groupings. The first group consisted of patients unable to understand any of the PB words. The second classification was made up of patients with very poor discrimination (from 2 to 30%). The third group classified patients with poor to moderate understanding (from 32 to 60%). The last category groups patients with moderate to excellent understanding (from 62 to 100%). This classification system follows the format of the 1964 study (9).

Patients with 0% discrimination account for one-fourth of the patients with speech test results. If patients with no hearing response are added to this group, 180 of the 499 cases had 0% discrimination.

The group of patients in the category for poor speech (2 to 30%) totals 15%. If we combine this group with the patients with 0% discrimination (including those with no auditory responses), nearly half of all patients in the study would be classified as having poor discrimination for speech. On the other hand, 44% of the testable patients fell in the category of good to excellent discrimination for speech. This is a marked change from earlier studies. In this recent series of cases, there are fewer patients with poor speech results and a larger number of patients with good to excellent test results.

The mean speech discrimination score for all the patients with speech tests was 47.2%.

Table 5. Speech discrimination results (418 cases)

Discrimination score	*N*	Percent of total
0%	102	24
2–30%	64	15
32–60%	70	17
62–100%	182	44

BEKESY AUDIOMETRY RESULTS

Bekesy audiometry was an important part of the early diagnostic differentiation of retrocochlear lesions. With the advent of impedance audiometry and electric response audiometry, Bekesy tests became less important. Today we rarely, if ever, use Bekesy audiometry in the differential diagnosis of the patient.

The standard procedure in Bekesy testing was to administer the test on the first visit to the office and on the preoperative visit. Sweep-frequency tracings were routinely run. If these results were not clear cut, discrete tracings were run for several frequencies. This was particularly applicable if differentiation between type II and type IV tracing proved difficult. Tracings that would not easily fit into the four patterns originally suggested by Jerger were not unusual. We concluded that, in Bekesy testing, the point of the gap between pulsed and continuous tracings was relatively unimportant, but that the size of that gap should determine its classification.

In this series, 313 patients received Bekesy tests. Classification of the Bekesy audiograms is shown in Table 6.

An analysis of the 313 cases reveals that roughly 40% were type III or IV. This may be compared with our first reports in 1964 of over 70% of the patients in the type III or IV Bekesy category. By far the largest category in the present series (over 50%) is the type II tracing.

Follow-up of a number of cases postponed or delayed for surgery revealed a dramatic change in Bekesy tracings. One case changed from a type II to type IV; several cases changed from a type IV to a type III.

From these data we concluded that Bekesy audiometry can no longer be considered definitive in the diagnosis of this type of problem.

SISI TEST SCORES

SISI tests, like Bekesy audiometry, are no longer consistently given to the suspected acoustic tumor patient. The positive results of SISI test

Table 6. Bekesy audiometry results (313 cases)

Type	*N*	Percent of total
I	21	7
II	163	52
III	70	22
IV	59	19

Table 7. SISI test scores (340 cases)

Discrimination score	N	Percent of total
0–30%	190	56
35–65	29	8
70–100	121	36

scores are higher than our Bekesy findings; nevertheless, there has been a dramatic change since the early reports on auditory findings in acoustic tumors. In the early studies, over 70% of all cases were classified as low SISI scores, compared to only 56% in this latest study. SISI test scores for 340 cases are shown in Table 7.

In administering the SISI tests, several frequencies were tested, because sometimes low SISI scores are produced at some frequencies and at other times high scores are produced at other frequencies. One patient responded with a 0% SISI score at 2,000 Hz and a 60% score at 4,000 Hz. In another example, 0% SISI scores were obtained at 500 and 1,000 Hz and a 90% score was obtained at 2,000 Hz. There were just enough cases of this type to make testing of two and usually three frequencies imperative.

SISI tests were routinely administered for higher frequencies, unless the audiogram of the patient prohibited testing for those frequencies. In this event, the test would be administered at 750 or 500 Hz.

In this study, more than a third of the patients scored in the high categories of 70 to 100%, that is, categories usually associated with cochlear type lesions. Only slightly more than half of the patients fell, as anticipated, in the category of 0 to 30%. We felt that this test, like the Bekesy test, was no longer of high significance in the differential diagnosis of the acoustic tumor.

TONE DECAY RESULTS

For the last 15 years we have routinely administered a tone decay test to every new patient with a unilateral sensorineural hearing impairment. This test, in addition to pure tone air and bone tests and speech tests, has been an integral part of the work-up of every new patient.

The tone decay procedure was based on Green's MTDT (14). This procedure is adequate as a screening device and is easily and quickly administered. Tone decay tests were carried out at two or more frequencies. The test results verified Owens' (15) report that tone decay was

Table 8. Tone decay test results (329 cases)

Tone decay	N	Percent of total
Negative	77	23
Partial	115	35
Complete	137	42

present at all frequencies tested when hearing loss was present. Tone decay results are shown in Table 8.

Forty-two percent of the patients had complete tone decay at the frequencies tested. An additional 35% of the patients had partial tone decay. Combining partial and complete tone decay, a total of 77%, or 252 patients, exhibited a degree of tone decay. The positive results on the tone decay test (partial and complete) were considerably higher than the positive results on the Bekesy tests. This is a deviation from previous acoustic tumor studies showing relatively good agreement between Bekesy tests and tone decay tests. All of the type III Bekesy cases did have complete tone decay. A number of patients, however, had both complete tone decay and partial tone decay that traced a type II Bekesy pattern.

Continuance of the tone decay test as a screening procedure in all new unilateral sensorineural impairments is desirable.

ABLB TEST RESULTS

The ABLB (Alternate Bilateral Loudness Balance) tests are no longer routinely carried out in suspected tumor cases. Approximately one-third of the patients in the early part of the series were given ABLB tests. The results of the ABLB tests are shown in Table 9.

The anticipated ABLB results of negative findings occurred in approximately 50% of the cases. It should be noted that 30% of the patients tested had complete recruitment on the ABLB tests. This is

Table 9. ABLB test results (148 cases)

Findings	N	Percent of total
Negative	73	49
Partial	30	21
Complete	45	30

consistent with the increased number of type II Bekesy patterns in this series and also with the 36% of the patients who established high SISI test scores.

IMPEDANCE AUDIOMETRY RESULTS

All patients suspected of having an acoustic tumor are currently tested with impedance audiometry. Because impedance audiometry was not available for approximately the first two-thirds of the patients in this series, a relatively small number of patients, 117, is discussed here. The acoustic reflex test (ART) is now established as an important part of the audiological test battery. After electric response audiometry, ART is the most positive audiological test.

The importance of this procedure is emphasized by a recent report (16) of 24 cases of normal or near normal hearing, symmetrical hearing impairment, and/or normal roentgenograms with absent or reflex decay. Impedance results are shown in Table 10.

It is not feasible for every office to have the equipment for ERA audiometry. Impedance audiometry, however, can and should be used in every otolaryngological office. As shown in results listed in Table 10, it is the most significant audiological test for positive findings. The acoustic reflex was present in less than 20% of the cases. If we combine the categories of reflex decay and absent reflex, more than 80% of the cases fall within these two categories.

CORRELATES OF AUDITORY TESTING

Examination of the correlates of various auditory tests for about 300 cases was possible. This was carried out to determine whether a distinctive pattern of results would emerge from this study. A comparison of the speech discrimination tests scores, Bekesy tests, and SISI tests with pure tone patterns is presented in Table 11. There was extensive scattering of auditory findings for all of the pure tone patterns. The low tone loss was

Table 10. Impedance audiometry results (117 cases)

Findings	*N*	Percent of total
Acoustic reflex	22	19
Reflex decay	65	55
Absent reflex	30	26

Table 11. Comparison of speech discrimination, Bekesy, and SISI tests with pure tone pattern (295 cases)

Speech Discrimination	Bekesy	SISI	Type of pure tone pattern				Total
			High	Trough	Low	Flat	
Poor	III,IV	Low	38	6	12	11	67
Poor	III,IV	Moderate	1	0	1	1	3
Poor	III,IV	High	5	0	0	1	6
Poor	I,II	Low	10	0	0	3	13
Poor	I,II	Moderate	2	0	0	0	2
Poor	I,II	High	7	1	1	10	19
Moderate	III,IV	Low	6	2	2	2	12
Moderate	III,IV	Moderate	2	0	0	0	2
Moderate	III,IV	High	5	0	0	1	6
Moderate	I,II	Low	12	0	0	2	14
Moderate	I,II	Moderate	1	0	0	1	2
Moderate	I,II	High	12	1	0	4	17
Good	III,IV	Low	11	2	1	4	18
Good	III,IV	Moderate	0	0	0	0	0
Good	III,IV	High	3	1	1	0	5
Good	I,II	Low	27	0	2	4	33
Good	I,II	Moderate	11	2	0	3	16
Good	I,II	High	38	4	2	16	60

more likely to produce completely consistent auditory results, with 55% of the cases resulting, as anticipated, in poor speech, type III or type IV Bekesy tracing, and low SISI score. Only 17% of the flat patterns resulted in completely consistent test results and only 3% of the trough patterns fell into this category.

The relationship of speech discrimination tests to types of Bekesy tracings and SISI scores is shown in Table 12. More than 80% of the patients with 0% speech discrimination scores produced type III or type IV Bekesy tracings. In considering all patients with poor discrimination of 30% or less, a total of 68% of those patients will produce a type III or

Table 12. Comparison of speech discrimination scores, Bekesy types, and SISI scores

Speech Discrimination	Bekesy				SISI		
	I	II	III	IV	Low	Moderate	High
0%	2	11	38	20	65	4	10
2–30%	3	22	13	12	33	3	16
32–60%	3	31	11	10	30	5	25
62–100%	13	98	7	17	61	17	69

type IV tracing. Eighty-two percent of the patients with 0% discrimination score had low SISI scores. When all patients with 30% or less on speech discrimination tests are combined, the number with low SISI scores remains approximately the same at 81%. On the other hand, 80% of the patients with good speech discrimination scores (62% to 100%) produced either type I or type II Bekesy tracings. Forty-seven percent of the same group of patients achieved high SISI scores.

Table 13 compares impedance tests scores with pure tone loss patterns and speech discrimination scores. All patients with 0% speech discrimination had an absent acoustic reflex. Of the 38 patients with very poor discrimination (0 to 30%), 37 had an absent reflex or reflex decay. Of the patients who did have an acoustic reflex, more than 90% had a good discrimination score (62 to 100%).

The relationship between the auditory tests and the size of the lesion is shown in Table 14. As is described in the Preface to this book, intracanalicular lesions were classified as small tumors. All tumors that resulted in cranial nerve involvement other than, or in addition to, the eighth nerve were classified as large tumors. Patients who had cerebellar ataxia or elevated intracranial pressure were also classified as having large tumors. All other tumors that extruded beyond the internal auditory canal and resulted in no neurologic findings other than eighth nerve findings were classified as medium-sized tumors. Sixty percent of all of the cases were considered to be medium size (301), while approximately 35% (173) were large tumors. Consequently, only 5% of the total (26) were classified as small tumors. Total hearing loss occurred in 78 of the cases and one patient without tests, so that audiometric data were available for 421 cases.

Table 14 relates results of various auditory tests to the size of the tumor. An analysis of this table shows that patients with large tumors produced the most consistent anticipated auditory results. Thirty-four of the patients with large tumors received impedance tests. Thirty-one of the thirty-four had an absent reflex or reflex decay. More than 80% of the large tumors exhibited complete or partial tone decay. About two-thirds

Table 13. Comparison of impedance test results, pure tone patterns, and speech discrimination scores

	Pure tone pattern				Speech discrimination			
Impedance	High	Trough	Low	Flat	0%	2–30%	32–60%	62–100%
Acoustic reflex	18	0	1	3	0	1	1	20
Reflex decay	25	1	0	4	0	3	8	19
Absent reflex	30	2	10	15	26	8	7	23

Table 14. Comparison of auditory findings and size of lesion

Test Results			Size of tumor Small	Medium	Large
Mean pure tone threshold		$N = 421$	59.35	60.31	77.68
Speech discrimination	0–30%	$N = 415$	8	100	57
	32–60%		4	44	21
	62–100%		12	126	43
SISI	0–30%	$N = 338$	9	117	63
	35–65%		1	19	8
	70–100%		7	84	30
Bekesy	I	$N = 311$	1	14	6
	II		9	112	41
	III		4	36	29
	IV		4	40	15
Tone decay	Complete	$N = 327$	8	85	43
	Partial		6	78	30
	Negative		5	52	20
Impedance	No reflex	$N = 117$	5	37	23
	Decay		1	21	8
	Reflex		0	19	3

of the patients with large lesions produced 0% or low SISI scores below 30%.

An examination of patients with small tumors shows that approximately half had high SISI scores, excellent speech discrimination, and type I or type II Bekesy tracings. On the other hand, none of the patients with small tumors who were given impedance tests had an acoustic reflex. All in this group had an absent reflex or reflex decay.

In patients with medium-sized tumors auditory results were more mixed. Approximately 40% (100) had poor speech discrimination. Thirty-seven percent (76) had a type III or type IV Bekesy tracing. Fifty-three percent scored low SISI scores (117). On the other hand, 75% (163) produced either complete or partial tone decay. Seventy-seven of the patients with medium-sized tumors received impedance tests; of them, 75% (58) had either an absent reflex or reflex decay.

Since a large number of cases (204) showed inconsistent results in one or more aspects of the auditory tests, a closer analysis of these inconsistencies was arranged in a total of seven groups. Results of this group analysis are shown in Table 15. Seventy-seven cases in one group (38%) demonstrated auditory findings typical of cochlear rather than

Table 15. Inconsistent results of auditory tests (204 cases)

Speech discrimination	Bekesy	SISI	*N*	Size of tumor Small	Medium	Large
Group I Mod-Good	I,II	High	77	7	54	16
Group 2 Mod-Good	I,II	Low	47	1	30	16
Group 3 Mod-Good	III,IV	Low	30	2	20	8
Group 4 Mod-Good	III,IV	High	11	0	9	2
Group 5 Poor	I,II	High	19	0	12	7
Group 6 Poor	I,II	Low	14	1	9	4
Group 7 Poor	III,IV	High	6	0	4	2

retrocochlear lesions. All of these cases produced moderate to good speech discrimination, type I or type II Bekesy tracings, and very high SISI scores. Seventy out of the seventy-seven cases were classified as large or medium-sized tumors. The 47 cases in group two were also consistent with expected results for cochlear problems, except for the low SISI scores. The 30 cases in group three were consistent with the expected auditory results for retrocochlear lesions, with a type III or type IV Bekesy tracing and a low SISI score, but were inconsistent with respect to the moderate to good speech discrimination scores. Group four consisted of 11 cases with type III or type IV Bekesy tracings with high SISI scores and good speech discrimination. Nineteen patients were classified as group five, consistent with cochlear lesions except for the very poor discrimination for speech. In group six, 14 cases had consistent findings for speech and SISI tests but with type I or type II Bekesy tracings. The 6 cases in group seven were consistent with retrocochlear problems as far as speech scores and Bekesy tracings were concerned, but high SISI scores were inconsistent.

COMMENT

Analysis of the data in these 500 cases further supports the contention that all unilateral sensorineural type hearing impairments need thorough investigation, including audiometric testing. Positive classic audiometric findings present strong evidence of an existing acoustic tumor. On the other hand, the absence of these results cannot rule out the possibility of a tumor. More than 200 cases in this study showed inconsistencies in the so-called classic audiometric indications.

Certain conclusions regarding auditory findings may be made on the basis of this group of 500 patients. Two-thirds of these patients had a high frequency pure tone loss configuration. Less than 10% of the total number could be classified as low frequency loss. This statistic has remained stable since the initial report in 1964 (9).

We may also conclude that speech discrimination testing is still of considerable importance in the differential diagnosis of retrocochlear versus cochlear involvement. Although a smaller percentage of patients have a 0% discrimination score and a larger percent have good scores of 62 to 100%, it is still an important part of the test battery.

We may further conclude that Bekesy testing no longer has a definitive role in the audiometric test battery. In earlier studies about 70% of the patients produced a type III or type IV Bekesy tracing. In this latest study only 41% fell in this category. This very likely reflects the increasing number of patients diagnosed early, while the tumor is smaller and before eighth nerve involvement is great. We would recommend retaining the modified tone decay test in the procedures as a screening device. It is easily administered, takes very little time, and can present helpful information in many cases.

As in the case of Bekesy audiometry, we are no longer routinely doing SISI tests on suspected tumor cases. Since only slightly more than half of the total cases in this series produced low SISI scores, it no longer appeared to be a definitive testing procedure.

Impedance audiometry has become a prime tool in evaluating these patients. Eighty-one percent of all patients given the acoustic reflex test had an absent reflex or reflex decay. This is the largest positive finding for any one test except for electric response audiometry. The advent of impedance audiometry and electric response audiometry in the differentiation of retrocochlear from cochlear loss has added a new dimension to diagnostic tests.

Rehabilitation of the Acoustic Tumor Patient

The patient who has just had an acoustic tumor removed is a prime candidate for hearing rehabilitation. We always recommend that the patient try the contralateral routing of off-side signals (CROS) hearing aid. The rental-trial of a CROS aid is recommended as soon as the wound is healed. The success rate in adapting to the CROS aid is greater in patients who try it immediately after surgery than in those who delay for weeks or months. Many patients will decide, following the trial period, that the aid plays an important part in their adjustment to the complete loss of hearing in one ear. Even the patients who eventually reject the use of the CROS aid are grateful for having been counseled and having had the opportunity for the CROS trial.

REFERENCES

1. Gradenigo, G. 1893. "Gehorstorungen infolge von direkten Lasionen des N. aucusticus durch intrakranielle Tumoren," In: Schwarzes Handbuch der Ohrenheilkunde, Vol. 2. F. C. W. Vogel, Leipzig.
2. Carhart, R. 1957. Clinical determination of abnormal auditory adaptation. Arch. Otolaryngol. 65:32–39.
3. Hallpike, C. S., and Hood, J. D. 1959. Observations upon neurological mechanism of loudness recruitment phenomenon. Acta Otolaryngol. 50:472–486.
4. Pestalozza, G., and Cioce, C. 1962. Measuring auditory adaptation: Value of different clinical tests. Laryngoscope 72:240–261.
5. Palva, T. 1964. Auditory adaptation. Acta Otolaryngol. 57:207–216.
6. Eggston, A. A., and Wolff, D. 1947. Histopathology of Ear, Nose and Throat. The Williams & Wilkins Co., Baltimore.
7. Cambon, K., and Guilford, F. R. 1958. Acoustic neurilemoma. Arch. Otolaryngol. 67:302–321.
8. Schuknecht, H. F. 1963. Meniere's disease: Correlation of symptomatology and pathology. Laryngoscope 73:651–665.
9. Johnson, E. W., and House, W. F. 1964. Transtemporal bone microsurgical removal of acoustic neuromas: Auditory findings in 53 cases of acoustic neuromas. Arch. Otolaryngol. 80:667.
10. Johnson, E. W. 1965. Auditory test results in 110 surgically confirmed retrocochlear lesions. J. Speech Hear. Res. 30:307–317.
11. Johnson, E. W. 1970. Auditory test results in 268 cases of confirmed retrocochlear lesions. J. Int. Audiol. 9:15–19.
12. Johnson, E. W. 1977. Auditory test results in 500 cases of acoustic neuromas. Arch. Otolaryngol. 103:152–158.
13. Hughes, R. L., Winegar, W. J., Johnson, E. W., and House, H. P. 1965. Tape recorded speech audiometry for the otolaryngologist. Trans. Am. Acad. Opthalmol. Otolaryngol. 69:335–337.
14. Green, D. S. 1963. The modified tone decay test (MTDT) as a screening procedure for eighth nerve lesions. J. Speech Hear. Disord. 28:31–36.
15. Owens, E. 1964. Tone decay in eighth nerve and cochlear lesions. J. Speech Hear. Disord. 29:14–22.
16. Sheehy, J. L., and Inzer, B. E. 1976. Acoustic reflex test in neuro-otologic diagnosis. Arch. Otolaryngol. 102:647–653.

Acoustic Tumors
Volume I, *Diagnosis*
Edited by W. F. House and C. M. Luetje

Chapter 10

Brainstem Electric Response Audiometry in Acoustic Tumor Detection

Weldon A. Selters, Ph.D.*

Audiologist, Otologic Medical Group, Inc., Los Angeles; also, Affiliated with the Ear Research Institute, Los Angeles

Derald E. Brackmann, M.D.*

Associate Clinical Professor of Otorhinolaryngology, University of Southern California School of Medicine, Los Angeles; also, Affiliated with the Ear Research Institute and the Otologic Medical Group, Inc., Los Angeles

Brainstem electric response audiometry, or BERA, has proven to be the best audiometric test for acoustic tumor detection. Our data show that BERA surpasses other screening tests for acoustic tumors because it has a higher detection rate and a lower false positive rate (1).

* Mailing address: 2122 West Third Street, Los Angeles, California 90057

The success of BERA depends upon the fact that acoustic tumors stretch or compress the auditory nerve, producing a delay in the response latency, which BERA can detect. This delay may occur in an ear with normal hearing.

Conversely, cochlear lesions have little effect on the brainstem response latencies until the hearing loss becomes severe. This point is illustrated later with two groups of patients with unilateral hearing impairments of varying degrees, one group having acoustic tumors, the other group not.

Brainstem electric responses recorded from scalp electrodes were described by Jewett, Romano, and Williston (2). They observed a series of peaks similar to those shown in Figure 1A, which for simplicity are called P_1, P_2, etc., in order of their occurrence. It is generally assumed that these peaks reflect the sequential activation of the auditory nuclei in the brainstem as the response travels up the auditory chain. The finding that acoustic tumors usually alter these responses is the subject of discussion in this chapter.

METHOD

The recording of brainstem responses is relatively simple, given proper equipment and testing conditions. The stimulus is a click from a TDH-39 earphone, which is driven by a brief, 160-μsec square wave, or dc pulse, delivered 20 times per second.

The intensity of the click is important. Tumor detection is best with as intense a click as possible, but this need must be balanced against the discomfort and risk to the patient's hearing at high intensities. Our standard click stimulus measures 121 dB peak SPL on an impact meter and 83 dB above average threshold for a group of 20 normal listeners. A lower intensity click will give poorer results in some cases, especially those with high frequency hearing losses exceeding 50 dB.

Electrical responses are recorded from silver, silver chloride electrodes taped to each mastoid and to the scalp vertex. The electrode area is prepared by a vigorous rubbing with gauze and alcohol or acetone. Conductive gel and skin abrasion reduce the contact resistance to 3,000 Ω or less; otherwise, the skin is abraded again. The vertex lead goes to the active input of a differential preamplifier, the ipsilateral mastoid lead to the reference input, and the contralateral mastoid lead to the ground input.

The amplified difference voltage seen between vertex and mastoid on the stimulated side is passed through a 30–3,200 Hz filter to reduce noise and is then further amplified. At this point the brainstem responses are

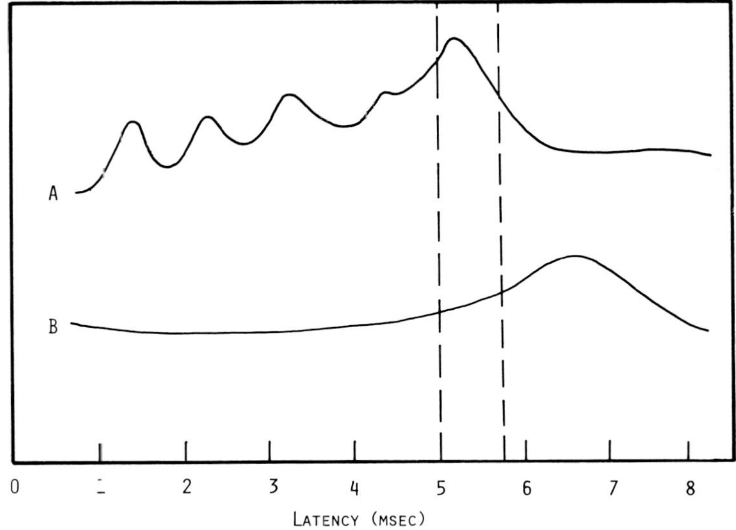

Figure 1. Brainstem auditory evoked potentials in (A) a normal ear and (B) an ear with an acoustic tumor.

still buried in electrical "noise" originating primarily from the muscles of the neck and head.

An averaging computer is used to extract the auditory responses from the random noise. This instrument stores or "remembers" the electrical activity that occurs during a brief time (10 msec) after each stimulus click presentation. As the click is repeated, responses that recur will grow in the computer memory. The muscle potentials and other potentials not time-locked to the click will be randomly positive and negative and will tend to cancel out in the summating process. For best results it is important to minimize muscular tension, which we do by making the patient comfortable in a reclining position. Many patients fall asleep during the half hour or so spent in recording; some find the 78-dB white noise used to mask the nontest ear soothing.

TUMOR EFFECTS ON RESPONSES

Desynchronization

Figure 1B shows a typical delayed P_5 response from a patient with an acoustic tumor. The delayed P_5 is also much broader than normal, which indicates less synchronization of the responding nerve fibers. It is presumed that tumor pressure delays some of the nerve fiber responses more than others. There could even be some cancellation of the electric fields emanating from the nerve fibers if some cells were repolarizing while others were firing.

This presumed desynchronization and cancellation could also explain the absence of the smaller peaks in Figure 1B. In fact, one-half of the tumor cases do not record an identifiable P_5 regardless of how good the hearing may be otherwise. This peculiar effect is best explained as resulting from desynchronization of the nerve fibers.

Latency Delay

The most important measure for tumor detection is the response latency. Peak amplitudes may be reduced by tumor pressure, but the effect is too irregular to be diagnostic.

Choice of which peak to monitor is arbitrary because tumor pressure will usually delay P_1, and this delay is passed along to all of the following peaks as well. P_5, the largest and the most recordable of the peaks, is the logical peak to monitor in most cases. If P_3 or some other peak gives a sharper and more easily measured latency, we occasionally use it instead of P_5 to determine a response delay.

What is a significant delay? The vertical lines in Figure 1 show the range of T_5, the P_5 latency, for 20 normal ears exposed to our standard 83-dB click. Most acoustic tumors will have a T_5 that is well above the upper limit of the normal range, as in Figure 1B. Approximately 10% of acoustic tumor cases have a T_5 within the normal range of 5 to 6 msec. A more sensitive measure is needed to detect a latency delay in these cases.

Measure of the T_5 for the opposite ear provides a means of improving the sensitivity of the test. A comparison of the left and right T_5's for a large number of normal listeners showed that the interaural difference for T_5 was O msec for most people. In no case was there more than a 0.2-msec difference between T_5's for an individual's two ears. Apparently the auditory brainstem is symmetrical neurologically.

It follows that a small delay in T_5 for one ear is best detected by a comparison with the T_5 for the opposite ear. If the interval difference, or IT_5, exceeds 0.2 msec, a delay has been detected.

IT_5 FINDINGS IN THE UNILATERAL HEARING LOSS

Non-Tumor Cases

Important questions are: How does sensorineural hearing loss affect the latency of P_5? Do cochlear lesions produce a delay, and if so, can this delay be distinguished from the delay produced by a tumor?

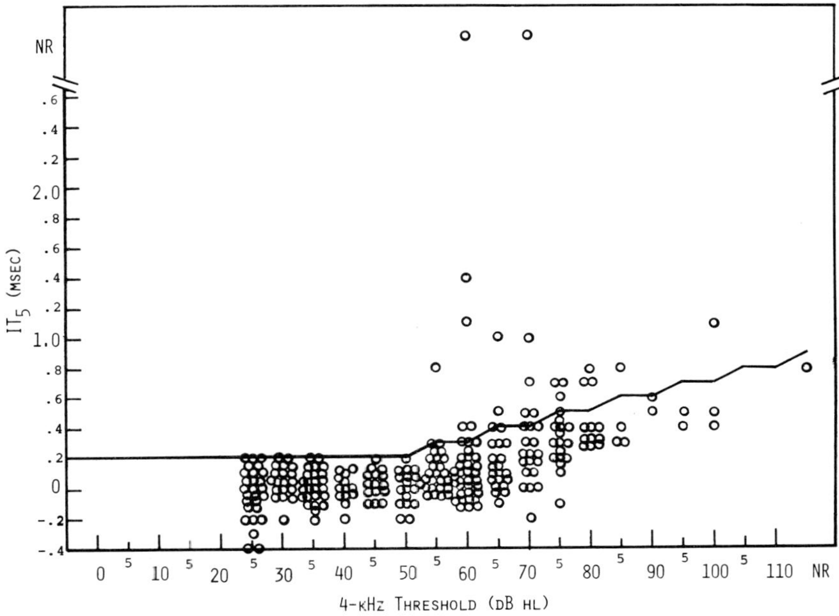

Figure 2. Interaural latency differences for 266 patients with unilateral sensorineural hearing losses (non-tumor).

Figure 2 shows the IT_5 values for 266 patients with unilateral hearing losses not caused by a tumor. The normal contralateral ear thresholds were 20 dB or less from 500 Hz through 4 kHz.

The selection criteria also specified pure tone thresholds of 75 dB or less at either 2 or 4 kHz. Ears with losses greater than 75 dB at both of these frequencies were excluded because they do not give reliable P_5 responses to the 83-dB click, making the test less useful.

An analysis of T_5 values as a function of thresholds by frequency showed the highest correlation between T_5 and the thresholds at 4 kHz. As illustrated in Figure 2, below 55 dB the 4-kHz hearing loss had no effect on IT_5, which averages 0 ± 0.2 msec. As the hearing loss at 4 kHz increases above 50 dB, IT_5 gradually increases, and a few cases appear with markedly increased IT_5s. More on these effects later.

Tumor Cases

Figure 3 shows the IT_5 values for 94 patients with unilateral hearing loss from surgically confirmed acoustic tumors. The audiometric selection criteria for this group were the same as for the preceding non-tumor

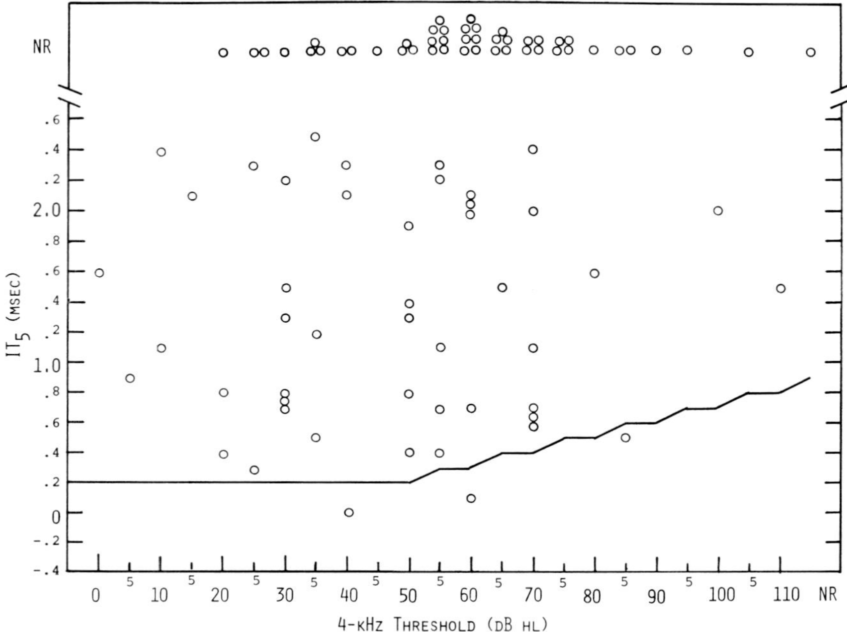

Figure 3. Interaural latency differences for 94 patients with unilateral hearing loss from acoustic tumors.

group; however, this group includes 8 patients with 4-kHz thresholds more sensitive than 25 dB.

One-half of the 94 tumor cases (50%) gave no P_5 response, which contrasts with only 2 no-response cases in the 266 of the non-tumor group (.08%). Desynchronization between individual nerve fibers producing cancellation of opposing electric fields is believed to be the cause for the disappearance of response after a tumor impinges on the auditory nerve.

The other half of the 94 tumor cases show latency delays ranging from 0 to 2.5 msec. Ninety-eight percent of the tumor cases have a delay greater than the 0.2-msec normal limit. However, in the non-tumor cases, 24% also have delays greater than 0.2 msec, which indicates that the 0.2-msec criterion for a positive retrocochlear finding may need adjustment to reduce the number of false positive findings.

Adjusting the IT_5 Criterion

The ideal test would separate tumor patients and non-tumor patients into two groups with no overlap. On the IT_5 scale the two groups do overlap, which means that whatever value of IT_5 is selected as the dividing criterion, there will be errors. The selection of a criterion will depend upon the relative importance of minimizing either the false positive or the false negative errors.

Figure 2 shows that most false positive errors occur with patients whose hearing loss exceeds 50 dB at 4 kHz. For instance, above 75 dB all of the IT_5s exceed the 0.2 msec normal limit. Obviously, some adjustment to the IT_5 criterion will be necessary for the test to be useful in patients with high frequency hearing loss.

The adjustment we have chosen is based on the hearing loss at 4 kHz as follows: above 50 dB, subtract from T_5 0.1 msec for each additional 10 dB or fraction thereof. Thus, 0.1 msec is subtracted with 4-kHz pure tone hearing loss of 55 or 60 dB and 0.2 msec for 65 or 70 dB, etc. (refer to Figures 2 and 3).

Evaluation of the Adjusted IT_5 Criterion

The adjustment to the IT_5 criterion reduced the false positive rate from 24% to 8% in the group of 266 with unilateral losses.

Figure 2 also shows that all of the false positives occurred in cases with a 4-kHz hearing loss greater than 50 dB. This shows that the test has greater validity when the 4-kHz threshold is 50 dB or less.

False negative cases, or patients with tumors that are not detected by BERA, are of much greater concern. In the group of 94 acoustic tumor cases shown in Figure 3, the criterion allowed three false negatives, a 2.3% rate.

In practice, the ratio of false positives to tumors discovered will determine whether the criterion is acceptable. This ratio will depend upon the incidence rate of acoustic tumors. Shaia and Sheehy (3) reported a 0.8% occurrence of acoustic tumors in a review of 1,220 cases of unilateral, sudden sensorineural hearing loss. Using 0.8% as an estimate for acoustic tumor incidence in unilateral sensorineural loss, and using 8% as the BERA false positive rate leads to the expectation of 10 false positive cases for every tumor case found.

Experience suggests further adjustment to the latency criterion. For instance, if the incidence rate for tumors decreased to only 1 per 500 cases of unilateral sensorineural hearing loss, BERA would be producing 40 false positives (8% $\times$ 500) for every tumor found. Then the criterion would need to be relaxed to reduce the false positive rate (which would also increase the false negative rate). Otherwise, confidence in a positive finding would decline to the point where a positive BERA would be ignored.

IT_5 COMPARED WITH OTHER TESTS

An additional group of 48 acoustic tumor cases increases the total to 142 patients with pure tone thresholds better than 80 dB at 2 or 4 kHz. These 48 had hearing losses in both ears.

Both left and right T_5's were adjusted by subtracting 0.1 msec for each 10 dB loss over 50 dB at 4 kHz before IT_5 was computed.

Most of the total group of 408 cases (142 tumor, 266 non-tumor) also had petrous pyramid x-ray films to check for enlargement of the internal auditory canals, electronystagmography (ENG) to check for a reduced vestibular response, and acoustic reflex tests (ART) to check for absence or decay of the crossed acoustic reflex. The percents of test failure are seen in Table 1.

TUMOR SIZE AND BERA FINDINGS

An earlier report (1) suggested that acoustic tumor size could be predicted from IT_5. Now, with a larger sample of cases, we find a lower correlation, which decreases the usefulness of IT_5 for predicting tumor size.

Large acoustic tumors press against the brainstem. Their expansion creates a deformation or shift of the brainstem that often can be detected by changes in P_5 on the opposite (non-tumor) ear. This effect is best detected by measuring the interval between P_3 and P_5 on the non-tumor ear. This interval, T_5–T_3, or $T_{5\text{-}3}$, will normally be 1.9 ± 0.1 msec. A $T_{5\text{-}3}$ of 2.1 to 2.8 msec was found in 71% of 55 cases having tumors 3 cm or larger in diameter. Most of these cases also demonstrated a weakening of the contralateral P_5 despite perfectly normal hearing in the non-tumor ear. In all cases of no brainstem shift, as in 43 tumors smaller than 2 cm, the contralateral $T_{5\text{-}3}$ was less than 2.1 msec.

A third clue to tumor size has a perfect prediction record so far. In 18 cases the only peak recorded has been P_1. In all 18 cases there was a large tumor in the cerebellopontine angle. This remarkable agreement may be explained this way: Most acoustic tumors originate within the internal auditory canal, press against the auditory nerve while still small,

Table 1. Four screening tests' failures (listed as percentages of tests performed)

	BERA	X-ray	ENG	ART
Percent false negative (tumor missed)	4	11	23	30
Percent false positive (false alarm)	8	27	28	28

and diminish P_1. Tumors that arise in the cerebellopontine angle expand medial to the canal, which explains the normal P_1. These tumors, because they are less confined, must grow to 3 cm to stretch the cochlear nerve sufficiently to produce desynchronization that obliterates the peaks after P_1. It is ironic, but not surprising, that these patients often have nearly normal hearing, but the size of the tumor precludes saving this hearing.

THE LATENCY—INTENSITY CURVE

A third factor, in addition to the retrocochlear lesion and the severe high frequency cochlear hearing loss, must be added to the list of causes for latency delay: conductive impairment. The latency of the auditory nerve response and, therefore, of the brainstem responses varies inversely with the intensity of the cochlear stimulation. That is, the greater the intensity of the stimulus, the shorter the latency of the responses.

Fortunately, it is easy to distinguish between a delay caused by a conductive loss and a delay caused by a tumor. To make the distinction, it is necessary to measure T_5 at several stimulus intensities. The slope of the latency-intensity curve will reveal a conductive versus a retrocochlear origin for the delay.

This point is illustrated by Figure 4, which shows latency-intensity curves for N, 20 normal ears; T, a tumor; C, a conductive loss; and S, a

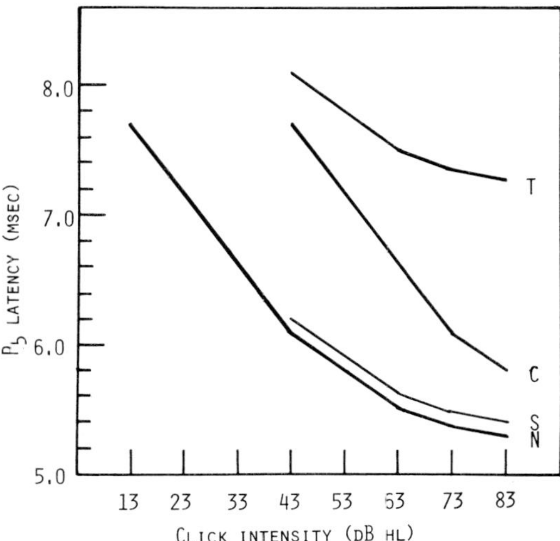

Figure 4. P_5 latency versus stimulus click intensity for T, acoustic tumor, C, conductive loss, S, sensory loss, and N, normal hearing.

sensory (cochlear) loss. Curves T, C, and S are fictional, for illustration only, but closely resemble actual curves. In each case a 30-dB hearing loss is assumed, so the three curves all begin at a click intensity that is 30 dB above the lowest click level on the normal curve. A conductive loss has the same effect as an equivalent reduction in stimulus intensity, so this curve, C, is shifted by 30 dB to the right of the normal curve. A tumor creates a delay that adds to the normal cochlear delay, so T is shifted from the normal curve by 2 msec. Finally, a 30-dB sensory loss, S, does not shift the normal curve at all, but merely has a higher threshold.

In practice we reverse this procedure. We plot the patient's P_5 latency-intensity curve on tracing paper and try to match this curve to the curve for his non-involved ear or with the normal curve if the other ear is not a good reference. Usually it is possible to classify the origin of the delay by this procedure.

The use of this technique can prevent the false prediction of a tumor when an unknown conductive loss causes a delay. For instance, ear canal collapse under earphones may introduce a misleading delay in P_5 that will be detected by this analysis.

SUMMARY

The finding of a delay in the brainstem electric response (BERA) to an 83-dB HL click is a simple, effective test for acoustic tumors. After allowance is made for delays due to severe high frequency cochlear losses and conductive impairments, the test has given a 96% tumor detection rate with an 8% false positive rate. Three other screening tests used for acoustic tumors have error rates at least three times higher than that of BERA.

Our routine evaluation of a tumor suspect has included petrous pyramid x-rays, ENG, and an acoustic reflex test. If the x-rays show definite enlargement of one canal, a contrast study is obtained, usually a CAT scan followed by a small dose Pantopaque polytome study if the scan is negative.

If the findings on x-ray are not definite, but the ENG or acoustic reflex test suggests a tumor, we usually obtain BERA. If that is positive, the contrast studies as described above are indicated.

Recently we have often used BERA as a primary screening test. In some cases the ENG and acoustic reflex test have been omitted because of BERA. In conclusion, BERA is a significant addition to the acoustic tumor detection test battery.

REFERENCES

1. Selters, W., and Brackmann, D., 1977. Acoustic tumor detection with brain stem electric response audiometry. Arch. Otolaryngol. 103:181–187.
2. Jewett, D., Romano, M., and Williston, J. 1970. Human auditory evoked potentials: Possible brain stem components detected on the scalp. Science 167:1517–1518.
3. Shaia, F., and Sheehy, J. 1976. Sudden sensorineural hearing impairment: A report of 1,220 cases. Laryngoscope 86:389–398.
4. Hecox, K., and Galambos, R. 1974. Brain stem auditory evoked responses in human infants and adults. Arch. Otolaryngol. 99:30–33.

Acoustic Tumors
Volume I, *Diagnosis*
Edited by W. F. House and C. M. Luetje

Chapter 11

Electronystagmographic Caloric Bithermal Vestibular Test (ENG): Results in Acoustic Tumor Cases

Fred H. Linthicum, Jr., M.D.*

Clinical Professor of Otorhinolaryngology, University of Southern California School of Medicine, Los Angeles; also, Affiliated with the Ear Research Institute and Otologic Medical Group, Inc., Los Angeles

Mohammed H. Khalessi, M.D.

Research Fellow, Ear Research Institute, Los Angeles (during the academic year 1974)

Diane Churchill

Chief Electronystagmography Technician, Otologic Medical Group, Inc., Los Angeles

---

The ENG (electronystagmographic test) is one of the battery of tests helpful in establishing the diagnosis of acoustic tumors. Any patient

* Mailing address: 256 South Lake Street, Los Angeles, California 90057

with a unilateral sensorineural hearing loss—or even a complaint of unilateral hearing difficulty in spite of a normal audiogram, tinnitus, or a balance disturbance—should have an ENG examination.

Vertigo is not a common symptom of acoustic tumors. It occurs in 15.4% of patients with small tumors and 18.6% of those with large tumors. Unsteadiness is a more common complaint, occurring in 57.6 to 80.8% of the cases, depending on the size of the tumor.

Visible nystagmus is a rare finding. Recordable nystagmus is found in only 10% of the cases. The direction of the beat is non-localizing, although it is more apt to beat away from the side of the lesion (80%).

FINDINGS

The ENG is found to be abnormal [30% reduced vestibular response (RVR) or more] in 82% of the cases. The percentage of cases with RVR is directly related to the size of the tumor. Ninety-five percent of patients with large tumors have RVR; 43% with small tumors have it (Figure 1).

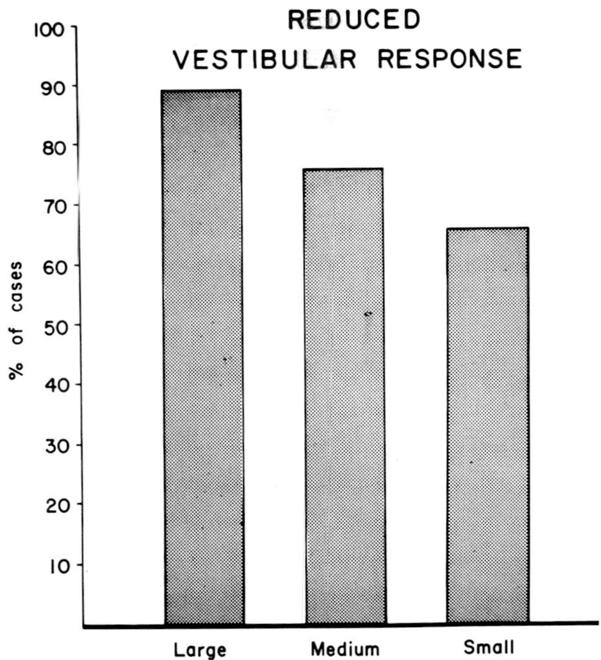

Figure 1. Relationship of tumor size to percent of patients with significant RVR.

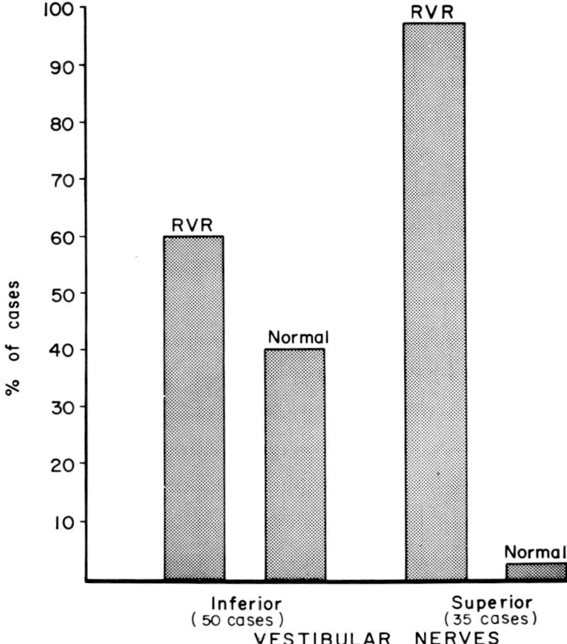

Figure 2. Correlation of percent of cases with RVR and origin of tumor.

In 97.2% of the cases of a tumor arising from the superior vestibular nerve, there was a significant RVR on the affected side. However, RVR occurred in only 60% of the cases of a tumor arising from the inferior vestibular nerve (Figure 2). It would appear, therefore, that the ENG is an accurate test for small tumors arising from the superior vestibular nerve, but not for those on the inferior vestibular nerve. Methods of investigating the response of the inferior vestibular nerve (supplied by the posterior semicircular canal and saccule) are currently under investigation.

There are, of course, many other causes of RVR, so this finding must be correlated with history, physical findings, and x-ray and auditory tests before it can be accepted as an indication of a possible cerebellopontine angle lesion.

NECESSITY OF BITHERMAL IRRIGATION

Several papers in the literature have advocated only-warm water stimulation. We feel that, because cold water irrigation may possibly induce a

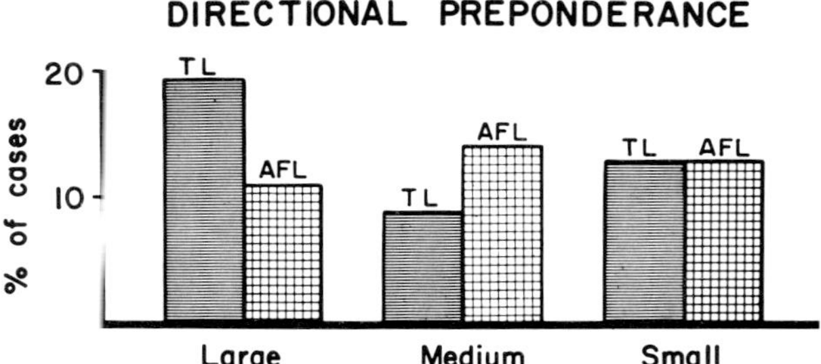

Figure 3. Cases with direction preponderence in addition to reduced vestibular response. Dependence on only one temperature would lead to incriminating the normal side in many cases. TL indicates nystagmus toward the side of the lesion. AFL indicates nystagmus away from the lesion.

latent nystagmus, it might be inaccurate, whereas the warm water test must overcome any latent nystagmus. Theoretically this is true. In fact it is not. Analysis of surgically proven tumor cases indicates that, in addition to an RVR, there is a directional preponderance toward the side of the lesion in approximately 50% (Figure 3). If only the hot water test is considered, the assumption is that the ear opposite the lesion has the reduced caloric response. Therefore, both cold and warm water irrigations should be used for accurate testing.

CONCLUSIONS

Eighty-two percent of patients with surgically verified acoustic tumors show a reduced vestibular response of 30% or more. The percentage of these patients is directly related to the size of the tumor. Small and medium tumors arising from the superior vestibular nerve produce an RVR in 97.2% of the cases, whereas tumors arising from the inferior vestibular nerve produce an RVR of only 60%. The ENG is a valuable test in establishing a diagnosis of cerebellopontine angle lesions. However, it must be correlated with audiologic and x-ray findings, usually including EMI scan and/or posterior fossa myelography, to establish a definte diagnosis.

Acoustic Tumors
Volume I, *Diagnosis*
Edited by W. F. House and C. M. Luetje

Chapter 12

Radiographic Findings in Cerebellopontine Angle Tumors

James A. Crabtree, M.D.*

Clinical Professor of Otology, University of Southern California School of Medicine, Los Angeles

Gale Gardner, M.D.†

Assistant Professor, Department of Otolaryngology and Maxillofacial Surgery, University of Tennessee Center for the Health Sciences, Memphis

---

The radiographic examination of the temporal bone has become an extremely important part of the neuro-otologic work-up in patients suspected of having acoustic tumors. Recently introduced diagnostic procedures, such as computerized axial tomography and brainstem electrical response audiometry, have further sharpened our ability to make this diagnosis. In seeking lessons to be learned as the result of our experience in the diagnosis and treatment of the 500 acoustic tumor patients who are discussed in this text, it is important to reassess the

* Mailing address: 1300 North Vermont #508, Los Angeles, California 90027
† Mailing address: 899 Madison—602A, Memphis, Tennessee 38103

value of temporal bone radiography. In this chapter we also review the historical aspects of this subject, as well as the techniques that we have found to be most useful.

HISTORICAL REVIEW

Equipment

The effort to design equipment capable of producing high quality temporal bone x-rays dates back to shortly after the discovery of x-rays by Roentgen in 1895. Much of this history is obscured by either failure to record the events in the first place, or failure to provide extensive translation.

Lysholm and Schonander (1,2) recognized the importance of proper centering of the central ray, head position, stereoscopy, and avoidance of scattering radiation through the use of diaphragms, tubes, and grids.

In 1928, Hodgson (3) in England described his efforts to overcome the unique problems associated with temporal bone radiography. The Franklin, General Electric, and Gianturko head units were the results of other efforts to provide high quality temporal bone x-rays.

The work of Gilbert Roy Owen (4) and Eugene Compere (4,5,6) resulted in the development of a head unit designed specifically 1) to ensure close but comfortable positioning of the patient's head in close relationship to the x-ray film; 2) to allow precise and repeatable positioning of the head by the technicians; 3) to avoid significant scattering of radiation by specially designed diaphragms, tubes, and a grid so as to allow a maximum of detail; and 4) to provide stereoscopic films.

Body section radiography (tomography, laminography) was developed in the 1930s. Ziedses des Plantes (7) in 1932 and Lemahieu (8) in 1952 made primary contributions. Sans and Porcher (9) in 1950 developed the Polytome, which was manufactured by the Philips Company. This unit produces a hypocycloidal trajectory so as to provide a maximum of sharp detail for the individual structures being examined. Frey (10) reported on the use of the Polytome for temporal bone radiography in 1956. Valvassori has reported extensively on the use of the Polytome in temporal bone diagnosis (11).

Technique

Compere's report in 1964 (5) provides an accurate bibliography of the development of the various projections that are useful for a demonstration of the temporal bone, types of film and screens that have been used, the most desirable techniques for film exposure, and methods of film processing. Dixon (12) has systematized these factors with the intent of making it practical for the otolaryngologist without special radiological training to perform temporal bone radiography in his office.

Acoustic Tumor Diagnosis

Only 17 years after the discovery of the x-ray, Henschen (13) demonstrated pathologic and radiographic evidence that acoustic tumors arise from the lateral end of the internal auditory canal, and suggested the possibility of x-ray diagnosis of this tumor.

In 1917, Carr (14) in Boston described the problems of accurate positioning necessary to obtain symmetrical projections and her efforts to solve this problem. Cushing (15), Carr's colleague, described his disappointment with the use of plain x-ray for even far-advanced acoustic tumors.

Chamberlain in 1926 demonstrated petrous pyramid erosion by a proven acoustic tumor by means of a fronto-occipital projection. This view, previously described by Grashey (5) in 1912 and reported on by Towne (16) in 1926, had a major impact on acoustic tumor diagnosis in this country (5).

Ebenius (17) in Stockholm in 1936 reported the radiographic findings of 34 patients operated upon by Olivecrona for acoustic tumors. He described six projections that he had used with the Lysholm-Schonander head unit, preferring the fronto-dorsal and axial. He noted the enlargement of the internal auditory canal in 27 patients (80%) in this series, and described the typical defect as being of a funnel configuration.

Camp and Cilley (18) in 1939, reporting on their work at the Mayo Clinic, stated a preference for the transorbital projection.

Beginning in the 1940s, the literature reflected a marked difference of opinion regarding the relative value of laminography and Polytomography versus the value of conventional or plain films for the diagnosis of acoustic tumors and other cerebellopontine angle tumors. Schwartz (19) in 1942 preferred laminography to conventional films.

In 1947, Revilla (20) reported on the x-ray results of 160 patients having had acoustic tumor surgery by Dandy. Base views with stereoscopy had been performed on 114 patients. Only 52 of these studies showed either enlargement or destruction of the internal auditory canal. Revilla concluded that the absence of x-ray findings did not constitute proof that a tumor was not present.

Lundborg's (21) extensive report of the Olivecrona series of 300 proven acoustic tumors in 1951 stated that of x-ray studies performed in 296 of these, 85% had shown internal auditory canal changes.

Lapayowker (22) reported on his use of tomography for acoustic tumor diagnosis, and concluded that this method was superior to plain films in detecting early bone changes within the internal auditory canal.

Compere (5,6) recommended the use of high quality conventional technique, using the head unit that he developed. He preferred 1) the sagittal posterior-anterior projection of Schuller, or transorbital projection; 2) the lateral skull view; and 3) the Stenver projection. He stated that the Chamberlain-Towne, or fronto-occipital of Grashey, was less valuable because of poor detail and distortion that resulted from the oblique angle and the length of object-to-film distance. He related most of the dissatisfaction over x-ray examination of the temporal bone to over-reliance on the Chamberlain-Towne projection.

Scanlan (23,24) in 1964 stated a preference for posterior fossa myelography for acoustic tumor diagnosis because of his disappointment with both conventional and laminographic technique.

Crabtree (25), House (26,27), and Sheehy (28) reported on their experience at the Otologic Medical Group with the diagnosis of first 54, and later 200 surgically proven acoustic tumors. Eighty-five percent of patients having tumors demonstrated abnormal findings with plain x-rays, using the method of Owen and Compere (4), and including the Stenver, Chamberlain-Towne, transorbital projection of Schuller or Caldwell, and lateral skull views. They concluded that plain films were superior to laminography for initial evaluation because erosion and canal size could be determined more easily.

Valvassori reported in a series of articles in 1974 and 1975 (11,29–39) his experience that with conventional films, superimposition of structures made precise identification of individual structures difficult and that foreshortening of the Stenver projection made it less useful. He preferred laminography, particularly Polytomography, and the frontal and lateral projections. In 181 surgically verified acoustic tumors, 78% had shown abnormal findings on preliminary tomographic films.

Naunton and Petasnick (40) in 1970 reported on six patients who had surgically proven acoustic tumors with normal preoperative tomograms. They emphasized that acoustic tumors may present initially with only cerebellopontine angle and not internal auditory canal findings. Crabtree had referred to this possibility in 1964 (25).

Goldman and Martin (41) from the M. D. Anderson Hospital in 1970, Wilner, et al. (42), from Henry Ford Hospital in 1970, and Brunner (43) from Copenhagen in 1971 all preferred Polytomography for initial examination of the temporal bone, rather than the use of plain films.

On the other hand, Etter (44,45) in 1972 and 1973 from Pittsburgh stated that conventional films provide equal results to more elaborate procedures (Polytomography). He reported that 90% of patients having acoustic tumors showed abnormalities of the internal auditory canal on plain films, but emphasized the necessity of carefully designed equipment and careful technique.

Wright and Taylor (46) in Indianapolis in 1973 reported that only 45% to 60% of patients having acoustic tumors can be diagnosed using plain films, but that the corresponding figure is 95% with Polytomography.

Osborn (47) in 1975, from Southampton, U.K., studied 56 acoustic tumor patients using both tomography and plain film. Tomography produced a slightly higher percentage of abnormal findings preoperatively (84% to 78.5%), but also produced a higher incidence of false positive results (10% to 3.5%). He concluded that plain films were of greater value for primary examination, and preferred tomography for uncertain situations.

Measurements

Several authors have reported measurements taken of the vertical diameter of the internal auditory canal of both normal patients and those having acoustic tumors. Table 1 demonstrates these findings. Compere (48) has recently stated that such figures must not be over-relied upon, feeling that preoccupation with numbers may produce errors in judgment

Table 1. Vertical diameter of internal auditory canal—normal range (six studies)

		Study[a]					
		1	2	3	4	5	6
Diameter	Max.	9 mm	11 mm	7 mm	8.5 mm	8 mm	10.5 mm
	Min.	5 mm	2.5 mm	3 mm	3.5 mm	2 mm	3 mm
	Average	6.3 mm	5.23 mm	—	—	4 mm	—
Bilateral Variation	Up to 1 mm	97%	75%	—	—	99%	100%
	1–2 mm	2%	23%	—	—	1%	—
	2–3 mm	1%	2%	—	—	—	—
	Max. Diff.	—	2.5 mm	—	1.5 mm	—	1.0 mm

[a] Studies are: 1, Ebenius (17); 2, Camp & Cilley (18); 3, Tarp (49); 4, Crabtree (25); 5, Valvassori (33); and 6, Lapayowker (22).

and result in failure to recognize pathology. It is important to realize that a number of factors may produce differences between the various groups of measurements. Different projections have been used, magnification factors have varied with the equipment used, and, while in some cases magnification has been corrected for mathematically, in others it has not. The actual technique of measuring and the points at which measurements were taken undoubtedly have varied considerably from one examiner to another.

Interpretation

Guidelines for interpretation of the x-ray appearance have been suggested by several authors. Valvassori (29), using tomography, considers the internal auditory canal to be abnormal whenever he finds 1) bone erosion of the canal, 2) a 2 mm or greater widening of the suspected canal, 3) shortening of the posterior wall by 3 mm or more, and 4) abnormal placement of the crista falciformis.

METHODS USED

The methods employed in the radiographic evaluation of the patients in this study include those techniques suggested by Owen and Compere (4). We use the head unit designed by Compere (5) and manufactured by the Continental X-ray Company of Chicago, Illinois. This unit features the use of "fine focus" tubes with the smallest possible cones and the grid diaphragm. We also position the head as closely as possible to the film. One petrous pyramid series includes the Stenver, Chamberlain-Towne, and the Schuller or Caldwell projections. Stenver's views are taken as a stereo pair. It is important to insist that if the exposure or positioning is not correct, the views must be repeated so as to ensure films of high quality (see Figure 1). In addition, a lateral view of the skull is taken. Film selection, exposure, and processing are carried out as discussed by Compere (5).

The clinical interpretation, after examination of these films, was based on three primary findings: 1) difference in the diameter of the internal auditory canals between the two sides; 2) difference in the contour of the two canals; and 3) some area of erosion either on the roof, floor, or posterior lip.

The extremely well-pneumatized petrous apex is the most difficult to evaluate. It is important that the cell walls be seen. With properly taken films, one can readily see the breakdown of the cell walls surrounding the internal auditory canal on the involved side.

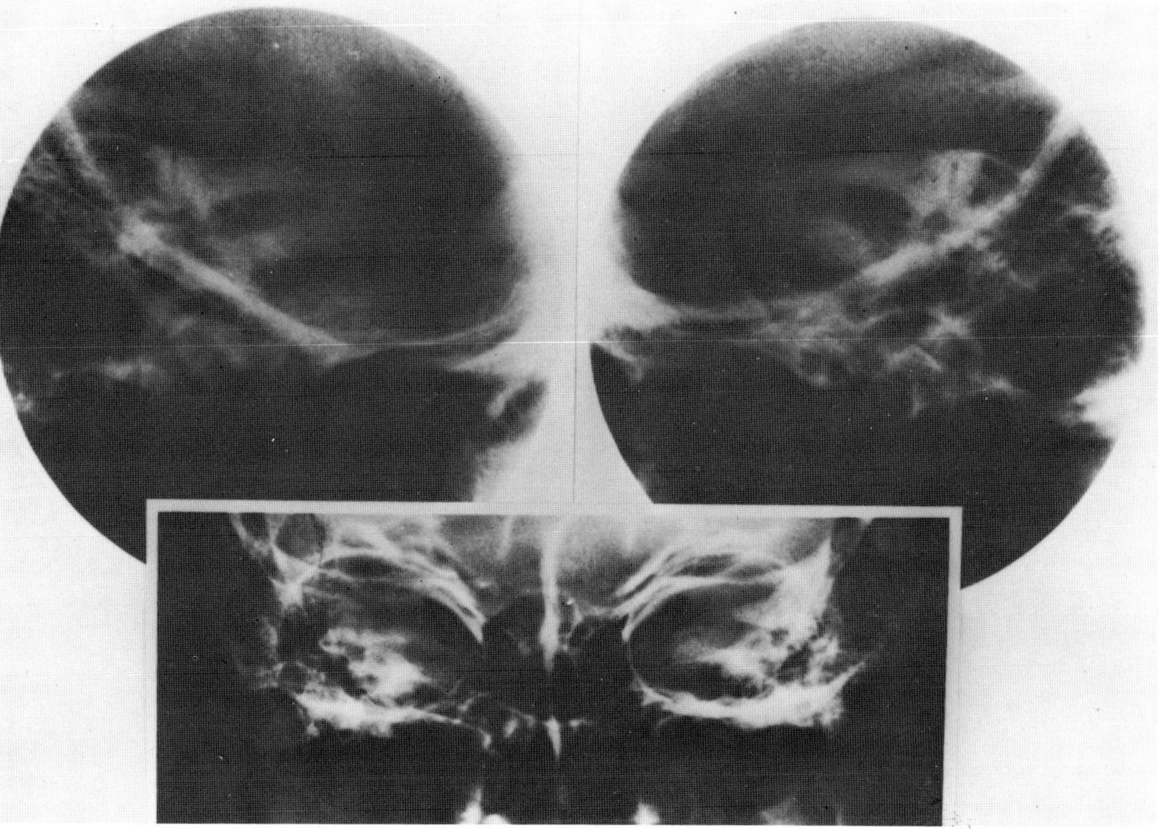

Figure 1. Stenver pair and transorbital (Caldwell) projection. Note enlargement and contour of left internal auditory canal.

MATERIALS AND RESULTS

We have reviewed the records of 500 consecutive patients having unilateral acoustic neuromas that were treated surgically between March 22, 1968, and January 31, 1975. Forty-three of these patients (8.6%) had petrous pyramid films that were interpreted as being normal.

In addition, we reviewed the records of the next 188 consecutive cases of patients having surgically proven unilateral acoustic tumors, who had preoperative plain films taken. This second series encompasses the time period between February 3, 1975 and July 20, 1977. Eighteen of these patients (9.6%) had normal petrous pyramid films.

Of the combined series of 688 patients, 61, or 8.9%, had normal petrous pyramid films.

DISCUSSION

No effort is made in this chapter to resolve the issue of conventional versus laminographic films for acoustic tumor diagnosis. Reports in the literature make it obvious that both techniques are capable of high quality, which will be attained proportionately to the interest and creativity applied to the technique used. The decisions to utilize temporal bone radiography as part of a neuro-otologic evaluation and to insist on high quality films are of much greater importance than the question of whether to depend on plain films or on laminographic films.

Our own experience, based on many comparative examinations, has been that in our hands adequate plain films provided us with more information. Erosion and size of the canal were much easier to recognize on properly taken plain films. For this reason, we have chosen not to depend on Polytomes for our initial radiographic examination. We have also felt that conventional technique has been more efficient from the point of view of both duration of the x-ray procedure and the cost to the patient.

We believe that the decision to use laminography versus conventional technique should depend on the setting within which an individual works. When an otolaryngologist is in close proximity to a radiologist who prefers to use laminography, it may be desirable to use this technique. It is important to insist that only films of high quality will be acceptable. This implies high quality equipment such as the Polytome, technicians who are allowed to specialize in this type of work as opposed to rotating among departments within the facility, a radiologist who is willing to develop a special interest in temporal bone radiography, and willingness on the part of the radiologist to insure prompt and efficient delivery of films to the otolaryngologist at reasonable cost.

From our own experience, we believe such arrangements are unusual. To deal with the problem in this way frequently leads to situations in which a complete radiographic examination is deferred, in spite of suspicion that an acoustic tumor is present. When this becomes the case, we suggest the practicality of the methods described in this study.

An earlier report (25) related the results of radiographic study of the first 200 patients treated surgically for unilateral acoustic tumors by the Otologic Medical Group.

In over half of these cases, the findings were so suggestive of a tumor that they were considered "diagnostic." The other cases, however, depended frequently upon subtle changes in the radiologic appearance, which, used in conjunction with other tests, led to the confirmation of tumor. False positive radiological findings occur almost exclusively in cases not considered "diagnostic."

The conclusions formulated in that paper appear to have stood the test of time, based on our experience with 688 additional acoustic tumor patients. These conclusions were:

1. Petrous pyramid x-rays made with the proper equipment, and correctly positioned and exposed, may give early evidence of acoustic neuroma.
2. The three views found to be most helpful in the diagnosis of acoustic neuromas are the Stenver, the Caldwell or transorbital, and the Chamberlain-Towne. Of these the Stenver is the most helpful.
3. A difference of 1 mm between the diameters of the two sides is considered suspicious. If the difference is accompanied by erosion or difference in shape of the two canals, the findings are strongly suggestive of an acoustic neuroma.

SUMMARY

In a review of 688 cases of surgically proven unilateral acoustic tumors, 8.9% had normal petrous pyramid studies preoperatively.

In spite of the addition of neurodiagnostic tests for acoustic tumors, such as computerized axial tomography and brainstem electrical response audiometry, the radiographic examination of the temporal bone using conventional technique remains as an extremely important part of the neuro-otologic work-up.

REFERENCES

1. Lysholm, E. 1928. Contribution to the technique of projection in roentgenological examination of pars petrosa. Acta Radiol. 9:54–66.
2. Lysholm, E. 1931. Apparatus and technique for roentgen examination of the skull. Acta Radiol. (Suppl.) 12.
3. Hodgson, H. G. 1928. The radiology of the normal and abnormal labyrinth. J. Laryngol. Otol. 43:92–97.
4. Owen, G. R., and Compere, W. E. 1959. Radiologic examination of the temporal bone. In: G. E. Shambaugh (ed.), Surgery of the Ear, pp. 83–118. W. B. Saunders Company, Philadelphia.
5. Compere, W. E. 1964. The radiologic examination of the petrous portion of the temporal bone. In: Radiographic Atlas of the Temporal Bone. American Academy of Ophthalmology and Otolaryngology, Publishers, St. Paul, Minnesota.
6. Compere, W. E. 1967. Conventional radiologic examination of the temporal bone. In: G. E. Shambaugh (ed.), Surgery of the Ear, Second Edition, pp. 99–136. W. B. Saunders Company, Philadelphia.
7. Ziedses des Plantes, B. G. 1959. Cited by Ole Tarp in: Tomography of the temporal bone with the polytome. Acta Radiol. 51:105–116.
8. Lemahieur, S. F. 1959. Cited by Ole Tarp in: Tomography of the temporal bone with the polytome. Acta Radiol. 51:105–116.
9. Sans and Porcher. 1962. Cited by Margaret J. McGann in: Plesiosectional tomography of the temporal bone. Am. J. Roentgenol. 88:1183–1186.
10. Frey, K. W. 1959. Cited by Ole Tarp in: Tomography of the temporal bone with the polytome. Acta Radiol. 51:105–116.
11. Valvassori, G. E. 1964. Laminography of the Temporal Bone. American Academy of Ophthalmology and Otolaryngology, Publishers, St. Paul, Minnesota.
12. Dixon, H. S. 1974. A Working Manual for Otolaryngologic Radiology. Instructional Course Material, American Academy of Ophthalmology and Otolaryngology.
13. Henschen, F. 1928. Cited by Erik Lysholm in: Contribution to the technique of projection in Roentgenological examination of pars petrosa. Acta Radiol. 9:54–66.
14. Carr, G. L. 1917. Roentgen ray findings in the skull in cases of brain tumors, with special reference to the porus acusticus. Am. J. Roentgenol. 4:405–410.
15. Cushing, H. 1963. Tumors of the Nervus Acusticus and the Syndrome of the Cerebellopontine Angle, pp. 1–13; 152; 159; 176; 177–209; 217; 237–241. Hafner Publishing Company, New York.
16. Towne, E. B. 1926. Erosion of the petrous bone by acoustic nerve tumor. Arch. Otolaryngol. 4:515–519.
17. Ebenius, B. 1934. The results of examination of the petrous bone in auditory nerve tumors. Acta Radiol. 15:284–290.
18. Camp, J. D., and Cilley, E. I. L. 1939. The significance of asymmetry of the pori acustici as an aid in diagnosis of eighth nerve tumors. Am. J. Roentgenol. 41:713–718.

19. Schwartz, C. W. 1942. Tumors of the acoustic nerve from a roentgenological viewpoint. Am. J. Roentgenol. 47:703–710.
20. Revilla, A. G. 1947. Neurinomas of the cerebellopontile recess. Johns Hopkins Med. J. 80:254–296.
21. Lundborg, T. 1951. Diagnostic problems concerning acoustic tumors. Acta Otolaryngol. (Suppl.) 99:1–111.
22. Lapayowker, M. S., and Cliff, M. M. 1969. Bone changes in acoustic neurinomas. Am. J. Roentgenol. 107:652–658.
23. Scanlan, R. L. 1964. Positive contrast medium (iophendylate) in diagnosis of acoustic neuroma. Arch. Otolaryngol. 80:698–706.
24. Scanlan, R. L. 1964. Roentgen diagnosis of acoustic neuroma with particular reference to the use of pantopaque. Laryngoscope 74:999–1003.
25. Crabtree, J. A. and House, W. F. 1964. X-ray diagnosis of acoustic neuromas. Arch. Otolaryngol. 80:695–697.
26. Hambley, W. M., Gorshenin, A. N., House, W. F. 1964. The differential diagnosis of acoustic neuroma. Arch. Otolaryngol. 80:708–720.
27. Hitselberger, W. E., and House, W. F. 1968. Polytome-pantopaque: A technique for the diagnosis of small acoustic tumors. Acta Otolaryngol. 65:555–564.
28. Sheehy, J. L. 1968. The neuro-otologic evaluation. Arch. Otolaryngol. 88:592–597.
29. Valvassori, G. E. 1969. The abnormal internal auditory canal: The diagnosis of acoustic neuroma. Radiology 92:449–459.
30. Valvassori, G. E. 1972. Myelography of the internal auditory canal. Am. J. Roentgenol. 115:578–586.
31. Valvassori, G. E. 1973. The diagnosis of acoustic neuromas. Otolaryngol. Clin. North Am. 6:391–400.
32. Valvassori, G. E. 1969. The diagnosis of acoustic neuromas. Semin. Roentgenol. 4:171–177.
33. Valvassori, G. E., and Pierce, R. H. 1964. The normal internal auditory canal. Am. J. Roentgenol. 92:1232–1241.
34. Valvassori, G. E. 1966. II. The contribution of radiology to the diagnosis of acoustic neuroma. Arch. Otolaryngol. 83:1104–1112.
35. Valvassori, G. E. 1966. The radiological diagnosis of acoustic neuromas. Arch. Otolaryngol. 83:582–587.
36. Valvassori, G. E. 1967. Tomography of the temporal bone. In: Surgery of the Ear, Second Edition, pp. 137–157. W. B. Saunders Company, Philadelphia.
37. Valvassori, G. E. 1969. The diagnosis of acoustic neuromas. Semin. Roentgenol. 4:171–177.
38. Valvassori, G. E. 1974. Benign tumors of the temporal bone. Radiol. Clin. North Am. 12:533–542.
39. Valvassori, G. E., and Buckingham, R. A. 1975. Tomography and Cross Sections of the Ear, p. 193. W. B. Saunders Company, Philadelphia.
40. Naunton, R. F., and Petasnick, J. P. 1970. Acoustic neurinomas with normal internal auditory meatus. Arch. Otolaryngol. 91:437–443.
41. Goldman, A. M., and Martin, J. E. 1970. Tumors involving the temporal bone. Radiol. Clin. North Am. 8:387–402.

42. Wilner, H. I., Fenton, J. L., Eyler, W. R., and Knighton, R. S. 1970. Tomographic evaluation of the internal auditory canal using positive contrast material. Radiology 95:95–99.
43. Brunner, S. 1971. Tumors of the temporal region. In: Fundamentals of Ear Tomography, pp. 204–211. Charles C Thomas, Springfield, Ill.
44. Etter, L. E. 1972. Roentgenography and Roentgenology of the Temporal Bone, Middle Ear and Mastoid Process, Second Edition. Charles C Thomas, Springfield, Ill.
45. Etter, L. E. 1973. Plain film demonstration of acoustic nerve tumors. Arch. Otolaryngol. 98:414–416.
46. Wright, J. W., and Taylor, C. C. 1973. Polytomography of the Temporal Bone. 5:97–98. Warren H. Green, Inc., St. Louis, Missouri.
47. Osborn, J. D. 1975. A comparative study of special petrous views and tomography in the diagnosis of acoustic neuromas. Br. J. Radiol. 48:996–999.
48. Compere, W. E. Personal communication.
49. Tarp, O. 1959. Tomography of the temporal bone with the polytome. Acta. Radiol. 51:105–116.

Acoustic Tumors
Volume I, *Diagnosis*
Edited by W. F. House and C. M. Luetje
Copyright 1979 University Park Press Baltimore

Chapter 13

Computed Tomography in Acoustic Tumor Diagnosis

Richard M. Witten, M.D.*

Department of Radiology, St. Vincent Medical Center, Los Angeles

Christina T. Wade, M.D.

Department of Radiology, St. Vincent Medical Center, Los Angeles

---

Computed tomography is a proven diagnostic procedure in acoustic tumor. When the cerebellopontine angle tumor is demonstrated by this study, other traditional and more hazardous studies may be omitted from the work-up. Positive contrast cisternography using iophendylate is no longer the definitive radiographic procedure in most patients. Currently, angiography, including jugular venography, is done only in unusual situations for special indications. Pneumoencephalography is rarely necessary.

Computed cranial tomography is an outpatient procedure and requires less exposure to x-ray than is necessary for routine skull films and radiographic tomography. The risk of serious reaction to the

* Mailing address: Department of Radiology, 2131 West Third Street, Los Angeles, California 90057

necessary use of iodinated intravenous contrast material is no greater than in routine intravenous urography, there being less than one death in 30,000 examinations (1).

Computed tomography yields information not routinely available in evaluation of patients suspected of acoustic tumor. Tumor size is more accurately determined by computed tomography than by any other method. Correct preoperative differential diagnosis of tumor histology is usually obtained.

Associated conditions, such as bilateral acoustic tumor manifestations of neurofibromatosis (Figure 1), cerebral atrophy, arachnoid cyst, and cerebral infarct, will be detected. Ventricular size and deformity are demonstrated. Hydrocephalus, when present, will be recognized. Other intracranial tumors and significant vascular abnormalities may be detected.

As with any diagnostic tool, computed tomographic examination for acoustic tumor must be carefully tailored and thoughtfully interpreted to produce optimum accuracy. In this chapter we set forth the details of our examination technique and the criteria used in interpretation, based on current practice, developed through our experience since April, 1975.

Computed tomography is undergoing rapid technological advance. It is certain that significant improvement in the accuracy of computed tomography will be realized in the near future.

TECHNIQUE OF EXAMINATION

All of our studies were done at St. Vincent Medical Center in Los Angeles using an EMI Mark I scanner with 160 × 160 matrix. The head is placed in the unit and positioned so that the scanning planes are 5–15° from the orbito-meatal line. Adjacent scans are done from near the foramen magnum upward through the lateral ventricles. Two scans producing four images through the posterior fossa are done using the 8-mm nominal section thickness. One or two higher scans producing two or four images are done using the 13-mm nominal section thickness.

At this time, the pre-infusion study is examined by the radiologist and technologist. Head position, freedom from artifacts, and accurate scan plan positioning are checked. Images showing the petrous pyramids are examined at the display console. Data manipulation to display only bone density structure is used to identify, resolve, and photograph the internal auditory canals. Despite earlier opinion (2), the internal auditory canals are shown in 90% of examinations. If the preliminary study does not show the canals, an additional scan, more accurately positioned, may

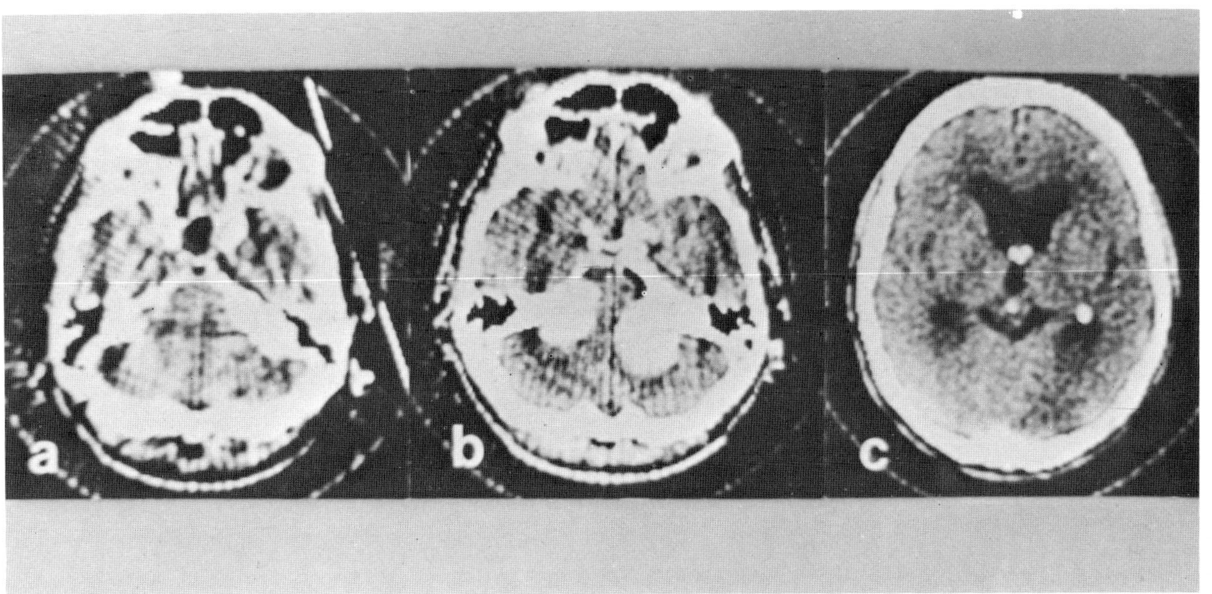

Figure 1. Example of bilateral acoustic neuroma with mild hydrocephalus. a: Tumors are not visible in pre-infusion scan because they have the same tissue density as brain. b: Tumors are visible after contrast infusion due to moderately intense enhancement of density. c: Mild dilation of the third and lateral ventricles is demonstrated.

be done. We have learned that, to demonstrate small lesions in the cerebellopontine angle cistern at the acoustic porus and in the internal auditory canals, it is imperative that the scan be accurately centered in the plane of the canals. Any other abnormality, such as hydrocephalus or mass shown in the pre-infusion study, is noted for further evaluation after contrast infusion.

The radiologist then gives an intravenous infusion of 300 ml of 30% iodinated contrast material. Several agents suitable for use are available. We are using diatrizoate meglumine injection USP prepackaged as 300-ml 30% solution (Reno-M-DIP, Squibb). In children and small adults the volume of infusion is appropriately reduced.

Postinfusion scanning begins when about one-half of the 300 ml has been delivered. We begin near the vertex of the skull and scan successively downward during and after infusion. Infusion usually is completed in 15 to 20 min. This procedure sequence ensures that maximum infusion effect will be present when the critical petrous region scans are being made.

The complete study, consisting of 12 to 16 images produced with 6 to 8 scan sequences, is then examined by the radiologist. Any necessary additional scans are done before the patient is released. A preliminary written report may be sent to the referring doctor or hospital with the patient. When examination is done in this way, patients are routinely examined in about one hour.

Since any head motion during the scan degrades the image, motion must be prevented. Mechanical head-holding devices are often required. Sedation may occasionally be useful. Anesthesia may be used but is rarely required. We have encountered several patients whose heads were too large to fit in our machine. Other machines do not have this size limitation. Some patients become claustrophobic and may not be able to tolerate the procedure. We consider a documented history of severe reaction to intravenous contrast material to be a relative contraindication to this procedure.

MATERIAL

We have included 158 patients with a computed tomographic diagnosis of acoustic tumor in this presentation. All examinations were done at St. Vincent Medical Center in Los Angeles from April, 1975, through December, 1977. This group is taken from a larger series of patients examined for symptoms or signs suggestive of acoustic tumor. We have also included 39 patients with non-acoustic cerebellopontine angle lesions. These are presented for the differential diagnostic features they demonstrate. False negative examinations are given separate analysis. When computed tomographic findings are equivocal or negative, suspect patients are then examined with positive contrast cisternography.

Of 158 computed tomographic diagnoses of acoustic tumor, 109 have been pathologically proven. Seventeen postoperative patients with known acoustic tumors have been shown to have persistent or recurrent tumor by computed tomography. Twenty-six patients with positive computed tomographic studies for acoustic tumor have not yet been proven. Six patients were incorrectly diagnosed as possible acoustic tumor. In three of these, positive contrast cisternography was negative. Three were found to be non-acoustic lesions. A few other patients were thought to have non-acoustic cerebellopontine angle lesions that were proven to be acoustic tumor. One of these had an associated arachnoid cyst larger than the tumor that led to the incorrect diagnosis of cholesteatoma. Occasionally, an unusally dense acoustic tumor may have been diagnosed as meningioma. One glomus jugulare tumor was initially called an acoustic tumor. In our experience since April, 1975, no patient has had surgical exploration because of a false positive computed tomography.

Of particular interest is the series of small tumors of less than 1.5 cm diameter. Twelve patients with tumors of less than 1.5 cm diameter have had negative computed tomography examinations. We have correctly diagnosed eleven patients with tumors of less than 1.5 cm diameter. It is apparent that approximately one-half of tumors of this small size are not being detected by computed tomography. Occasionally, tumors of more than 1.5 cm diameter will not be demonstrated. Above 2 cm diameter, only unusual tumors are missed. In one instance, an acoustic tumor considered greater than 4 cm diameter at surgery was not visible even in retrospect in the computed tomographic examination. This lesion was equal in density to brain and exhibited no recognizable contrast enhancement on infusion. The internal auditory canal was not widened.

It is our opinion that it is possible to diagnose 90% of acoustic tumors greater than 1.5 cm diameter by computed tomography. Smaller tumors, less than 1.5 cm diameter, are being detected in about one-half of the cases. The least likely to be detected are acoustic tumors that are truly limited to the intracanalicular region.

FALSE NEGATIVE STUDIES

In our total series, 23 patients with negative computed tomograms have been proven to have acoustic tumor. We realize there may be other patients with negative computed tomographic diagnosis in whom acoustic tumor may later be proven. Some factors that lead to incorrect negative computed tomographic study have been recognized. Early in our experience, we failed to examine in the correct plane. On review of these cases, it is clear that we had not imaged the plane of the internal auditory canals. Artifacts due to motion or equipment dysfunction or Pantopaque droplets have obscured a few tumors. One patient with an acoustic tumor 3.5 cm in diameter at surgery had a negative pre-infusion scan. Because of a previous reaction to contrast material, no infusion study was done.

CHARACTERISTICS OF ACOUSTIC TUMOR

The computed tomographic studies of 158 acoustic tumors have been analyzed (Table 1). The features observed have been classified as criteria for the diagnosis of acoustic tumor. These features are useful in the differential diagnosis of other cerebellopontine angle lesions.

Internal Auditory Canal Findings

The computed tomographic appearance of the internal auditory canals is usually symmetrical. The canals can be displayed to appear cylindrical (Figure 2). When acoustic tumor is present, the canal containing the tumor is usually widened and flared toward the porus with diverging anterior and posterior walls. The abnormal canal is usually wider than the normal canal (Figure 3). A few larger tumors have not widened the internal auditory canal (Figure 4).

Direct comparison of the findings from computed tomography with plain film and routine tomographic findings is difficult. The canals are viewed in a trans-axial plane, more like the sub-mental vertex radiographic projection in standard tomography. The image is produced in a different way and may be varied by data display adjustment. It is our experience that canals containing tumors that appear only slightly eroded, widened, or funnel-shaped on radiographic tomography may appear more distinctly abnormal by computed tomography.

It has been stimulating to speculate why the canals sometimes appear more abnormal in computed tomograms than in radiographic tomograms. Computed tomography analyzes bone tissue density more sensitively than radiographic tomography. We wonder whether these studies are detecting and displaying the presence of a change in bone character adjacent to the internal auditory canal that precedes radiographic evidence of erosion and widening.

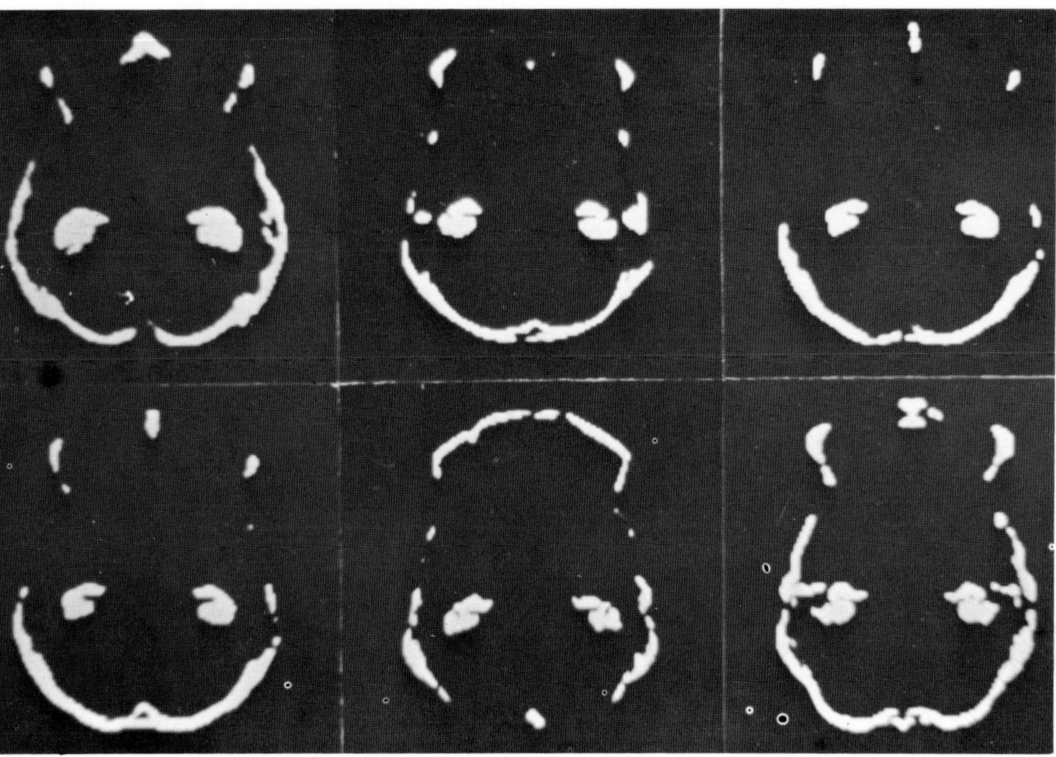

Figure 2. The internal auditory canals are detected by data display manipulation to show only bone density structures. The normal appearance of internal auditory canals is shown in six patients.

Table 1. Analysis of computed tomographic findings in acoustic neuroma

	CT[a] Detection of Acoustical Neuroma			Widened IAC[b] Acoustical Canal		Widened Ipsilateral Cistern		Hydrocephalus Found	
	No. Correct	No. Missed	Percent Correct	No.	Percent	No.	Percent	No.	Percent
Total Series	158	23	87	133	84	48	33	19	12
Analysis by Tumor Size									
Less than 1.5 cm	11	12	47	7	63	0	0	0	0
1.6 to 2.0 cm	27	6	81	21	77	9	33	1	3
2.1 to 3.0 cm	71	2	97	59	83	21	30	4	5
3.1 to 4.0 cm	33	2	94	31	93	9	27	8	24
Larger than 4.0 cm	16	1	94	15	93	9	56	9	56

[a] Abbreviation CT indicates computed tomography.
[b] Abbreviation IAC indicates internal auditory canal.

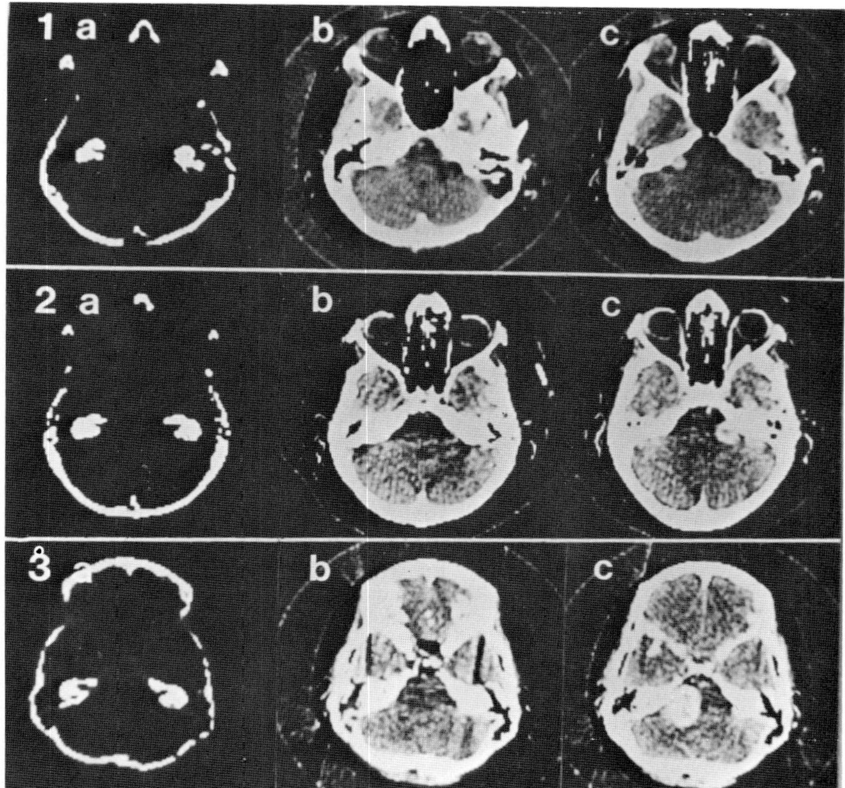

Figure 3. Three patients with acoustic neuroma. 1. 0.9-cm acoustic neuroma. a: The canals are not enlarged but slight asymmetry is suggested. b: Tumor not visible in the preinfusion scan. c: The tumor is demonstrated by density enhancement after contrast infusion. 2. 1.5-cm acoustic neuroma. a: Widened canal with flared porus. b: Commonly seen artifacts between the petrous bones obscure structures, including the normal pons. c: Moderately intense non-homogenous enhancement of tumor density after contrast infusion. 3. 3.0-cm acoustic neuroma. a: Widening of the internal auditory canal. b: Tumor not visible. Fourth ventricle not detected. c: Non-homogenous enhancement after contrast infusion.

Tumor Density

Acoustic tumor is characteristically about the same density as normal brain tissue. Before contrast infusion, it is usually difficult to see the tumor as a structure separate from brain tissue. Occasionally the tumor may be bordered by a halo of lesser density thought to be due to edema in the brain tissue adjacent to the tumor. In several cases the tumor

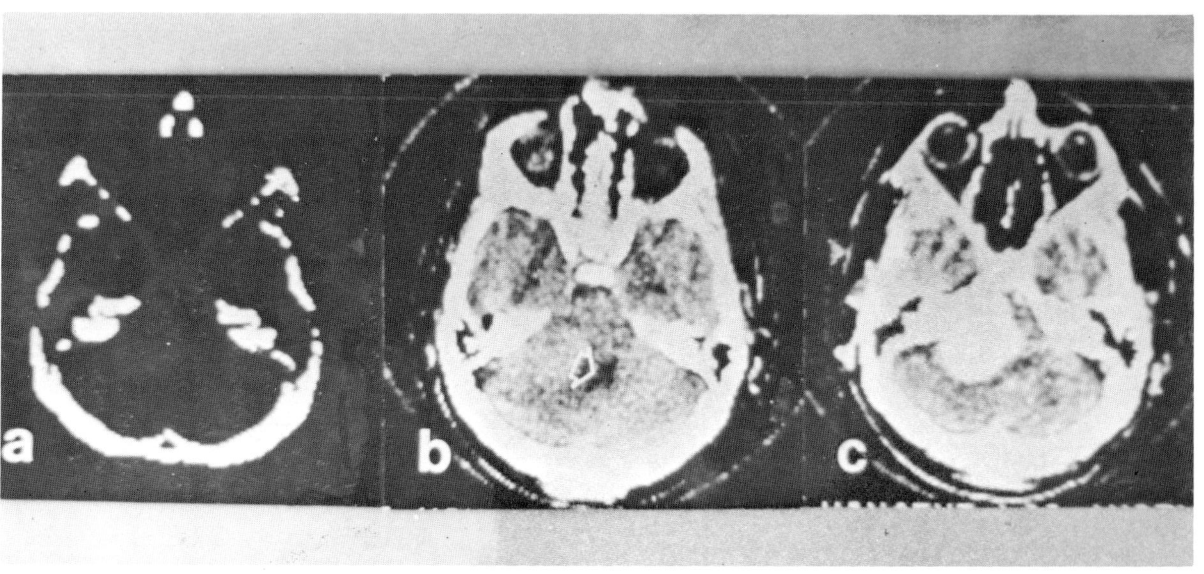

Figure 4. 4.0-cm acoustic neuroma. a: This tumor did not demonstrate widening of the canal. b: Displacement and distortion of the fourth ventricle (arrow). c: Intense tumor density enhancement after contrast infusion.

appeared slightly more dense than brain. Tumor density may be non-homogenous. The areas of lesser density within the tumor appear to correlate with the presence of cystic areas within the tumor (Figure 3).

Contrast Enhancement

After intravenous infusion of contrast material, acoustic tumors exhibit moderately intense enhancement of density. The density enhancement is non-homogenous through the tumor substance. Again, this appears to be due to non-enhancement of cystic components (Figure 3).

The intensity of contrast enhancement is influenced by several factors. Enhancement increases with larger amounts of contrast material. Density enhancement also appears to increase with time during the 10–20 min after completion of contrast infusion. This observation, along with other information, suggests that there is diffusion of contrast material beyond the intravascular spaces into tumor tissue. There is some variability in intensity of contrast enhancement among acoustic tumors (Figure 5).

Tumor Position

Acoustic tumor typically grows concentrically outward from the internal acoustic porus. A tumor that is situated even slightly eccentric to the porus is unlikely to be an acoustic tumor.

Asymmetry of Cisterns

With growth of acoustic tumor in the cerebellopontine angle, the brainstem and pons are displaced away from the tumor. The effect of this displacement widens the cerebrospinal fluid space between bone and brain on the tumor side and narrows the cistern on the contralateral side. This asymmetry is recognized in about one-third of the cases (Figure 5). The effect is not seen in the smallest tumors. With larger tumors the effect may not be seen, since cisternal space may be compressed or obliterated bilaterally (Figures 3 and 6).

Fourth Ventricular Findings

The fourth ventricle shows some abnormality in nearly one half of the cases. The typical alteration is slight displacement from the midline away from the tumor (Figure 6). Slight distortion in the configuration of the fourth ventricle is more difficult to evaluate. Slight bowing or slight rotational distortion is sometimes suggested. More subtle findings are not considered reliable, including questionable decrease in the size of the fourth ventricle and failure to demonstrate the fourth ventricle.

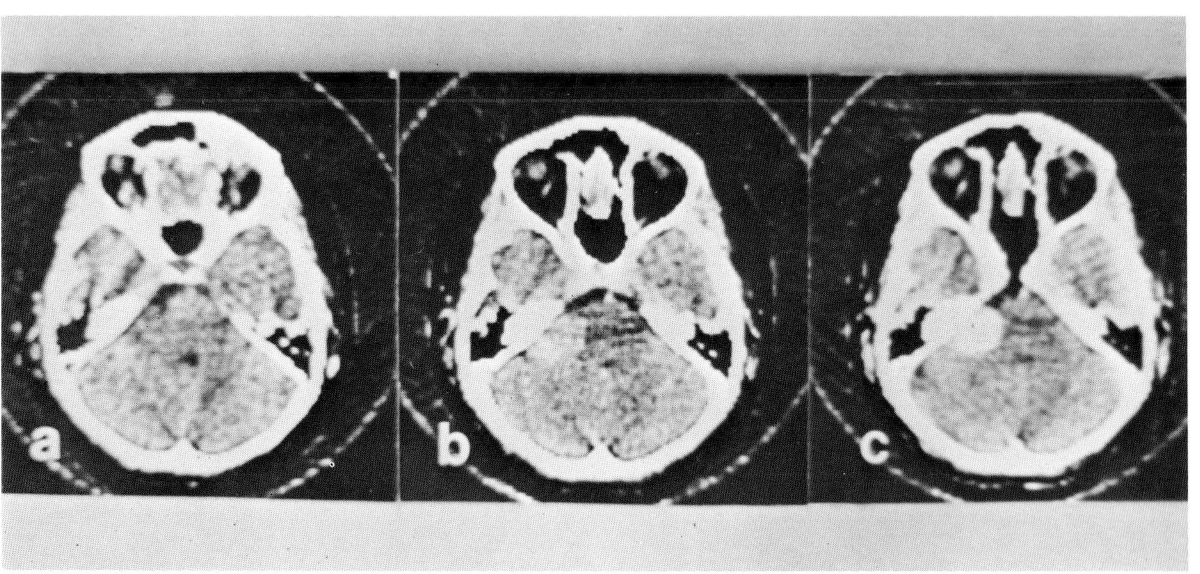

Figure 5. 2.4-cm acoustic neuroma. a: Widening of the ipsilateral cerebellopontine cistern is shown. b: Moderate enhancement is present at the conclusion of infusion. c: Increased tumor density enhancement is demonstrated in a scan done 10 min after b.

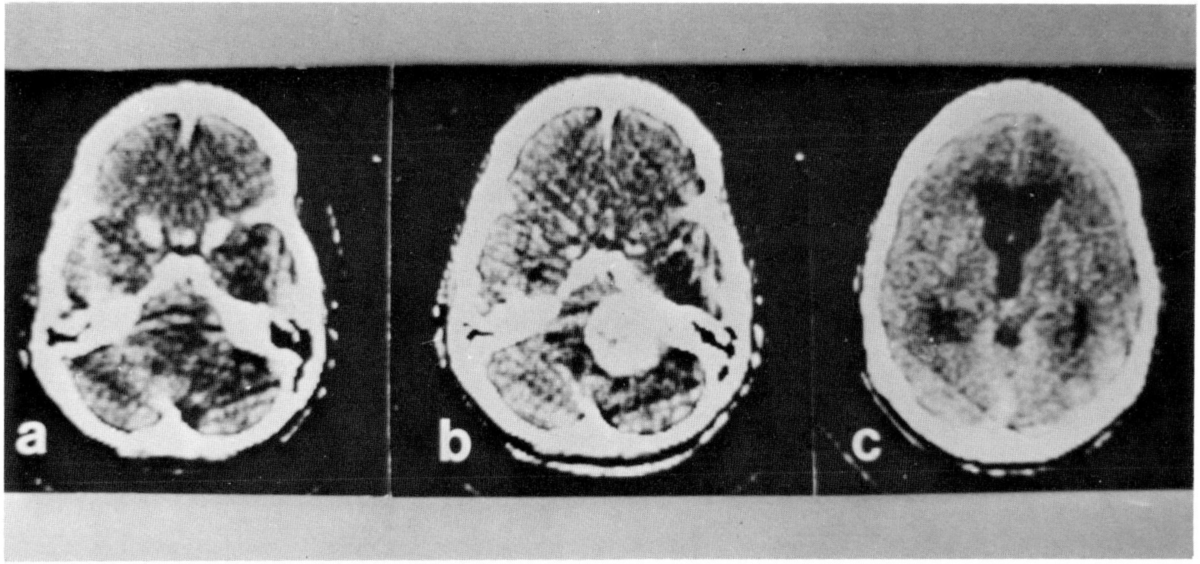

a

b

c

Figure 6. 3.5-cm acoustic neuroma. a: Cisterns compressed bilaterally. b: Moderately intense non-homogenous density enhancement after contrast infusion. c: Mild hydrocephalus is shown.

Hydrocephalus

Acoustic tumors cause dilation of the third and lateral ventricles. There is good correlation between tumor size and the probability of hydrocephalus. An apparent threshold for the possibility of production of hydrocephalus appears to be reached when tumors become 3 cm or greater in diameter. We have encountered only one patient with hydrocephalus in the presence of an acoustic tumor of less than 2 cm diameter. Only four patients with acoustic tumors less than 3 cm diameter had hydrocephalus. In a series of 44 patients with acoustic tumors larger than 3 cm diameter, 17 had hydrocephalus (Figure 6).

Computed tomography demonstrates ventricular size in all patients. Hydrocephalus, when present, is now routinely detected in every patient. The possible need for ventricular shunting as a step in the treatment can be evaluated.

Arachnoid Cyst

Occasionally, an arachnoid cyst occurs with acoustic tumor. Such cysts, containing cerebrospinal fluid, may be recognized in addition to the tumor (Figure 7). Rarely, such cysts may be larger than the acoustic tumor. The presence of a cyst should not confuse the diagnosis of acoustic tumor. Arachnoid cyst in the cerebellopontine angle without acoustic tumor occurs, but it is rare.

NON-ACOUSTIC CEREBELLOPONTINE ANGLE TUMORS

Non-acoustic cerebellopontine angle tumors may present with symptoms and signs suggestive of acoustic tumor. Computed tomography may show mass effects similar to those of acoustic tumor such as asymmetry of cisterns, displacement and distortion of the fourth ventricle, and hydrocephalus. Our 39 non-acoustic tumors are presented for the features they demonstrate. These characteristic features usually permit accurate preoperative differential diagnosis.

Meningioma

We have examined 16 patients with pathologically proven cerebellopontine angle meningioma. The tomographic findings in meningioma are distinctive even when the tumor is a rounded mass in the cerebellopontine angle. Meningiomas are more dense than brain tissue, as is seen in pre-infusion scans. After contrast infusion, meningiomas show intense homogenous density enhancement throughout the tumor.

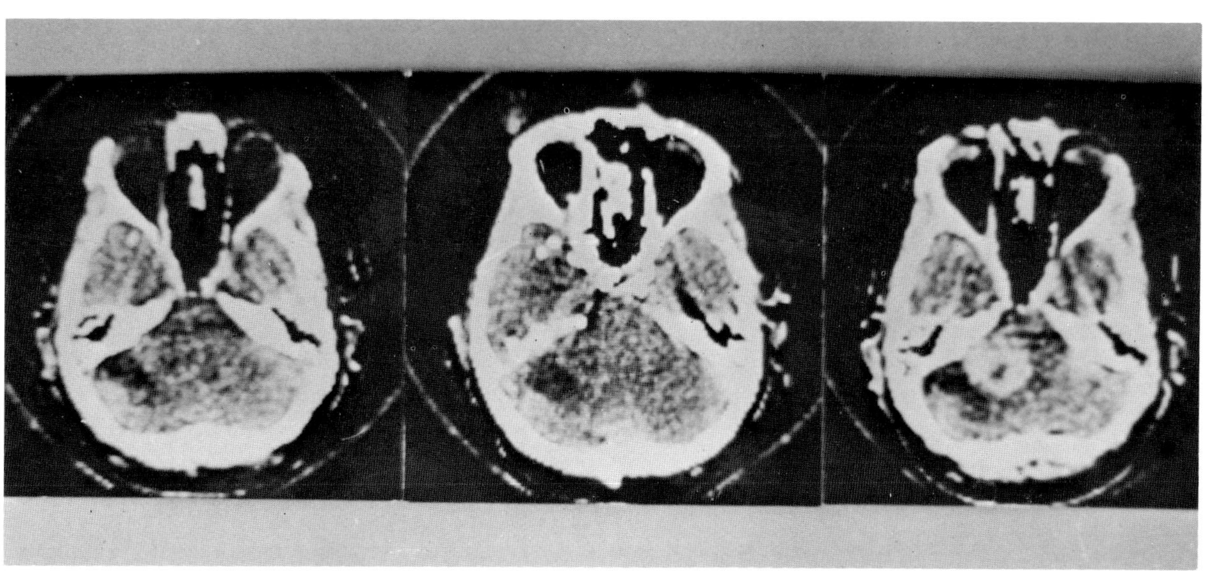

Figure 7. 2.9-cm acoustic neuroma with arachnoid cyst. a and b: Tumor density is equal to brain. The less dense structure adjacent to the tumor was found to be an arachnoid cyst at surgery. c: Non-homogenous density enhancement after contrast infusion.

The internal auditory canal has not been widened by meningioma (Figure 8). Other meningiomas involving the cerebellopontine angle are less likely to be mistaken for acoustic tumor due to their tendency to involve bone and to extend widely along the petrous pyramid and adjacent regions. Some meningiomas are heavily calcified and can be seen in radiographic examinations. These may be as dense as bone on computed tomograms (Figure 9).

Cholesteatoma

We have examined seven patients with cerebellopontine angle cholesteatoma. These lesions varied in size up to 5 cm diameter. Cholesteatoma is typically much less dense than brain. Contrast enhancement is negligible or absent, and when suggested, the questionable enhancement has been limited to the peripheral margin of the mass. The internal auditory canal is not widened. There may be typical sharply defined erosion of bone in the petrous apex. These tumors tend to extend medially on to the clivus and may displace or envelop the vertebral and basilar arteries. Superior extension into Meckel's cave and the tentorial notch occurs frequently (Figures 10 and 11).

Glomus Jugulare Tumor

Glomus tumors appear slightly more dense than brain before contrast infusion. They show modest homogenous contrast enhancement. Glomus tumors typically invade bone and present in the cerebellopontine angle slightly inferior to the acoustic porus. With display manipulation the tumor may occasionally be seen growing within the petrous bone (Figure 12).

Tumors of Other Cranial Nerves

We have encountered two fifth nerve neuromas, one seventh nerve neuroma, and one ninth nerve neuroma. Preoperative differential diagnosis from acoustic tumor depends upon tumor location and the appearance of the internal auditory canal. The seventh nerve neuroma was indistinguishable from acoustic tumor.

Miscellaneous Lesions

Other lesions are mentioned only as possibilities when the findings on computed tomography are not characteristic. A few metastases have mimicked acoustic tumor clinically. An eccentric pontine glioma was mistaken for acoustic tumor. An eighth nerve astrocytoma had computed tomographic findings typical of acoustic tumor. An arteriovenous mal-

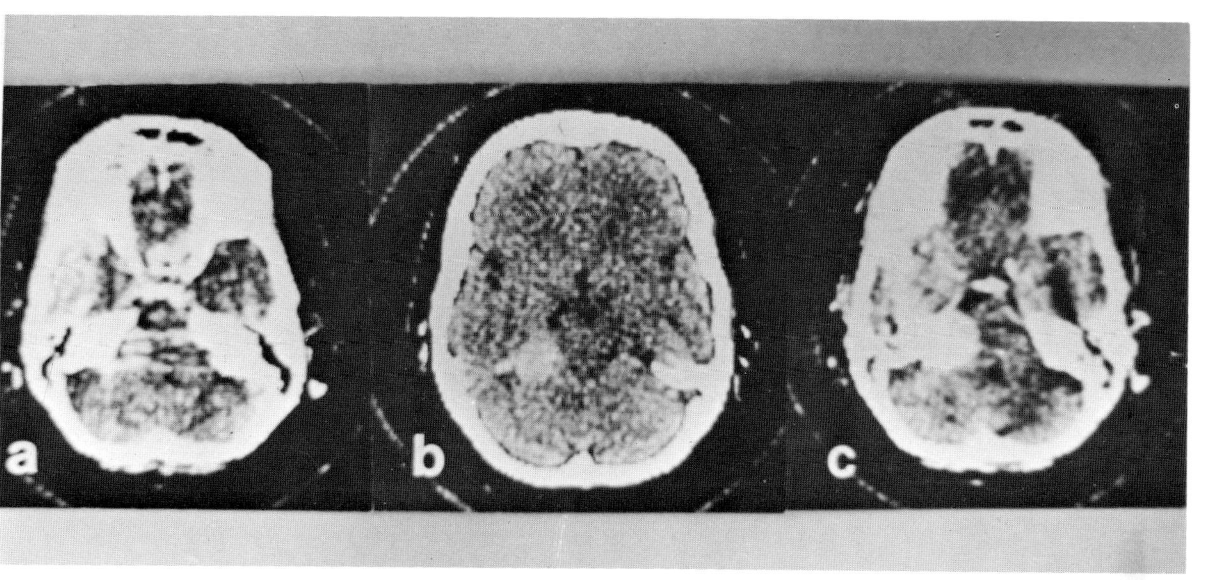

Figure 8. 2.8-cm meningioma in the cerebellopontine angle. a and b: Tumor density is typically greater than brain density in the pre-infusion scan. The tumor is centered slightly above the acoustic porus. c: Intense density enhancement after contrast infusion. An area of lesser density in the tumor image is caused by artifacts, such as are seen in a. Asymmetry of cisterns and displacement of the fourth ventricle are shown.

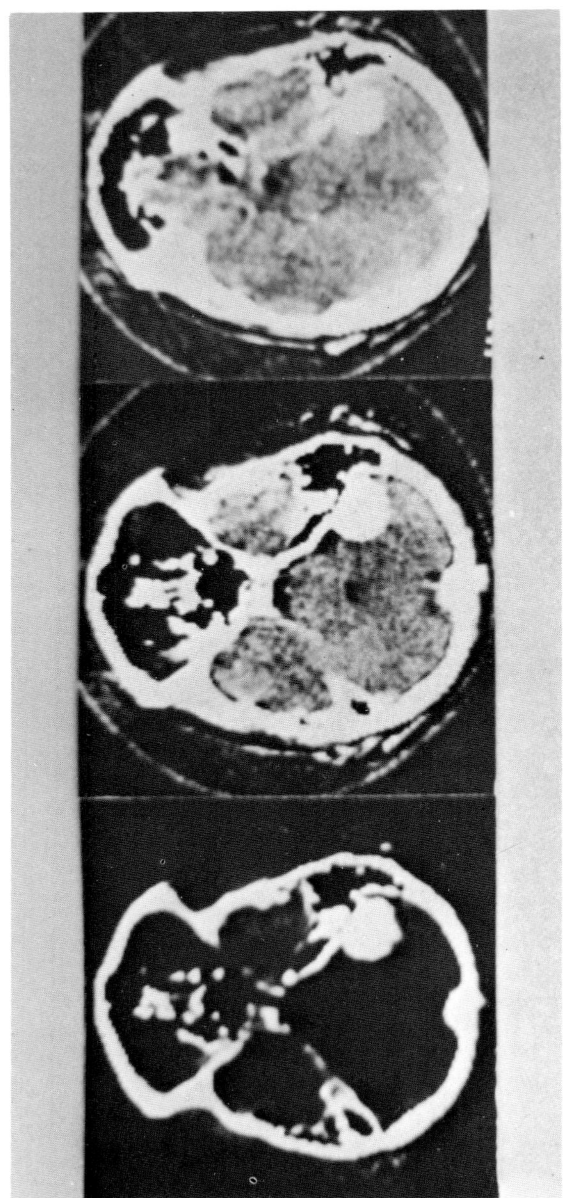

Figure 9. A calcified meningioma located posterior to the internal acoustic porus. Slight asymmetry of the cisterns is shown.

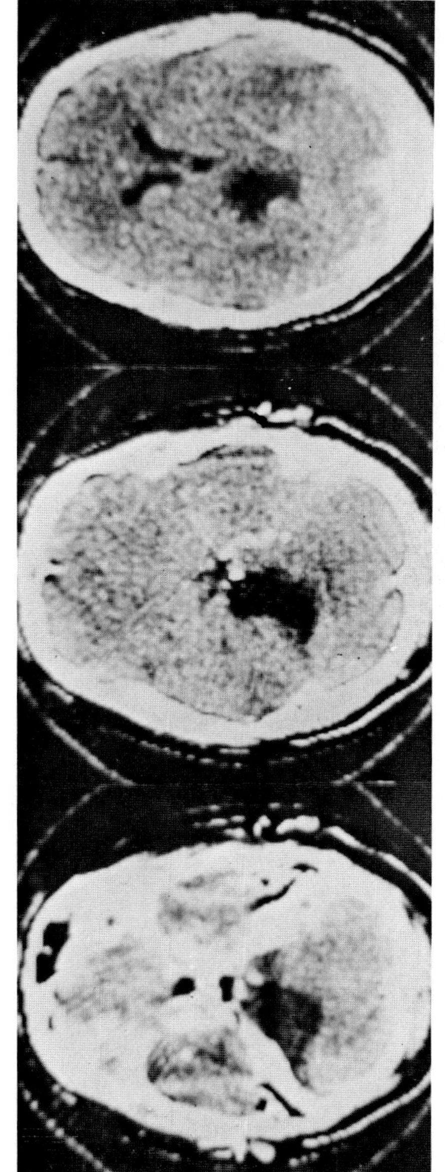

Figure 10. Cerebellopontine angle cholesteatoma showing extension along the petrous pyramid and upward into Meckel's cave and the middle fossa. The typical low density of cholesteatoma is shown.

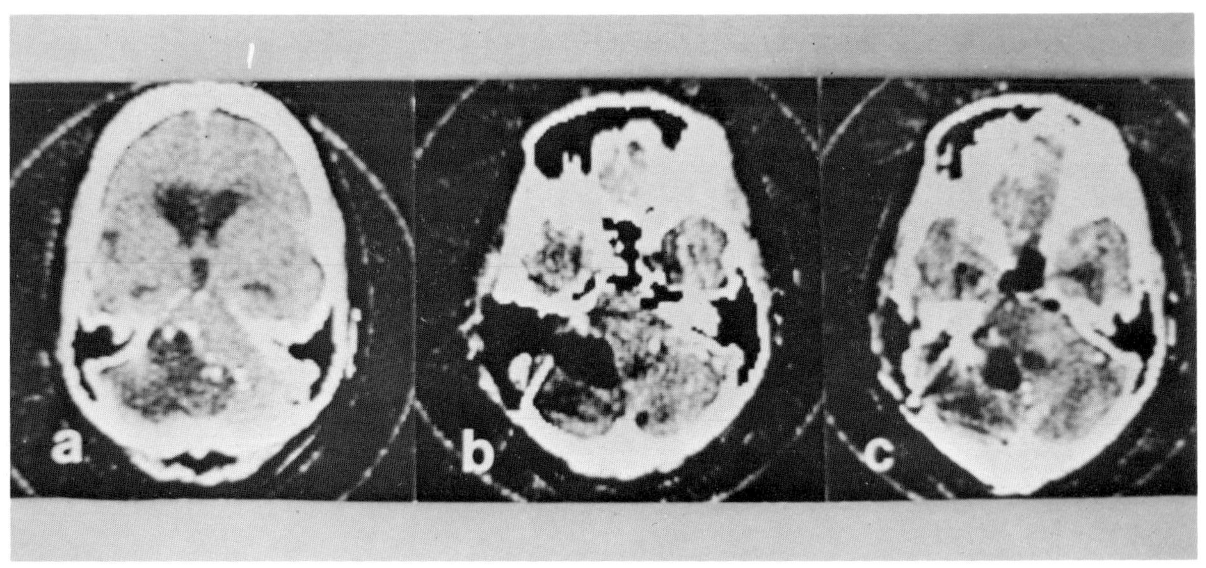

Figure 11. a: Very large cholesteatoma with scattered droplets of oil from a positive contrast cisternogram. The tumor was removed through a translabyrinthine approach. b and c: Fat was used to pack the operative labyrinthine surgical defect. The fat can be seen herniating through the bone defect and extending into the posterior fossa.

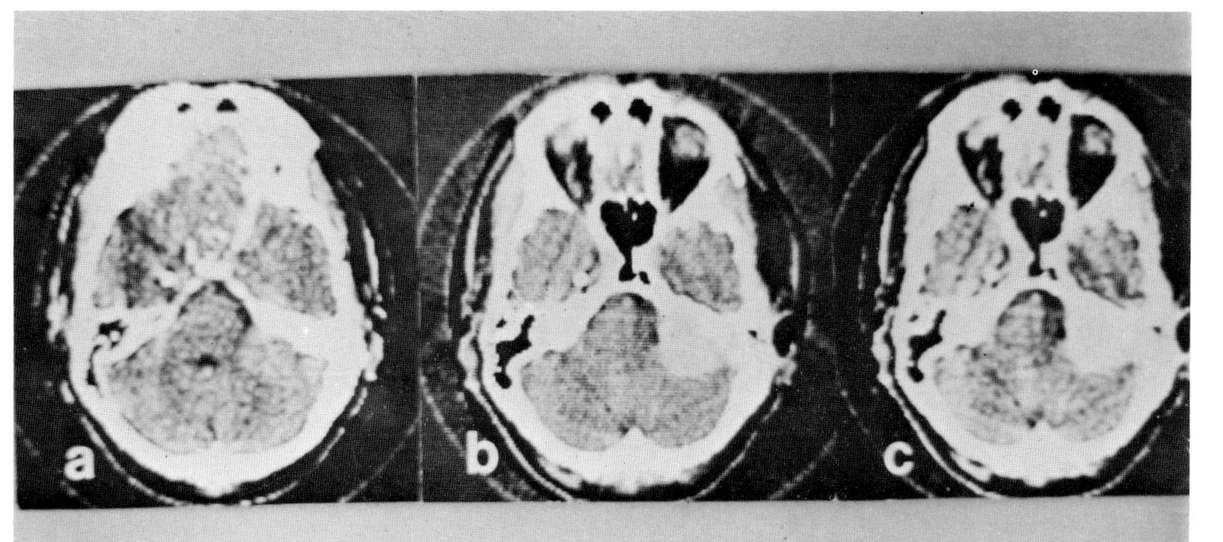

Figure 12. Glomus jugulare tumor. a: The tumor is slightly more dense than brain in the pre-infusion scan. b: Tumor invasion of bone is demonstrated. b and c: Moderately intense homogenous enhancement after contrast infusion.

formation with the cerebellopontine angle was encountered that produced widening of the internal auditory canal.

COMPUTED TOMOGRAPHY IN POSTOPERATIVE PATIENTS

This technique has been especially valuable in patient evaluation and follow-up after treatment for cerebellopontine tumors. The effect of surgery can be documented and evaluated. The effect of radiotherapy can be monitored when applicable, as in glomus tumors.

The Acute Postoperative Period

When patients have postoperative difficulty, computed tomography may be helpful. Computed tomography can be done as needed in the immediate postoperative period. It may be necessary to remove bulky or air-containing bandages to eliminate artifacts. Problems like hemorrhage, hydrocephalus, subdural hematoma, fluid collections, and cerebral infarct or edema may be detected.

One patient was examined on the third postoperative day because of signs of increasing intracranial pressure. Fat, a tissue of very low density, was recognized in the posterior fossa. Subcutaneous fat had been used to pack a large surgical defect in the petrous bone. The fat had herniated inward through the bone defect and produced cerebrospinal fluid obstruction. Prompt improvement followed removal of the pack (Figure 11).

Long-term Follow-up

The course of hydrocephalus is easily followed. The function of ventricular shunts can be monitored as needed by repeat computed tomography.

In those cases treated with subtotal resection of tumor, a postoperative baseline study can be obtained at the time of discharge from the hospital after surgery. By comparison with the postoperative study, the possibility of re-growth of tumor can be accurately assessed in the course of follow-up examinations (Figure 13).

Positive contrast posterior fossa cisternography should be done in patients with findings consistent with acoustic tumor when the computed tomographic study is negative or equivocal. Small tumors and intracanalicular tumors will not be missed if this sequence is followed. Computed tomographic study should be done before positive contrast cisternography, since residual oil droplets in the posterior fossa produce artifacts in the computed tomographic images.

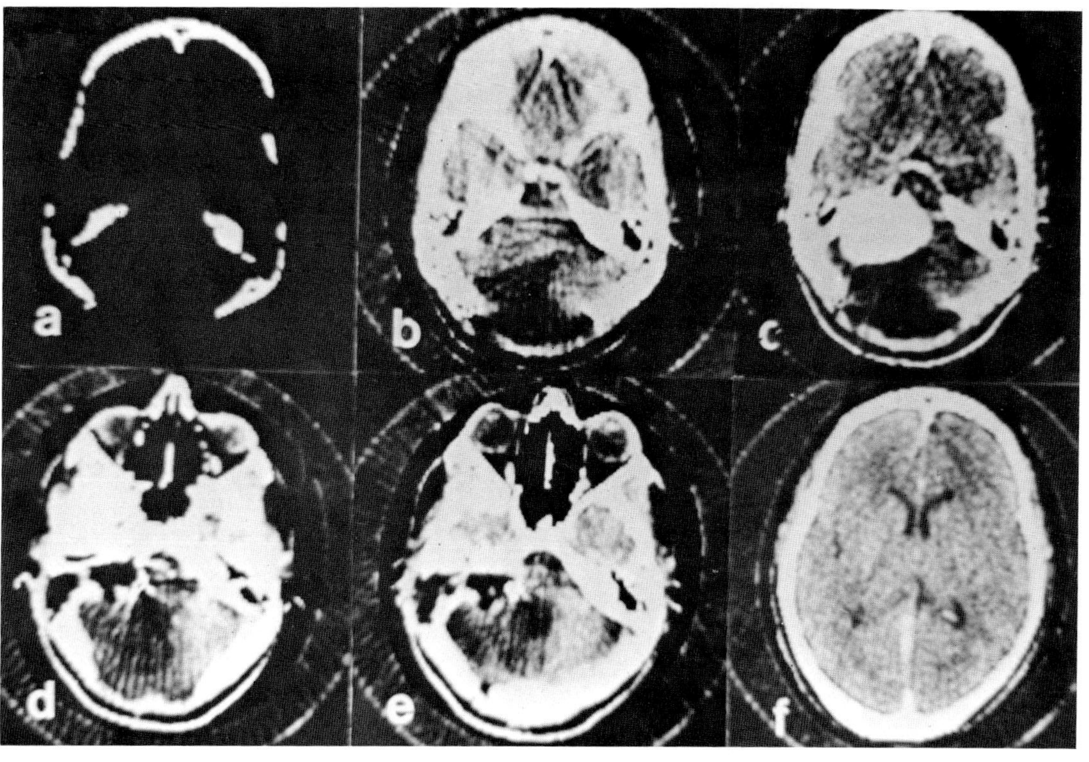

Figure 13. 4.0-cm recurrent acoustic neuroma. a and b: A surgical defect in the occipital region is seen. Abnormal brain density in the cerebellum is shown. c: Recurrent tumor shows enhancement after contrast infusion. d, e, and f: Examination 2 months after translabyrinthine removal of the recurrent tumor shows no evidence of residual tumor. f: The ventricles are normal in size and shape.

Angiography and pneumoencephalography can be avoided in most cases. When meningioma or glomus tumor or possible vascular abnormality is suggested, angiography is selected as the next radiographic study. Information about ventricular size and associated intracranial abnormalities is routinely obtained. Usually, non-acoustic cerebellopontine angle tumors producing symptoms of acoustic tumor can be correctly diagnosed. Tumors showing unusual features may require angiography and/or positive contrast cisternography. Pneumoencephalography is rarely needed.

CONCLUSIONS

Computed cranial tomography is a powerful tool for detection of cerebellopontine angle tumors. Accurate differential diagnosis of histologic type is usually possible. When studies are tailored for cerebellopontine angle diagnosis, acoustic tumors of greater than 1.5 cm in diameter are being demonstrated in about 90% of the cases. Acoustic tumors of less than 1.5 cm in diameter are being detected in about one-half of the cases.

Computed cranial tomography is indicated in any patient with findings suspicious for acoustic tumors. After plain films of the skull and petrous pyramids and radiographic tomography of the temporal bones, computed tomography should be done. The technique should include scans of the internal auditory canals for evidence of asymmetry or widening of the acoustics porus. Tumor enhancement with intravenous contrast material is important in recognition and differential diagnosis. The intensity and homogeneity of enhancement are significant differential diagnostic features.

Technological improvements are being made rapidly in the field of computed tomography. Images having better spatial resolution, and fewer artifacts will be produced by these improved devices.

In this chapter we present observations and recommendations drawn from our experience with computed tomography. We hope our experience will encourage more confident use of computed tomography in the diagnosis of cerebellopontine angle tumors.

ACKNOWLEDGMENTS

This report is the result of the combined efforts of each of the radiologists at St. Vincent Medical Center: Richard P. Storrs, M.D., William W. M. Lo, M.D., Franklin H. Shimizu, M.D., E. Michael McMonigle, M.D., and A. K. Raja

Rao, M.D. The contributions of special procedure technologists are recognized: B. Zink, R.T., B. Akiyama, R.T., C. Imamura, R.T., M. McGuire, R.T., J. Carvajal, M.A., R.T., X. Nagy, R.T., and E. Stone, R.T.

REFERENCES

1. Witten, D. M., Hirsch, F. D., and Hartman, G. W. 1973. Acute reactions to urographic contrast medium. Am. J. Roentgenol. 119:832–840.
2. Bergeron, R. T., Cohen, N. L., and Pinto, R. S. 1977. Role of computerized tomography in the diagnosis of acoustic neuromas. Acta Otolaryngol. 103:314–317.

Acoustic Tumors
Volume I, *Diagnosis*
Edited by W. F. House and C. M. Luetje

Chapter 14

Iophendylate Examination of the Posterior Fossa in Diagnosis of Cerebellopontine Angle Tumors

B. Hill Britton, M.D.*

Associate Clinical Professor of Otolaryngology, University of Southern California School of Medicine, Los Angeles

---

Of all diagnostic modalities enlisted to aid in the early diagnosis of acoustic tumors, the development of Pantopaque posterior fossa myelography appears to be one of the most significant. Over the past decade, numerous articles have appeared concerning the use of this radiopaque contrast substance, its safety, its indications, and its diagnostic accuracy. In this chapter, the historical aspects of the development of this examina-

* Mailing address: 1300 North Vermont Avenue, #508, Los Angeles, California 90027

tion, as well as important factors regarding interpretation and technique, are reviewed. A brief statistical review of important findings demonstrated in this survey of 500 surgically verified acoustic tumor cases is also presented.

In the past several years another radiographic examination has at times supplanted the use of Pantopaque myelography. This, of course, is the use of computerized tomography. The exact role of computerized tomography is covered in a separate chapter, and is only briefly discussed here as it pertains to decision-making regarding the evaluation of an acoustic tumor suspect.

HISTORICAL ASPECTS

One of the earliest reports concerning the use of iodides within the subarachnoid space was made by Sicard and Forestier in 1922 (1,2). They pointed out that the first demonstration of its possible usefulness was noted upon accidental injection of iodized poppy seed oil into the subarachnoid space. They later reported use of it within the epidural and subdural spaces and in the cerebral ventricles (3). Among the early difficulties encountered were the high vascularity of this oil and its irritation to the arachnoid tissues.

The use of iophendylate (Pantopaque) was reported in the literature in 1944 by Ramsey, French, and Strain (4) and by Steinhausen et al.(5). Iophendylate contains 30.5% iodine by weight and has a specific gravity of 1.26. It is absorbed much more readily than iodized poppy seed oil, and since the initial reports it has been generally considered to be the most useful of the iodine oils. Following its introduction and more widespread use, a number of reports have appeared concerning possible inflammatory reactions with it (6–9). In 1968, Shapiro (2) reported that the possibility of arachnoiditis was enhanced by blood within the subarachnoid space. Since that information became available, it has been accepted that if bleeding was encountered with the lumbar puncture to introduce iophendylate, the procedure should be terminated and repeated at a later date. The possibility of hypersensitivity reactions to this substance has been considered; however, this possibility has been extremely difficult to verify. Certainly patients with a prior history of true iodine sensitivity should not have Pantopaque, but should have pneumoencephalography combined with tomography.

In 1952 a fatality following Pantopaque myelography caused by hydrocephalus secondary to severe adhesive arachnoiditis was reported (10). This case may well be germane to two cases, which are reported in more detail later in this chapter, in which severe post-Pantopaque reactions occurred.

In the author's experience over the past 10 years of utilizing posterior fossa myelography, these have been the only two cases noted of severe complications following the use of Pantopaque. The incidence of post-Pantopaque headache and backache of a severe degree has been limited, occurring in less than 5% of the cases.

The technique of using Pantopaque in the posterior fossa was described in 1955 by Brown and Aye (11). Referring to the use of iophendylate in the foramen magnum, they felt that its use was safe within the cranium, contrary to prior reports in the literature.

In 1963, Baker (12) at the Mayo Clinic described 204 cases, including 13 cerebellopontine angle tumors, of posterior fossa myelography using 9–12 cc of iophendylate. Scanlan (13,14) in 1964 reported his experience with 100 patients using the technique of Baker.

It was at approximately this time that some sources of diagnostic error using standard fluoroscopic technique were re-evaluated. The most concerning among these was the possibility of overlooking a small intracanalicular tumor because of the lack of fine bone detail of the internal auditory canal on films taken at fluoroscopy. Hitselberger and House (15) at this point reported on the use of 1-cc aliquot of dye in combination with the Polytome unit, enabling study of the fine bone detail of the internal auditory canal, as well as its relationship to the radiopaque dye column. The use of the 1-cc Pantopaque examination on an outpatient basis, utilizing the Polytome or a head unit, was further reported by Britton et al., from 1968 to 1977 (16–18).

TECHNIQUE AND INTERPRETATION

The anatomy of the cerebellopontine cistern is variable in regard to its exact shape as well as its exact size. Acoustic tumors within the cerebellopontine angle are spherical or egg-shaped, and, depending on their size, a variable amount of dye may surround the lesion. If the dye can surround only a portion of a large tumor due to limitation of the cistern by the mass, an erroneous reading may be made (Figure 1). This results in underestimating the exact size of the lesion. It cannot be overemphasized that it is necessary to obtain multiple radiographic views during fluoroscopy, utilizing not only standard frontal and lateral projections but also basilar or transantral projections. Visualization of the area of the otic capsule and the internal auditory canal is necessary to arrive at correct conclusions regarding the filling or non-filling of the canal. A finger-like projection of dye above or below a tumor mass may be misinterpreted as dye within the internal auditory canal if the canal is not well seen (Figures 2 and 3). The most common source of diagnostic error is inadequate films because an inexperienced radiologic technician or physician performed the examination.

Spill of the dye column through the tentorial notch into the frontal fossa may produce severe headache for the patient. It can be avoided by using care when the dye column enters the posterior fossa. As in all areas

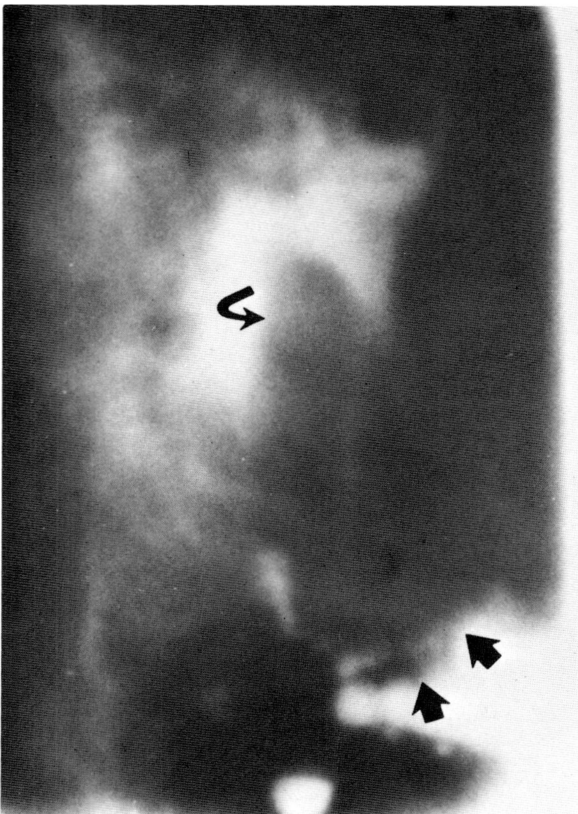

Figure 1. A Polytome Pantopaque study in the Stenver's projection. There is incomplete outline of the tumor mass with a small aliquot of Pantopaque (1 cc). The tumor mass was estimated to be approximately 2 cm in diameter; however, at the time of surgery, it was noted to be 4 cm in diameter. The inferior extent of the tumor was not adequately visualized with this study. The curved black arrow indicates the floor of the internal auditory canal. The wide black arrows show the tumor margin.

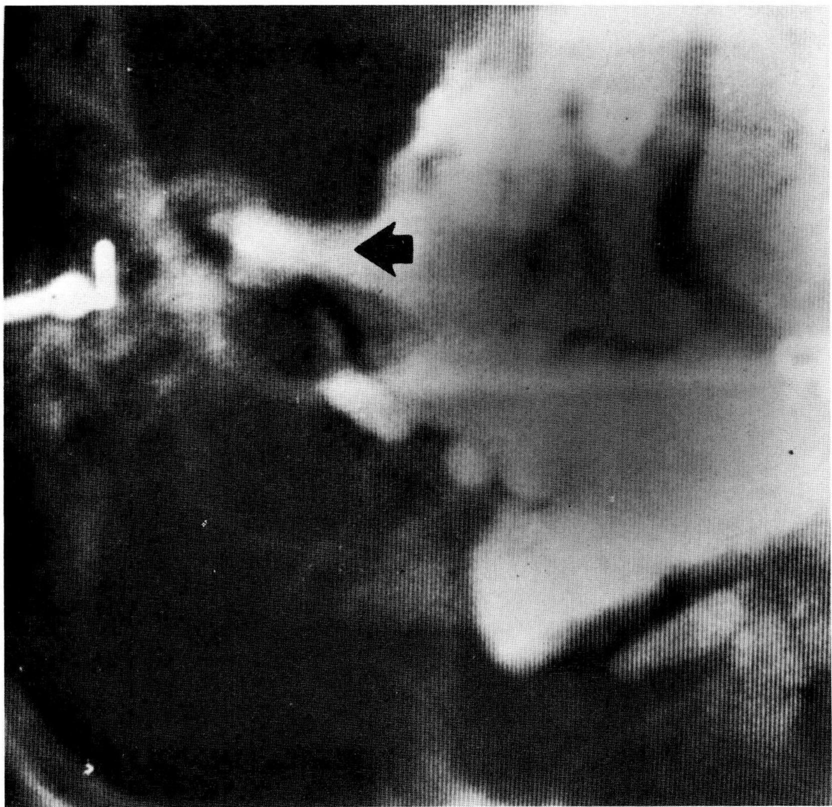

Figure 2. Normal filling of the internal auditory canal on a fluoroscopic spot film in a position similar to the Stenver's projection. The small opaque marker is in the external auditory canal. The black arrow points to the dye column filling the internal auditory canal. Compare this illustration with Figure 3.

of radiology, carefully positioned and carefully performed radiographs, with attention to exact details, are of utmost importance. Pursuing these ideals of careful radiographic technique will greatly reduce the chance of diagnostic error.

CASE REVIEW

The purpose of this review is to study the 500 verified acoustic tumor patients who had radiographic examinations. Of this group, 484 patients

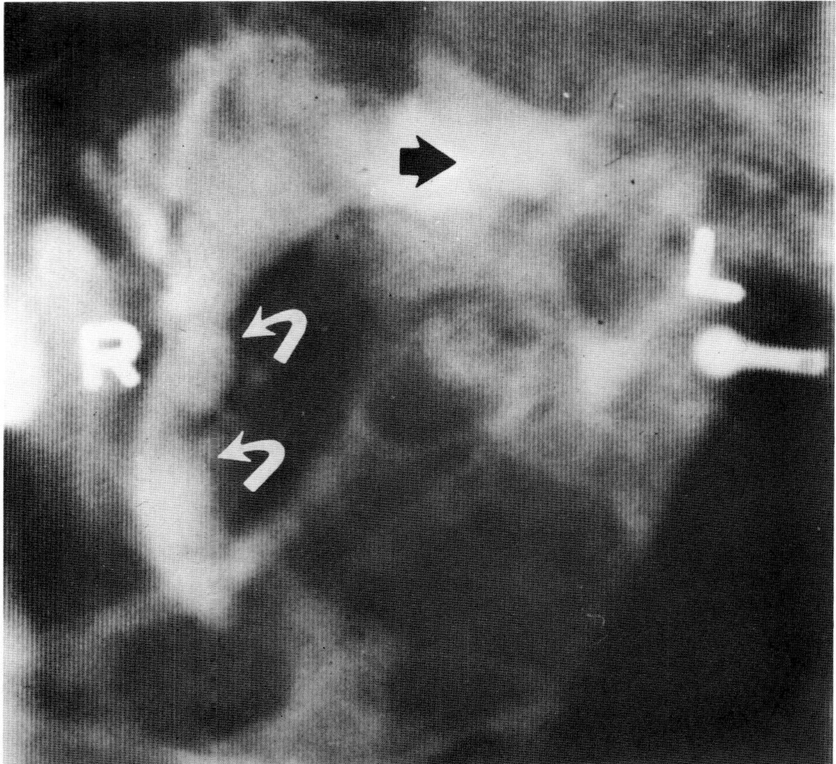

Figure 3. A similar projection and appearance to Figure 2. One can easily be misled into assuming that the finger-like projection above the internal auditory canal indicated by a black arrow is actually filling the internal auditory canal. In fact, this is dye above a tumor and the main bulk of the tumor mass is below this area, as indicated by the curved white arrows. Compare with Figure 2 for similarity in appearance.

had Pantopaque studies; 16 did not. However, during the same time interval, approximately 2,000 normal or negative Pantopaque studies were done, resulting in a positive examination rate of approximately 20%. In essence, therefore, this is a review of about 2,500 cases of Pantopaque examination.

Of the 16 patients who did not have a Pantopaque examination, the following breakdown can be made. In 11 patients, the diagnosis was confirmed with routine brain scan; therefore, Pantopaque examination was deemed unnecessary. Two patients had definitive diagnosis established by cerebral arteriography. One patient had the diagnosis confirmed by brain scan and cerebral arteriography, and one patient had pneumoencephalography in combination with tomography because of a history of iodine dye sensitivity. In one patient an acoustic tumor was found at the time of middle fossa decompression of the internal canal; the tumor had not been expected preoperatively. A Pantopaque study was not performed in this patient prior to his definitive tumor removal.

Within the group of Pantopaque examinations, there were no false negatives. There was one false positive study, which revealed non-filling of the internal auditory canal with no tumor mass definitely outlined. Upon middle fossa exploration of the internal auditory canal, diffuse arachnoid adhesions were found, presumably due to old tubercular meningitis. No known infections following Pantopaque examination have occurred in these 2,500 cases.

COMPLICATIONS

Severe headache and backache were complications of the Pantopaque examination in less than 5% of the cases. Two patients, M.C. and J.H., discussed below, had severe post-Pantopaque complications.

M.C.

The first patient, M.C., a 53-year old female, complained of imbalance and a falling sensation, which she had noted for 5 years prior to being seen. She also noted a progressive left-sided hearing loss, which was sensorineural in type. An office Polytome Pantopaque study was performed, revealing a left cerebellopontine angle filling defect with a vertical dimension of approximately 3 cm. Medrol was not instilled into the subarachnoid space following the Pantopaque injection. The tumor was thought to be large, since it extended to the jugular foramen. The spinal fluid protein analysis at the time of Pantopaque examination was 62 mg/100 ml. Several days after the examination, the patient developed severe headaches that progressed to left-sided focal motor seizure and then a grand mal seizure. Arteriograms at that time showed obstructive hydrocephalus, confirmed on pneumoencephalography. The patient's condition deteriorated. An urgent ventricular atrial shunt was done. This resulted in a reversal of her acute symptoms and a slow but steady improvement for several months. The patient subsequently had a translabyrinthine removal of a 4.5-cm acoustic tumor and had a relatively uneventful recovery postoperatively.

J.H.

The second patient, J.H., was initially seen with a complaint of a slight left-sided hearing loss noted for approximately 6 years, with a sudden and precipitous drop in the hearing on the left side noted a month prior to being seen. This patient had undergone a fluoroscopic Pantopaque examination elsewhere using 3 cc of dye 10 days prior to being seen. Subsequent to the examination, he had difficulty with urination, moderately severe headaches, and decreased vision in the right eye for 2 days prior to being seen. Films taken at the initial fluoroscopy revealed a 2.5-cm cerebellopontine angle mass on the left side consistent with an acoustic tumor. At the original procedure, it was noted that dye removal was incomplete: approximately 2 cc of the Pantopaque remained. Three weeks following the initial examination with Pantopaque, repeat fluoroscopy revealed that the dye droplets were freely mobile. A repeat lumbar puncture was performed, removing the residual Pantopaque dye. Opening pressure was 120 mm of cerebrospinal fluid in the reclining position. Eighty milligrams of methylprednisolone acetate and 80 mg of hydrocortisone were injected into the intrathecal area at that time. The patient was also given Decadron intramuscularly for the first 48 hr, followed by an oral dosage schedule. The patient improved following the use of cortisone. Analysis of the spinal fluid taken at the time of the repeat tap revealed CSF protein of 209 mg/100 ml. Electrophoretic studies showed an increased gamma globulin fraction. Two months following the initial Pantopaque examination, the patient complained of severe headaches, nausea, and vomiting. Examination at that point revealed the first evidence of papilledema, and bilateral Babinski reflexes and a left lateral rectus palsy were present. A radioactive iodinated serum albumin study revealed the majority of activity within the basal cisterns after 28 hr. After 48 hr the activity was within the ventricular system but not over the convexities. Preoperative diagnosis was made of communicating hydrocephalus, and a ventricular atrial shunt was carried out. Arachnoid biopsy at that time showed evidence of chronic arachnoiditis. The patient steadily improved. Four months after the initial Pantopaque examination, the patient underwent a left translabyrinthine removal of a 2.5-cm acoustic tumor. This case, J.H., has been previously reported by Mortara and Brooks (19).

Both of these cases appear to be similar, with development of subsequent increased intracranial pressure and hydrocephalus following the use of Pantopaque. Whether or not this was specifically related to the presence of a tumor and some alteration in cerebrospinal fluid flow dynamics is a moot point. There have, however, been no similar reactions noted in non-tumor patients. These reactions do not seem to be related to the size of the tumor, since the first patient had a very large lesion and the second patient had a medium-sized lesion. Interestingly, these cases occurred in 1970, within 4 months of each other.

CONCLUSIONS

Despite the disadvantages of possible resultant backache and/or headache, which are self-limiting, and the several reported cases of severe intracranial reactions, Pantopaque myelography remains an extremely important tool in the early diagnosis of acoustic tumors. Currently it is the most accurate test for the definitive diagnosis of acoustic tumors. It is hoped, through better screening tests prior to consideration of Pantopaque myelography or computerized tomography, that the negative-positive ratio can be changed from a 20% positive rate to, ideally, a 70 or 80% positive rate. Among the more accurate screening tests on the horizon is the use of brainstem evoked response audiometry.

Computerized tomography (CT) of the cerebellopontine angle is an important and welcomed step forward in the radiographic diagnosis of acoustic tumors. At the present time, however, it has an inherent, high false negative rate on tumors less than 1.5 cm in size. Because of this, a negative CT scan cannot at this point be considered synonymous with the absence of a tumor. Several clinical investigations regarding the integration of Pantopaque myelography and computerized tomography are being undertaken. One of these is to perform Pantopaque myelogram on all tumor suspects who have negative computerized tomography test results. A second investigation is to perform Pantopaque studies on all small tumor suspects and computerized tomography on all large tumor suspects. Again, even if the computerized tomography is negative on large tumor suspects, follow-up with Pantopaque myleography should be done. It is not clear at the present time which system of diagnostic investigation will eventually be preferred.

In conclusion, Pantopaque myelography, particularly in regard to its accuracy in the diagnosis of acoustic tumor, remains useful despite marked advances with computerized tomography. It is hoped that further refinements in the use of computerized tomography may supplant the use of invasive diagnostic study. The future of radiography of the cerebellopontine angle is exciting indeed.

REFERENCES

1. Camp, J. D. 1950. Contrast myelography past and present. Radiology 54:477–505.
2. Shapiro, R. 1968. Myelography, Second Edition, pp. 11–24, 98–106, 119–124, 391–396. Year Book Medical Publishers, Chicago.
3. Sicard, J. A., and Forestier, J. 1926. Roentgenologic exploration of the central nervous system with iodized oil (Lipiodol). Arch. Neurol. Psych. 16:420–434.
4. Ramsey, G. H., French, J. D., and Strain, W. H. 1944. Iodinated organic compounds as contrast media for radiographic diagnoses IV. Pantopaque myelography. Radiology 43:236–240.
5. Steinhausen, T. B., Dungan, C. E., Furst, J. B., Plati, J. T., Smith, S. W., Darling, A. P., Wolcott, E. C. 1944. Iodinated organic compounds as contrast media for radiographic diagnoses III. Experimental and clinical myelography with ethyl iodophenylundecylate (Pantopaque). Radiology 43:230–235.
6. Peacher, W. G., and Robertson, R. C. L. 1945. Pantopaque myelography: Results, comparison of contrast media, and spinal fluid reaction. J. Neurosurg. 2:220–231.
7. Tarlov, I. M. 1945. Pantopaque meningitis disclosed at operation. JAMA 129:1014–1016.
8. Fisher, R. L. 1965. An experimental evaluation of Pantopaque and other recently developed myelographic contrast media. Radiology 85:537–545.
9. Bull, J. 1971. Myelography. Neuroradiology 2:1–2.
10. Erickson, T. C., and Baaren, H. J. 1952. Late meningeal reaction to Pantopaque used in myelography (report of a case which terminated fatally). Trans. Am. Neurol. Assoc. 134–137.
11. Brown, F. M., and Aye, R. C. 1955. Myelographic demonstration of the basilar artery. Am. J. Roentgenol. 73:32–34.
12. Baker, H. L. 1963. Myelographic examination of the posterior fossa with positive contrast medium. Radiology 81:791–801.
13. Scanlan, R. L. 1964. Positive contrast medium (iophendylate) in diagnosis of acoustic neuroma. Arch. Otolaryngol. 80:698–706.
14. Scanlan, R. L. 1964. Roentgen diagnosis of acoustic neuroma with particular reference to the use of Pantopaque. Laryngoscope 74:999–1003.
15. Hitselberger, W. E., and House, W. F. 1967. Acoustic neuroma: The adaptation of polytomography and iophendylate to the early diagnosis of acoustic tumors. Am. Surg. 33:791–796.
16. Britton, B. H., Hitselberger, W. E., and Hurley, B. J. 1968. Iophendylate examination of posterior fossa in diagnosis of cerebellopontine angle tumors. Arch. Otolaryngol. 88:608–617.
17. Britton, B. H., and Fluitsma, B. 1974. Iophendylate examination of the posterior fossa. Rad. Clin. North Amer. 12:431–439 (December).